BIOMEDICAL ETHICS

A Multidisciplinary
Approach to Moral
Issues in Medicine
and Biology

EDITED BY DAVID STEINBERG, M.D.

UNIVERSITY PRESS OF NEW ENGLAND
HANOVER AND LONDON

Published by University Press of New England,
One Court Street, Lebanon, NH 03766
www.upne.com
© 2007 by David Steinberg
Printed in the United States of America
5 4 3 2 1

Library of Congress Cataloging-in-Publication Data
Biomedical ethics : a multidisciplinary approach to moral issues in medicine and biology /
edited by David Steinberg, M.D.
    p. ;   cm.
Articles reprinted from Medical ethics.
Includes bibliographical references and index.
ISBN-13: 978-1-58465-643-2 (paperback : alk. paper)
ISBN-10: 1-58465-643-3 (pbk. : alk. paper)
1. Medical ethics. 2. Bioethics. I. Steinberg, David, 1940–
II. Medical ethics (Burlington, Mass.)
[DNLM: 1. Bioethical Issues—Collected Works. 2. Bioethics—Collected Works. WB 60 B6157 2007]
R724.B4914 2007
174'.957—dc22   2007011147

To my wife, Sharon

CONTENTS

PART THREE: NOVEL TECHNOLOGIES

PART FOUR: IN THE CLINICAL ARENA

This anthology includes writings by the most accomplished scholars in the various disciplines devoted to examining and resolving the ethical conundrums of biology and medicine. I'm grateful to our authors for accepting the invitation to write for the *Lahey Clinic Journal of Medical Ethics,* especially since our publication is based in a medical center rather than the ethics department of a large university or a free-standing ethics institute. I often wondered whether prospective authors had any idea that my telephone solicitations were sandwiched between visits with patients who had leukemia, lymphoma, Hodgkin's Disease or some other serious illness.

Lahey Clinic was founded in Boston in 1923 by Frank H. Lahey, one of the most distinguished surgeons of his time. Dr. Lahey had the vision to appreciate the value of physicians from various medical and surgical specialties working closely together in an environment that also stressed the importance of education and research. Lahey Clinic is one of the original models for multispecialty group practice and has become world famous. In 1980 it moved from Kenmore Square in Boston to its current campus in Burlington, Massachusetts, just outside Boston. Some of the most vexing ethical dilemmas arise in the treatment of patients; therefore, it isn't as improbable as it may first sound that a medical center would be the source of a scholarly publication devoted to biomedical ethics.

The mission of the Lahey Clinic Medical Ethics Newsletter—its original name—is to bring scholarly writings in biomedical ethics to professional ethicists, people in the health and related professions, patients and the general public. Our authors are asked to write at a high level of scholarship but in language accessible to the general reader. The relative brevity of our columns must have been a challenge for our writers, who are accustomed to the more generous space allotment of traditional ethics journals; however, short articles that efficiently inform are a blessing for the busy reader. For readers who want to explore a topic in greater depth references have often been provided. (References and quotations not listed in Notes are from this volume.) When it was pointed out to me that our "newsletter" contained no news the publication's formal name was changed to the *Lahey Clinic Journal of Medical Ethics.*

I've often been asked how I managed to get so many prominent people to contribute to the journal. It was relatively easy. I simply asked them to write on some aspect of their field of interest and expertise. It's a testament to their academic generosity that our authors agreed to do so. Unfortunately, because of space constraints many superb articles from the *Lahey Clinic Journal of Medical Ethics* could not be included in this volume. (They can be found at our Web site, http://www.lahey.org/ethics.)

The conundrums of biomedical ethics have varied implications and demand examination from many perspectives. Philosophers examine these problems using reason as their tool. The humanist explores how ethical dilemmas affect people. The lawyer thinks about these matters in terms of statute, case law and regulations. Theologians and the clergy apply religious doctrine and seek understanding from a spiritual perspective. Healthcare professionals become ethics experts because they can't avoid ethical dilemmas in their clinical practice. The defining feature of this collection of writings is its multidisciplinary character. Our writers include philosophers, healthcare professionals, lawyers, medical historians, anthropologists, scientists, writers, humanists, psychologists, theologians and sociologists. A unique feature of this volume is its exploration of biomedical ethics with a multidisciplinary lens.

The articles in this book are reprinted from five sections of the *Lahey Clinic Journal of Medical Ethics:* the Feature story, the Dialogue section, Ask the Ethicist, the Legal Column, and Humanities. The Dialogue section is devoted to discussion of the Feature Story of the previous issue. In Ask the Ethicist a specific case is presented to an ethicist for his or her opinion. Humanities is devoted to books, theatrical productions or movies that illuminate the experience of illness. Most of our legal columns are written by academically based lawyers who study the role of law in meeting the ethical challenges encountered in biology and medicine.

The organization of this volume in six sections is largely arbitrary. The imposition of structure was a frustrating experience because most of the articles could reasonably be classified under several different headings. The compensation for this difficulty is a collection of writings by the best minds devoted to the challenging and intellectually fascinating ethical dilemmas of biomedicine—dilemmas that should demand our attention for their intellectual and emotional content and because few of us will avoid them in our personal lives.

Although the oldest article reprinted in this anthology was first published in 1995 the writings in this book are not dated. Many ethical issues have been debated for centuries so it shouldn't be surprising that the articles in this anthology, even if a few years old, remain as relevant now as they were when first published.

I owe an enormous debt of gratitude to James L. Bernat, MD, associate editor of the journal, professor of Neurology at Dartmouth Medical School and a neurologist on the staff of the Dartmouth-Hitchcock Medical Center. The *Lahey Clinic Medical Ethics Journal* is published in collaboration with the Dartmouth-Hitchcock Medical Center. Jim has not only facilitated publication of this anthology, he has also provided vital editorial and administrative assistance in the production of the journal. He has also been a source of wise counsel and has provided invaluable support to me in my at times lonely job as editor.

I am grateful to the people who over the years have served as members of our editorial board and helped sustain the high quality of the journal. They include: Allan M. Brandt, PhD; Dan W. Brock, PhD; Daniel Callahan, PhD; Kenneth M. Dolkart, MD; Bernard Gert, PhD; Paul Gross, MD; Diane M. Palac, MD; Thomas J. Prendergast, MD; Paul Reitemeier, PhD; Paul L. Romain, MD; James A. Russell, DO; and Andrew G. Villaneuva, MD. I would also like to thank our legal editor, David M. Gould, Esq, and I am grateful to Paul Reitemeier, PhD, and Patricia McTiernan for their helpful reviews of my introductory articles. I'm also grateful to Ralph Fuller, former director of the Lahey Clinic Public Affairs Department, who had sufficient faith in me to take a chance and publish the first issue of our journal in July 1994.

I am grateful to Lahey Clinic for its generous support of the journal; special acknowledgment should be given to its chief executive officers—Robert E. Wise, MD; John A. Libertino, MD; and David M. Barrett, MD—who, despite the budgetary problems of today's hospitals and clinics recognized the critical importance of medical ethics and supported the journal's mission to bring ethics education to the community.

I also owe an incalculable debt of gratitude to Stephen R. Karp. Support from the Karp Family Foundation given in memory of Harold Karp has made this volume and much of my work in biomedical ethics possible. Vital early support also came from the Robert E. Wise Foundation and Pamela and Renke Thye.

Editing an ethics publication while taking care of very sick patients with complex illnesses can be tiring and stressful. I would not have survived the experience without the invaluable assistance and support of our managing editors. For more than eight years Patricia Busacker did a highly professional job of managing the *Lahey Clinic Journal of Medical Ethics*. She skillfully edited the majority of articles in this volume. Her death was an enormous personal and professional loss for all of us. I'm also grateful to Nancy Knoblock Hunton who skillfully took over following Patricia's death and to our current managing editor, Jeanne Zimmerman. I also owe a great debt of gratitude to my secretary, Bonnie Neacy, for her steady and invaluable help.

I owe a special thanks to my wife, Sharon, whose calming influence, valuable suggestions and support made this volume possible. That she did this while courageously undergoing treatment for breast cancer is remarkable.

PART ONE

The Nature of Biomedical Ethics

DAVID STEINBERG, MD

Introduction: The Nature of Biomedical Ethics

Webster's dictionary defines ethics as the discipline concerned with what is right and what is wrong and what is good and what is bad. Philosophers offer differing versions of the meaning of ethics. Singer[1] defines ethics as being about how we ought to live and what our goals ought to be. Veatch[2] defines ethics as the analysis of choices; to pursue a particular choice is to decide it is better than available alternatives. Gert[3] says ethics is "a public system applying to all rational persons governing behavior that affects others and which has the minimization of evil as its end." That the basic definition of ethics[4] is subject to various interpretations serves as a sentinel warning that the geography of ethics may be somewhat hazy. Gert notes, "If one starts by saying morality is. . . . nothing one says afterward seems quite right."

The substance of ethics is values. Ethics is devoted to the promotion of intrinsically important values. How to clone a human is a scientific and technical matter; whether it is right or wrong to clone a human is ethics. How to most humanely and efficiently perform euthanasia is a medical and technical matter; whether euthanasia is right or wrong is ethics. That there is disagreement on their hierarchical ranking when, in specific situations, values clash, is evidence that the discipline of ethics does not rest on solid bedrock. It lacks the luxury of empirical proof that observation affords scientific inquiry.[5]

Ethics is pertinent to all fields of human endeavor. Ethical questions emerge in public, professional and personal affairs. They exist in business, science, law, engineering, politics, agriculture, and military affairs. This volume is devoted to ethical dilemmas in the practice of clinical medicine (medical ethics) and related biological and technological fields (bioethics). These areas may overlap; both arenas are encapsulated in the term *biomedical ethics*. Although their deliberations may on occasion take a turn into obscure alleys, medical ethics and bioethics are not esoteric theoretical activities because they intimately affect our lives and the lives of the people we care about. The ability to remove your dying grandmother from a mechanical ventilator that would only prolong her suffering, your protection against becoming a research subject without having given informed consent, and your ability to obtain a fairly allocated organ for transplantation are recognized rights as a consequence of antecedent ethical debate. It is virtually certain that some matter of biomedical ethics either has or will intimately affect your life.

The articles in this section ponder the nature of ethical knowledge. What theory or technique should be used to solve ethical problems? Although ethical dilemmas may be difficult to resolve they can't be ignored because ethical decisions often cannot be avoided. If your father's doctor advises a do-not-resuscitate order a decision must be made one way or the other. Whether a sixteen-year-old boy should be permitted to die because his Jehovah's Witness parents refuse blood transfusion must be decided one way or the other. Whether human embryonic stem cell research should be permitted must be decided one way or the other. Although many philosophical issues have been debated for centuries, in the practical world of biomedical ethics decisions cannot proceed at a glacial pace. The moral conundrums of biology and medicine must be confronted because they are often unavoidable; but, as the articles in this anthology demonstrate, they also warrant serious attention because they present fascinating and potentially rewarding intellectual challenges.

Because ethical dilemmas are multidimensional and can be considered from a variety of perspectives they engage the interest of many disciplines. For centuries religions have taught basic rules of behavior; the Ten Commandments is a venerable set of ethical principles. The complexity of biomedical dilemmas has beckoned theological and philosophical analysis and, Jonsen claims, the first modern bioethicists were philosophers and theologians. The law has a stake in biomedical ethics and in an ideal over-simplified world would allow what is ethical and prohibit what is unethical.

Brandt, a historian of medicine, notes that bioethics is shaped by the social and political conventions of the times. The humanist is involved because what is debated by bioethics often intimately affects people. Jonsen approvingly notes that the discipline of bioethics has stimulated a vigorous discussion by a concerned general public initiating a process he calls the "discourse of bioethics." A comprehensive exploration of biomedical ethics requires a multidisciplinary approach and explains why the writers in this anthology include philosophers, historians, theologians, lawyers, medical humanists, healthcare professionals and various other academics.

According to "cognitivists" reason can define moral judgments as either true or false; "emotivists" adopt a contrary position and believe moral judgments are neither true nor false but simply reflect our likes and dislikes. Leon Kass mingled reason and emotion when he said, "In crucial cases, however, repugnance is the emotional expression of deep wisdom, beyond reason's power fully to articulate it."[6] Kagan and Shweder separate reason and emotion and debate the relative roles of each in the development of a uniquely human moral sense. They ask whether reason is "the guardian of conscience" or whether morality is less gloriously rooted in a desire to avoid the unpleasant feelings of guilt and shame. Kagan speculates this question will be answered when a drug is developed that eliminates the discomforts of conscience but leaves reason intact. Magnus and Callahan also confront the relative roles of reason and emotion in their discussion of genetically modified organisms.

Zoloth declares a secular bioethics based on rationality and objectivity barren. Because religion advocates for charity, humility, and the most vulnerable she calls it the missing ingredient in bioethics. In response Callahan says theological ethics has done a better job of putting ethics in the larger framework of life and human destiny. Callahan may be modest; many of the matters that, according to Zoloth, require the religious voice have been explored by Callahan, an acknowledged atheist.

Secular ethical theories no less than religious dogma are predicated on assumptions; in that sense they are also faith based. Utilitarians believe actions are right or wrong based on their consequences. Deontologists believe in rules logically derived from principles and judge human actions right or wrong for reasons other than their consequences; for example, the moral philosopher Immanuel Kant expressed in his "categorical imperative" the belief that we ought to act only according to maxims we would will to become a universal law.

Principlism, a popular approach to ethics is derived from the belief that a common morality exists antecedent to ethical theory and "all persons who are serious about living a moral life already grasp the core dimensions of morality." This common morality is postulated as the universally shared set of moral beliefs that exist independent of local customs or religious dogma and apply in all societies at all times.

Principlism has translated common morality into four prima facie binding principles. These have most famously been expressed by Beauchamp and Childress as respect for autonomy, nonmaleficence (do no harm), beneficence (benefit others), and justice (fairness).[7] Gert's parallel translation of common morality is expressed as basic moral rules presumably acceptable to "all impartial rational persons." These include: Don't Cause Death; Don't Cause Pain; Don't Cause Loss of Ability; Don't Cause Loss of Freedom; Don't Cause Loss of Pleasure; Don't Deceive; Don't Cheat; Keep Your Promise. If a common morality exists, a code of ethics that could universally be accepted by reasonable and moral people is feasible.

Turner claims proponents of a common morality are overly sanguine because there is no empirical anthropological, historical or sociological evidence to support their claim. He points to violence against innocent people as " a damming staple of human history" that belies existence of a shared morality. Bioethics, according to Turner, fails to recognize the challenges posed by plural moral traditions in multicultural and multifaith societies.

Wilson and Haig challenge the conventional views of religion and many secular intellectual traditions by rooting morality in Darwinian biology.

Their message is that both moral and immoral behaviors are selected by evolutionary processes when they confer a survival advantage. That human moral systems are fundamentally biological may be disconcerting because it reminds us, as Edward O. Wilson has said, "however exalted in self-image, we were descended from animals."[8]

Difficulty determining the relative weight of ethical principles in specific circumstances is a common reason for ethical uncertainty and conflict. When a patient refuses treatment that is in his or her best medical interest the physician's conflict is not between right and wrong but between two morally valid principles on a collision course. The doctor wants to respect the patient's autonomy over his own body and at the same time honor the obligation of beneficence and help the patient recover. Although values may not be as neatly divided between the sexes as feminists suggest, the exchange between Tong and Meilaender on the relative weights due a "feminist" ethic of care that emphasizes social relationships and personal responsibilities and a "masculine" ethic that stresses autonomy, individual rights, and contractual duties illustrates that in practice, ethics often calls for the judicious balancing of conflicting obligations.

Perhaps morality is subject to various interpretations because it is a human construct that does not exist in the palpable world where its nature could more accurately be examined. Regardless of the reason, the often devilish ambiguity of biomedical ethics demands humility and an openness to conflicting opinion. At the same time we must remember that some actions are clearly right and others clearly wrong. As the articles that follow illustrate, a critical component of biomedical ethics is the struggle to make these distinctions.

NOTES

1. Singer Peter. *Ethics.* Oxford University Press Oxford New York, 1994.

2. Veatch Robert M. *Medical Ethics.* Jones and Bartlett Boston Portola Valley, 1989.

3. Gert Bernard. *Morality: A New Justification of the Moral Rules.* Oxford University Press, 1988.

4. I will use the words *ethics* and *morals* interchangeably

5. Despite its greater apparent certainty science rests on the assumption that the universe tomorrow will behave according to the same laws as the universe today.

6. Kass Leon. The Wisdom of Repugnance. *The New Republic* June 2, 1997 pages 17–26.

7. Beauchamp Tom L and Childress James F. *Principles of Biomedical Ethics.* Oxford University Press Fourth Edition, 1994.

8. Edward O. Wilson. Intelligent Evolution *Harvard Magazine* November–December, 2005.

ALLAN M. BRANDT, PHD

Bioethics: Then and Now

From the viewpoint of a medical historian looking back at the last quarter of the 20th century, the rise of bioethics as a movement and a discipline is nothing short of remarkable. During this period, an intensive medical and public discourse emerged that identified and debated critical moral dilemmas in medical care and research. The signs of this bioethics "revolution" are all around us. Hardly a day goes by when some moral conundrum of medicine is not aired on the front page, or, even more significantly, on television or the Internet. In our clinical institutions, the impact of bioethics is readily apparent: IRBs (Institutional Review Boards) actively assess the ethics of virtually all proposed human subjects research; the Joint Commission on Accreditation of Healthcare Organizations has mandated that hospitals have a mechanism for resolving ethical dilemmas. Most American medical schools teach medical ethics, and national board exams test candidates for their understanding of key ethical principles. And now, interactive sites on the Internet provide immediate instruction and counsel for vexing ethical dilemmas.[1]

This impressive set of activities marks an opportune moment to briefly assess the historical origins of bioethics, as well as its effectiveness in addressing contemporary moral problems in American medicine. As recently as 1970, the world of medicine was sacrosanct; its considerable cultural and political authority made it almost unthinkable that so much in medicine would become open to public debate, and that patients might reclaim authority over medical decisions and practice. In this respect, many observers of the rise of bioethics have declared it a dramatic victory in the name of moral progress.[2]

Bioethics offered a sharp critique of the insular world of medical research and a paternalistic tradition in medical practice. Among the most powerful triggers for the emergence of bioethics were a series of public revelations of gross abuses of human subjects who had been unknowingly coerced into participation in dangerous, nontherapeutic research. The Tuskegee Syphilis Study, the Willowbrook Hepatitis Study, and a long list of studies identified in anesthesiologist Henry Beecher's heroic 1966 analysis[3] are but the most prominent examples of tragic failures within research medicine to respect basic human rights. These and similar revelations exposed a research culture in which the interests of subjects had been fundamentally disregarded in the name of science.[4] Rising concern about research ethics also pointed to more fundamental questions about the character of medical authority within clinical medicine. Informed consent soon became the most basic premise for both research *and* clinical care.[5] The rise of bioethics can only be fully understood in the broader context of the rights-based movements for self-determination in the 1950s and 1960s; these include the civil rights movement, the rise of a new women's rights movement, and the early patient rights activities focused principally on psychiatric issues of civil commitment and the right to refuse treatment.[6] Bioethics led to a new patient-centered ethic, often advocating patients as genuine participants in their care rather than only the objects of diagnosis and treatment.

Assessing the deeper impact of bioethics in medical and research practice is, however, no easy task. A much-needed fuller assessment would require considerable historical and sociological investigation of a range of variables that are under any circumstances quite difficult to measure. Do patients today really exercise more autonomy over medical decision making? Are research subjects better protected from the intensive and competitive demands of new scientific knowledge? Just as we might assess equity in access to medical care, we might ask if all patients have had equal access to the advantages of new ethical precepts. Is there a socioeconomic gradient? Do better-educated patients, for example, benefit more significantly from informed consent than less well-educated ones? No doubt much changed over recent decades, but there are still significant problems. And indeed, some critics have argued that bioethics, regardless of its progressive intent, has actually had the effect of enhancing medical power over patients and research subjects by legitimate medical institutions and practices. To cite but one example, the consent form—in both research and therapeutic contexts—is often viewed by subjects and patients as but a legal apparatus to protect researchers and physicians from liability.

In short, bioethics as it evolved in the last decades of the 20th century is historically *contingent;* it reflected—and responded to—a series of specific contemporary critiques of biomedical practice and was fundamentally shaped by the social and political conventions of the time in which it emerged. Therefore, the bioethics that emerged in this period may no longer be a particularly good "fit" for the range of moral and ethical dilemmas currently confronting American medicine. Informed consent, the hallmark of bioethics, takes physicians' authority as a given. The prevailing assumption was that if physicians adequately respected patients' autonomy, their considerable authority would pass (through knowledge) back to their patients. Patient autonomy, therefore, rested upon an *a priori* physician autonomy. Bioethics in this form rarely considered the broader social and institutional contexts in which this ethical transaction occurred.

But today we see the authority and autonomy of the provider under attack. Importantly, if patient autonomy was at the center of discussion over the past decades, today physician autonomy seems to be the critical issue. A brief and perhaps typical clinical vignette illustrates aspects of this problem:

A patient with moderate back pain of relatively short duration comes to see her primary care physician. Following a careful history and physical examination, the physician recommends ibuprofen and rest. He explains that if there is no improvement in the next week the patient should let him know so that they can follow up. The patient asks if she needs an MRI. He explains that it currently isn't indicated, but that if she doesn't improve they can pursue other diagnostic options, perhaps including an MRI. The patient then asks if he is not ordering the MRI now because of financial incentives. The doctor is troubled by this exchange and what it represents about his relationship with his patient.

This vignette indicates that forces external to the doctor-patient interaction have altered the character of the relationship. Even though the doctor may believe that he would never compromise a patient's care regardless of financial incentives, his patient is concerned. The quality of trust has been altered, perhaps permanently. The patient worries that the doctor has lost his *authority* to care, and that his autonomous capacity to act in the patient's interest is eroded by new and often hidden rules and financial incentives. Such issues are, of course, not new to managed care. Physicians have always operated under the influence of considerable external (sometimes hidden) incentives. The point here is that bioethics—as it came to be constituted in the 1970s and 1980s—offered little in the way of analyzing such forces, be they economic, cultural or psychological.

As bioethics evolved over recent decades, the central question for healthcare providers confronted with an ethical dilemma was typically "what *should* I do?" Today, many of the dilemmas of medical care focus on the question: "what *can* I do?" This question recognizes essential constraints on clinical and moral choices and reflects an important historical shift in assumptions about agency within our healthcare system.

Although the parameters of a new bioethics are far from clear, several broad questions are already clearly apparent.[7] We will need more empirical research on practices associated with ethics both in patient-provider relationships and in our healthcare institutions and systems. Medical ethics is moving beyond the assertion of critical principles to assess concretely the obstacles that may inhibit our ability to realize them. This agenda requires a wide range of disciplines from clinical caregivers to the humanities and social sciences, as well as stronger assessment of the relationship of health policy to medical ethics. Only a complex dialogue that helps to reveal consensual social and moral values in a diverse culture—a dialogue among experts and the many constituencies doing medical work and seeking medical care—is likely to result in a new and effective medical ethics. In this respect it seems likely that as medicine changes, so too must our medical ethics.

NOTES

1. www.nih.gov/sigs/bioethics

2. Rothman DJ. *Strangers at the Bedside.* New York: Basic Books, 1991.

3. Beecher HK. Ethics and clinical research. *N Engl J Med* 1966;274(24):1354–60.

4. Jonsen AR. *The Birth of Bioethics.* New York: Oxford University Press, 1998.

5. Faden RR, Beauchamp TL. *A History and Theory of Informed Consent.* New York: Oxford University Press, 1986.

6. See e.g., Kluger R. *Simple Justice: the History of Brown v. Board of Education and Black America's Struggle for Equality.* New York: Knopf, 1975; Echols A. *Daring to Be Bad: Radical Feminism in America. 1967–1975.* Minneapolis: University of Minnesota Press, 1989; and Filene PG. *In the Arms of Others: a Cultural History of the Right-to-Die in America.* Chicago: I.R. Dee, 1998.

7. Kleinman A, Fox, RC, Brandt AM (eds). Bioethics and beyond. *Daedalus* 1999;128(4).

☰ ☶ ☶ ☰

ALBERT R. JONSEN, PHD

Bioethics: Then and Now

Bioethics appeared in the world of medicine in the early 1970s, and as Allan Brandt rightly notes, has grown into a remarkably vigorous discipline. Professors of bioethics exist in most medical schools, courses are taught not only to medical students but to undergraduates, and a continual stream of books and articles is devoted to the topics of the field: death and dying, experimentation with humans, genetics and reproductive technology.[1] I must agree with Brandt that the form it has taken since its beginnings has stressed the relationship between physicians and patients, to the neglect of the structure of the institutions within which that relationship occurs. He proposes that "the bioethics that emerged in this period [from the 1970s until today] might not be a particularly good 'fit' for the range of moral and ethical dilemmas currently confronting American medicine." I will, in this short commentary, explain why bioethics took the route that it did and suggest the route it must take in the coming decades if it is to become a better "fit" in the world of medicine and healthcare.

Brandt correctly identifies the starting point of bioethics' journey: the "insular world of medical research and a paternalistic tradition in medical practice." Persons encountered the medical world as patients or, much less frequently, as subjects of research. In both, physicians exercised great power. They held what one scholar called "professional dominance," that is, they could decide what constituted disease, who might have access to treatment and whether that treatment was only for the patient's benefit or for the advancement of science.[2] Although physicians have been paternalistic and authoritarian throughout the history of medicine, the extraordinary transformation of medicine by science and technology has reinforced these traits. This was due, perhaps, to the very nature of science and technology. Science is arcane; scientists are masters of intricate information expressed in private languages. Technology is complex; only those with exact skills can apply it. Scientific knowledge and technical skill insures that decisions about its use and application will become the prerogative of its possessors.

Also, as medical knowledge became more scientific, it became incorporated in the insistent movement of science to acquire more, and more certain, knowledge. The practice of medicine was wrapped into the practice of research, and patients became, usually without their knowledge and consent, the subjects (or objects) on which the hypotheses of the scientists and the new treatments of physicians were tested. Medicine, through the first half of the 20th century, was proud that it had become "scientific," and certainly patients were the beneficiaries of many innovative discoveries that were translated into care. At the same time, those patients remained outside the process of decision-making that ultimately affected them deeply.

The occurrence of certain highly visible events, such as the Nazi concentration camp experiments and the American Tuskegee studies, were catalysts for debate over the ethics of experimentation. At the same time, many patients felt oppressed by the technology that prolonged rather than alleviated their suffering. Certain innovative interventions could save and prolong their lives, but at the same time, imposed severe constraints on the quality of those lives. Renal dialysis was one of these two-edged swords. Introduced in the early 1960s, it saved from certain death patients with permanently failed kidneys but confined them to a regimen of perpetual dependence on a machine and recurrent bouts of fatigue and dialysis-related illness. Many persons gladly bore these inconveniences; others found life with them to be intolerable. Some patients committed "dialysis suicide" by terminating or neglecting their regular treatment. New ventilatory techniques sustained life and breath but sometimes the light of life, in the mind and the affections, was dimmed or gone. The miracle technologies were not "fixes." They often imposed changes in the quality of life that persons felt they should decide to accept or reject. Gradually, in medical care and in research, the idea of informed consent emerged as a legal standard. The technology that had reinforced the paternal authority of physicians became an instrument that patients could decide to employ in their own behalf.

Bioethics appeared within that social context: technology giving physicians more power to treat than they had ever possessed; patients feeling the need to control the effects of that power in their lives. However, the initial bioethicists were not, for the most part, physicians. They were theologians and philosophers: scholars with a knowledge of academic ethics but only observers of medicine (except when they, like most mortals, became patients). They appreciated the need for scientific advance but deplored the depreciation of the freedom of persons who were the sources of that advance, namely, the experimental subject.

Theologians of note, such as Paul Ramsey of Princeton, and philosophers of repute, such as Hans Jonas of the New School of Social Research, undertook to revise the ethics of medicine in ways that would counteract medical authoritarianism and paternalism.

These scholars, and those who followed them, introduced into medical ethics a quite novel view. Those who practiced medicine had constructed medical ethics. These practitioners reflected on the personal and social conditions that would conduce to a successful healing and a successful practice. Only rarely did they employ the concepts and the methods of the philosophers and theologians who ruminated on the moral life. However, the first bioethicists were formally trained in those concepts and methods and explicitly brought them to the analysis of the new questions about medical authority and about life and death.[3] Ramsey drew on theological notions of covenant, the mutual compact between Yahweh and the People of Israel, to frame a notion of covenantal fidelity between doctors and their patients, research scientists and their subjects. Jonas imported notions of classical European philosophy into his development of the ethics of responsibility between scientists and subjects. Other theologians and philosophers who entered the bioethical debates evoked ethical arguments from their disciplines. In general, those arguments emphasized the freedom, authenticity and responsibility of individuals. They slighted the broader settings of politics, economics and culture within which human actions take place because, at that time, their disciplines attended much more to personal action and inter-personal relationships than to social structures and institutional structures.

In the ensuing years, the perception of the nature of the problems of bioethics has shifted from the interpersonal (which is still important) to the institutional. The authority of medical managers has usurped the authority of physicians and the rights of patients. The use of technology is contingent on policy and financing as much, or more, than on medical need. The rights of patients are debated now, not just by philosophers, but also by congressmen whose opinion is deeply colored by political ideology. It is clear that the broader social and institutional contexts are crucial to understanding and ameliorating ethical problems. Contemporary bioethicists have recognized the overemphasis on the ethics of autonomy and desire a richer appreciation of the ethics of justice. They are working at the reconstruction of a discipline that will have stronger conceptual tools to pry open the problems created by the social and economic structures of modern health care. However, this is a work in progress and, with few exceptions, bioethics does not yet "fit" these problems in the same way that the early bioethics "fit" the problems of emerging technology.

I have written about bioethics as a discipline, that is, the work produced by scholars employing shared methods of analysis and using specialized terminologies to express the results of their analysis. However, there is another bioethics. It exists in the media, in political debates, in the meetings of hospital committees, in the anxious discussions of patients, families and doctors over treatment and care, in the corporate planning of biotechnology companies and in many other places. This is not a bioethics of formal concepts and analytic methodology. It borrows bits and pieces from disciplinary bioethics, talking about informed consent, risks and benefits, equity, rights, and the like. It knows something of the issues, such as physician-assisted suicide, genetic therapy and cloning. But it is a bioethics carried on by concerned people, aware of the problems and desirous to see them resolved in some fashion. This is the discourse of bioethics rather than the discipline. The questions asked by Brandt about the deeper impact of bioethics are, as he said, answerable only by a fuller assessment. However, it seems to me that these questions are much more vigorously discussed in the many settings of bioethical discourse than ever in the past. Some of that discourse has led to specific social change, such as the enactment of Oregon's law about physician-assisted suicide and the same state's policies on the rationing of healthcare resources. But even where specific evidences of change are absent, the problems are broadly and openly and intelligently discussed. In the long run, bioethics as a discipline is justified to the extent that it introduces into public discourse ideas and ideals that, through the means open to a democratic society, move social, institutional and economic powers in directions that better reflect those ethical ideas and ideals.

NOTES

1. Jonsen AR. *The Birth of Bioethics*. New York: Oxford University Press, 1998.

2. Freidson E. *Professional Dominance: the Social Structure of Medical Care*. New York: Atherton Press, 1970.

3. Jonsen AR. *A Short History of Medical Ethics*. New York: Oxford University Press, 2000.

☷ ☷ ☷ ☷

JEROME KAGAN, PHD

The Nature of Morality

One of the important facts of evolution is that each species can possess unique characteristics. Snakes shed their skin, spiders build webs, bears hibernate. Humans evaluate their actions and themselves as good or bad and, as a consequence, experience a distinctive emotion whenever they behave in ways that are inconsistent with their understanding of the way a good person behaves. These two properties define the human moral sense.

Philosophers, psychologists and biologists have grappled with two questions related to human morality. Why do humans, but no other animal, judge events as good or bad? Second, what factors determine the particular characteristics that will be judged good or bad within a particular culture? This brief essay addresses these two profound issues.

THE EMERGENCE OF A MORAL SENSE

The first signs of a moral competence can be observed in every home with young children. A 2-year-old looks warily toward a parent after spilling juice on the floor. The child's face and posture announce that she knows she has committed an act that violates what she knows to be proper.

Although the infant younger than 1 year perceives the changes in face and voice that communicate parental displeasure with an action, the infant is not mature enough to infer that breaking objects, dirtying clothes and crying at the dinner table, although followed by disapproval, belong to a category of bad acts. In order to infer this evaluation, the child must discover the connections among three different events—her actions, the outcomes of those actions and the parents' subsequent reactions. The ability to make inferences based on a temporal sequence of events is fragile in the first year; the infant is not mature enough to discover the concept "punishable behavior."

However, this competence does not explain why 2-year-olds impose a good/ bad label on punished actions. Answering that question requires a bit of speculation. Evocation of a state of uncertainty to an unexpected event that cannot be understood is a biologically prepared reaction that invites a name when children become aware of their feelings at the end of the 2nd year. When the uncertainty pierces awareness, the child is motivated to name it. The symbolic label applied is close in sense meaning to the adult understanding of the word *bad*.

Children also create representations of the normal appearances of objects and notice those that are deviant. A child who sees a broken toy on the floor assumes that some action by another person must have caused the flaw. Because breaking toys is a bad act, the broken toy is also bad.

The ability to empathize with another in distress, which also emerges in the second year, has obvious relevance for morality. Two-year-olds can infer some of the thoughts and feelings of another and show signs of tension if they see that another individual is hurt. They may even offer penance if they were the cause of the other's distress. As a result, an intention to hurt another produces an anticipation of the unpleasant feelings the other might experience and therefore suppression of the intended asocial act.

When the awareness of self emerges by age 2, children apply the labels good and bad to themselves as they have done for objects and to their behaviors. If self is regarded as a bad object, the child is vulnerable to the same unpleasant feeling states that are linked to actions that were classified as bad. Hence, children try to avoid accruing evidence suggesting that the adjective bad is appropriate for them. The child understands that if he is a bad object, he will evoke unpleasant feelings in others, in the same way that bad actions produce unpleasant feelings in the self and will infer that others will avoid him.

A desire to avoid or to deny the labeling of self as bad increases with age and, in time, will take precedence over fear of punishment as the primary determinant of proper behavior. A few years later, when the child is 6 or 7, a new cognitive ability will permit the emotion of guilt. The older child can rerun a behavioral sequence mentally and decide whether the damage he caused could have been prevented. If the child concludes he could have avoided breaking a vase or hurting another, he is likely to experience guilt.

THE CONTENTS OF MORALITY

Although all humans possess a moral sense, they differ, with one exception, in the acts, thoughts and feelings they judge as good or bad. The exception is the moral standard on hurting another without justification. This restraint on unprovoked aggression is due to the emergence of the feeling of empathy for another in the 2nd year.

It is more difficult to defend the natural inevitability of any other moral standard, including standards on individual freedom from the demands of others, justice, loyalty, honesty or self-interest. Many monks and nuns voluntarily gave up their personal freedom in order to serve God. Contemporary American lawyers who have just joined a large firm do not regard loyalty to the institution as a moral imperative because their culture has persuaded them that concern with one's self-enhancement is the primary standard one should obey.

An important change in Western society over the last few centuries has been an erosion of the ethical constraints on behavior that are linked with membership in particular social categories, especially gender, place of residence, type of work, class and religion.

A person who is identified with one or more of these categories accepts the constraints linked to membership in return for the feeling of virtue and self enhancement that membership provides.

For example, forms of work—soldier, priest, banker, feudal landlord or scribe—were regarded as lifelong roles that brought pride and responsibilities in Renaissance Europe. Most contemporary Americans and Europeans do not regard their vocation as a source of distinctive pride or special responsibility. Teachers, plumbers, clerks and machinists do not enjoy the same self-enhancement as 17th century Boston silversmiths or ministers. However, humans require feelings of enhancement and virtue. I suggest that attainment of personal status, wealth and power, as well as a satisfying love relationship, serve that function in modern society. But these goals do not require one to worry about the feelings or needs of large numbers of fellow citizens.

A second change, perhaps more significant, is a result of America's need to make our society more egalitarian and to persuade minority citizens, especially those who are poor and of color, that the playing field is sufficiently even that they have a fair chance of worldly success. Persuading citizens of this fact required Americans to remove the symbols of virtue that had been attached to family pedigree, ethnicity, religion, marital status and even sexual preference.

As a result, behaviors and beliefs that, in the past, were regarded as having some sacredness have lost this quality for large numbers of Americans, but especially for those under 30 years of age. Self-enhancement and loyalty to one's immediate family are the primary standards that retain some power. The virtue that comes from a desire to nurture members of one's society even though they are strangers which had a moral imperative earlier, has been weakened considerably.

A QUESTION FOR THE FUTURE

Discoveries in molecular biology and neuroscience suggest that during the next half century scientists will discover a drug that eliminates the feeling components of guilt and remorse while leaving intact the semantic knowledge that certain behaviors are ethically improper. An individual who took this drug regularly would continue to know that deceiving a friend, lying to a client and stealing from an employer were morally wrong, but would be protected from the uncomfortable feeling of remorse that normally accompanies violation of a personal standard. Hence, it is reasonable to wonder whether our society will be changed in a major way if a majority of our citizens were protected from guilt. This question addresses a long-standing debate on the basis for ethical actions and the criteria individuals apply when they are faced with a moral choice.

Most Western philosophers, but especially Kant, made reason the bedrock of conscience. People acted properly, Kant believed, because they knew the behavior was morally right. This argument for reason as the guardian of conscience has considerable merit. All individuals wish to regard the self as virtuous and try to avoid the uncertainty that follows detection of the cognitive inconsistency created when one behaves in ways that are not in accord with one's view of a good person. Dostoevsky was imprisoned for five years in an isolated Siberian outpost with peasant convicts who rejected him because of his middle-class origins and moral premises. Although it would have been expedient for Dostoevsky to have adopted, temporarily, the values of his debauched fellow prisoners, he continued to honor the standards he brought to this harsh setting. Kant would have understood his inability to act in ways he thought were immoral.

On the other hand, some philosophers—Peirce and Dewey are two examples—have argued that anticipation of feelings of anxiety, shame or guilt motivate continued loyalty to one's moral standards.[1,2] A person who was certain that he was protected from these emotions might find it easier to ignore the moral imperatives acquired during childhood.

The tension between these two positions is especially clear in modern industrialized societies where the balance between the feeling of virtue that follows enhancing another and the pleasure that follows the enhancing of self has shifted toward a more consistent favoring of the latter state. A spouse with young children caught in a marriage that has grown stale must decide whether the ethical demand to maintain family integrity should take precedence over the desire to feel happier, more excited and challenged. A young scientist eager for a promotion, a higher salary and a brief moment of fame must decide whether to visit a sick parent or continue working on a book.

The conflict 19th century adults experienced over this choice has been replaced, in Western society, with a growing consensus, almost universal among the young, that self's pleasures and potency come first. The awarding of priority to self-enhancement in deciding whether one is happy has eroded an earlier habit of also relying, occasionally, on the judgment that one is loving, charitable, loyal, honest and nurturing, and has diluted the power of Kant's argument. Although it is not obvious that a drug that blocks remorse will eliminate the mutual social obligations that make a society habitable, nonetheless, a posture of vigilance is appropriate for, unlike gorillas, humans can hold for a very long time representations of envy, anger and dislike toward those they have never met. Hence, the anticipation of guilt and shame helps to restrain rudeness, dishonesty and aggression. We will have to wait for history to resolve this question.

NOTES

1. Peirce CS. *Collected Papers.* Cambridge, MA: Harvard University Press, 1932.
2. Dewey J. *Human Nature and Conduct.* New York: Holt, 1922.

☷ ☲ ☲ ☴

RICHARD A. SHWEDER, PHD

The Nature of Morality: The Category of Bad Acts

Three types of questions about the nature of morality can be distinguished: (a) philosophical, (b) psychological and (c) epidemiological. The philosophical question asks whether (and in what sense) "goodness" and "badness" are real or objective properties that particular actions possess in varying degrees. The psychological question asks, what are the mental states and processes associated with the human classification of events as good versus bad? The epidemiological question asks, what is the actual distribution of moral judgments across time (developmental time and historical time) and across space (for example, across cultures)? With such questions in mind, I develop a limited critique of Kagan's "The Nature of Morality," while at the same time fully endorsing his central message that the study of moral psychology benefits greatly from the study of the emotions. Vice versa, I also suggest that an understanding of the cognitive side of moral judgment is a necessary precondition for a full understanding of the psychology of the emotions.

"Cognitivists" (Plato is perhaps the most famous) answer the philosophical question in the affirmative. They believe that any particular moral judgment, like scientific judgments, must thus be either true or false. They conclude, moral competence amounts to discovering the truth of the matter by means of either secular or theological modes of reasoning.

In contrast, philosophical "emotivists" (Hume is perhaps the most famous) argue that there really is no real property "out there" to be represented or described with such terms as "good" or "bad." According to the emotivists, moral judgments are neither true nor false. They are merely expressions of personal or collective choice. Judgments of "good" and "bad" just express likes and dislikes, positive and negative feeling states, tastes and aversions. What you should not do, say the emotivists, is ask whether likes, preferences or tastes are accurate estimations of what is truly "good" (or "bad"), because those moral terms are merely labels for our feelings.

Kagan suggests answers to the epidemiological and psychological questions. (1) The moral sense is unique to our species and universal across cultures and history. (2) Doing harm to others without reason is the only action considered immoral in all societies. (3) Moral judgments about particular actions do not converge over time or space. (4) In contemporary Western society a morality emphasizing autonomy (having the things you want, preference maximization) is superceding a morality emphasizing duties and obligations related to membership in social categories. (5) Adults experience their moral judgments both as "cognitive" judgments and "emotive" judgments; both reason and feeling play their part in moral psychology around the world. Nevertheless, Kagan believes, moral judgments are motivators of action primarily to the extent that they produce in human beings feelings of repugnance, guilt, indignation and shame; and he doubts the cognitive side of our moral nature is sufficient to motivate moral action.

He also tells this story about moral development. "Good/bad" categories, mostly devoid of meaning, are already (innately?) available to the neonate and then get "imposed on" experience and filled in with content. This happens once the child has the intellectual capacity to notice and remember connections between actions and their consequences, negative subjective states (uncertainty, feelings of tension, unpleasant emotions) and parental disapproval. With the exception of "arbitrary assault," Kagan seems to suggest that the connection between any action and its classification as "bad" is almost entirely mediated by parental reactions and the experience of negative feeling states. Here his fondness for emotivism seems most apparent.

My admiration for Kagan's research on morality and emotion is great and some of my own work[1,2,3] is strongly supportive of his observations about crosscultural variability in moral judgments. In the places in India where I do research the category of "bad acts" includes a widow eating fish, a woman having a conversation with her husband's elder brother, and parents refusing to sleep in the same bed with their children.

I have also proposed that on a worldwide scale there is a "big three" of morality. There is an "ethics of autonomy" based on moral concepts such as harm, rights and justice, which is designed to protect individuals in pursuit of the gratification of their wants. There is an "ethics of community" based on moral concepts such as duty, hierarchy and interdependency, which is designed to help individuals achieve dignity by virtue of their role and position in a society. There is an "ethics of divinity" based on moral concepts such as natural order, sacred order, sanctity, sin and pollution, which is designed to maintain the integrity of the spiritual side of human nature. These ethics vary in their centrality and distribution both across and within groups.

I offer the following limited critique of Kagan's position: First, the prohibition on arbitrary assault is not the only "natural" or universal moral standard.

There are many others, including the moral imperative to "treat like cases alike," to protect the vulnerable, to avoid incest, to reciprocate in social exchanges, to be grateful for gifts, to honor promises. I would add to the list many of the "virtues." Of course, as Kagan well knows, the rub with all such universal standards, including the norm against hurting others "without a reason," is that they are too abstract to determine moral decisions about particular cases. For example, even in cases of genocide or acts of "martyrdom" by terrorists, the killers typically believe they are acting in "self-defense" (that is, with reason) against some perceived threat to their group or way of life.

Secondly, a question arises. Is Kagan a soft cognitivist who believes, as I do, that human reason has limits and leaves room for fully rational and morally decent people to disagree in their moral judgments? Or is he an emotivist who believes that the experience of a negative feeling state is sufficient reason to classify almost anything as morally bad? One tenet of soft cognitivism is that normal human beings are intuitively philosophical cognitivists. As Arthur Lovejoy has noted,[4] when someone says, "The conduct of Adolf Hitler was wicked," they "do not in fact conceive of themselves merely to be reporting on the state of their emotions." They mean to be saying something more than "I am very unpleasantly affected when I think of it." Any viable cultural system provides its members with "good reasons" for seeing this or that event in such a way that it can be locally experienced as a concrete instance of some abstract moral standard. This process of filling in with "good reasons" the gap between abstract universal moral standards and concrete local actions may involve many parochial concepts and beliefs, but it is very cognitive. I also suggest that one reason there is disagreement across cultures about which actions are good is because there are so many universal abstract moral standards (justice, loyalty, benevolence, duty, respect, liberty) that they are in conflict and cannot all be maximized simultaneously. A choice must be made about which "goods" take precedence. Hence one can be a soft cognitivist while granting that emotional experiences in childhood may play a big part in signaling which of the virtues is most important on the local cultural scene.

Thirdly, "Western society" is big enough to accommodate many different types of groups with many different types of ethics. Lene Jensen discovered that liberal and fundamentalist Protestants in the USA both endorse an ethics of community, despite Robert Bellah's concerns about excessive individualism.[5] The liberals also accept an ethics of autonomy while the fundamentalists don't. How these ethical ratios are playing themselves out is more complex than some of the critics of Western individualism and hedonism have suggested.

Finally, it seems to me that reason and feeling have never had symmetrical parts to play in moral psychology. Reason can justify our moral reactions (and if you are a fully rational person, motivate them as well) while feelings can only motivate behavior, but never justify it. Upon analysis, many emotions seem to contain within themselves a moral core. "Fear" is associated with issues of safety and harm and motivates us to eliminate the conditions that produce it. "Anger" and "indignation" are associated with issues of fairness, equity and just deserts and motivate us to eliminate injustice from the world. "Love" and "compassion" are associated with protection of the vulnerable and motivate us to take care of others. In each case, our emotional reactions can be justified by the good reasons (the "cognitive appraisal conditions," e.g., the threat to safety, the injustice, the vulnerability) that produced them. They can't be justified by simply pointing to the motivating feeling states (e.g., the heat or tension or uncertainty) that "drive" us to act. It would be quite insufficient to translate "I am angry at him" as only meaning "I have been unfairly treated by him." "I have been unfairly treated by him" is in the domain of reason. It is a proposition about a state of the world that can be judged true or false. If it is false, one should not be angry if one is a reasonable person. Yet, "anger" is more than its cognitive core. It is also the feeling state. And, of course, human societies have never been entirely populated by fully rational persons—those who are motivated to do all things only for good reasons. Which is why one suspects Kagan is right that without the feelings that go with guilt, shame, disgust, righteous indignation and the anticipation of stigma we would live in a less moral world.

NOTES

1. Shweder RA, Mahapatra M, Miller JG. Kagan J, Lamb S eds. Culture and Moral Development. In *The Emergence of Morality in Young Children.* Chicago: University of Chicago Press, 1987:1–83.

2. Shweder RA, Jensen L, Goldstein W., Goodnow JJ, Miller P, Kessel F eds. Who Sleeps By Whom Revisited: A Method for Extracting the Moral "Goods" Implicit in Praxis. In *Cultural Practices as Contexts for Development.* San Francisco: Jossey-Bass, 1995.

3. Shweder RA, Much NC, Mahapatra M, Park L., Brandt A, Rozin P. eds. The "Big Three" of Morality (Autonomy, Community, Divinity), and the "Big Three" Explanations of Suffering. In *Morality and Health.* New York: Routledge, 1997.

4. Lovejoy A. *Reflections on Human Nature.* Johns Hopkins University Press, 1961:253,255.

5. Jensen L. Different worldviews, different morals: America's culture war divide. *Human Development* 1997;40:325–344.

☰ ☷ ☷ ☰

DAVID SLOAN WILSON, PHD

The Biological Basis of Morality

Evolution and morality often seem to occupy opposite corners of human thought. After all, words such as "bestial" refer to the very worst things that people do to each other. If we are mere beasts, what is to prevent us from behaving in a bestial fashion? So many people are reluctant to accept the theory of evolution, or to connect it to anything relevant to their own lives, for fear of the perceived dire moral implications if it were true.

The actual relationship between evolution and morality is more complex and interesting. Evolution can explain our capacity for moral behavior in addition to our capacity for immoral behavior, and understanding the biological basis of moral systems can make them stronger rather than weaker.

Every year I explain the biological basis of morality by asking my students to tell me what they associate with morality. One side of the blackboard becomes filled with their suggestions: charity, generosity, altruism, forgiveness, courage, honesty. There is very little disagreement about what constitutes goodness, at least on a broad scale. Then I ask for immoral traits and I can barely write fast enough to list their suggestions on the other side of the board: selfishness, deception, murder, cowardice, hypocrisy.

"What will happen if we place the epitome of a moral person and the epitome of an immoral person together on a desert island?" I ask my class. The answer is a no-brainer. The moral person will become shark food within days. Then I ask a second question: "What will happen if we put a group of moral people on one desert island and a group of immoral people on another desert island?" The answer to this question is also a no-brainer. The moral people will work together to escape the island or turn it into a little paradise, while the immoral people will turn their island into a living hell. Now my third and final question: "What will happen if we add a few immoral people to the moral island and a few moral people to the immoral island?" The answer to this question is not so easy, but is some messy combination of the decisive answers to the first two questions.

As simple as this class exercise might seem, it shows that there is nothing unbiological about the golden rule, the ten commandments, and all the other virtues preached by religious and ethical traditions around the world. Societies that adopt these virtues will survive and reproduce fabulously well and usually are encouraged to do just that by the injunction to be fruitful and multiply. The main problem with explaining morality as a biological adaptation[1] is its vulnerability to subversion from within. What we call immoral is parasitic and predatory on what we call moral. There's trouble in paradise as soon as the first immoral person paddles over to Virtue Island.

The formal version of my class exercise is called multilevel selection theory. Natural selection can operate among individuals within social groups (within-group selection), but it can also take place among social groups within a larger population (among-group selection).

Within-group selection tends to favor the traits that we associate with immorality, that benefit the self at the expense of others and the group as a whole. Among-group selection tends to favor the traits that we associate with morality, which benefit others and the group as a whole, often at the expense of the self.

Species differ in the degree to which their properties have been molded by within- vs. among-group selection. Social insects (bees, wasps, ants and termites) are famous for their altruism and service to their colonies. What this means in evolutionary terms is that most traits in social insects evolved by increasing the fitness of the entire colony, relative to other colonies (among-group selection), rather than by increasing the fitness of the individual insect, relative to other insects within the same colony (within-group selection). However, some traits in social insects have evolved by within-group selection, such as workers laying their own eggs rather than participating in the economy of the hive. Other traits have evolved to prevent these "cheating" behaviors. Despite the many differences between social insect colonies and human social groups, the mix of cooperative, exploitative and policing activities in social insect colonies has an unmistakably human appearance.

Biological systems consist not merely of two tiers (individuals and groups) but many tiers. Individuals are themselves groups of lower-level units such as genes and cell lineages, and social groups are nested within larger groups and multispecies ecosystems. When multilevel selection theory is applied to the entire multitier hierarchy, striking discoveries result that cause our own moral systems to be seen as part of a much larger picture. For example, most genes and cell lineages evolve by increasing the fitness of the whole organism, relative to other organisms, but some evolve by spreading at the expense of other genes and cell lineages within the same organism. Just like cheating bees and individuals regarded as immoral in human groups, these "selfish" elements are favored by natural selection within their collectives but undermine the collective as an adaptive unit. We regard them as diseases but they are not foreign organisms that have invaded our bodies; instead they are a part of us that succeed at the expense of the rest of us, rather than by contributing to the communal effort! Examples include cancers and genes that subvert the usually fair process of meiosis. In the case of meiosis, division usually assures that all genes comprising an individual have the same chance of being represented in the gametes. The phenomenon of meiotic drive involves genes that "cheat" by subverting the "fair" rules of meiosis, getting into more than 50 percent of the gametes, but often decreasing the fitness of the individual as a result. Similarly, evolution in foreign disease organisms can favor traits that cause some strains to succeed at the expense of other strains within the same host, or by causing the entire disease population within the host to spread to new hosts. These examples of multilevel selection have important medical implications, in addition to their relevance to the study of morality.

Until very recently (by evolutionary standards) our ancestors lived in small groups who hunted and gathered for a living. Just as for bodies and beehives, traits could evolve by benefiting individuals at the expense of others within the same group, or by benefiting the whole group relative to other groups. Both levels of selection have been important in human evolution, which may well explain our morally ambivalent nature. We are capable of perceiving what is good for others and acting accordingly at least some of the time, but we are also sorely tempted to behave in ways that are regarded as immoral. We have a passion for evaluating the moral conduct of those around us and often judging them more harshly than we judge ourselves. Finally, even our limited capacity for morality has a disturbing way of stopping at the boundaries of our groups, giving way to behaviors such as genocide that are judged as the ultimate in immorality by the members of other groups.

Cultural evolution can be a multilevel process in addition to genetic evolution. A few years ago I encountered a religious passage written 350 years ago that stated "True love means growth for the whole organism, whose members are all interdependent and serve each other ... We see the same thing among the bees, who all work with equal zeal gathering honey." This comparison between a body, a beehive and a religious community made me wonder if multilevel selection could make as much sense of religious groups as the other collective units of life. I believe that the answer is "yes."[2] In addition, the same evolutionary principles can explain other human social organizations—such as politically and ethnically defined groups—leading to a truly general theory of "unifying systems" in our own species and in life in general.

The possibility that human moral systems (religious and otherwise) can be explained as a product of evolution has only recently become an active field of inquiry and will surely be regarded as controversial against the background of previous intellectual traditions, religious and secular alike. In addition to challenging conventional views of religion, it also challenges major paradigms in the social sciences, such as individual self-interest as a grand explanatory principle. However, far from threatening basic moral values, an evolutionary theory of "unifying systems" can strengthen them and lead to practical solutions to modern societal problems. After all, if morality is an adaptation that can evolve under appropriate social and environmental conditions, and if evolution can take place by fast-paced cultural processes in addition to slow-paced genetic processes, then by establishing the appropriate conditions we can influence the future course of moral evolution.

NOTES

1. Moral behavior, such as members of a group altruistically helping each other, confers an evolutionary survival advantage. Moral systems have therefore evolved through natural selection and are deeply rooted in biology rather than simply in reason or religious revelation.

2. Wilson D S. *Darwin's Cathedral: Evolution, Religion, and the Nature of Society.* Chicago, University of Chicago Press, 2002.

SUGGESTED READING

Boehm C. *Hierarchy in the Forest: Egalitarianism and the Evolution of Human Altruism.* Cambridge, MA: Harvard University Press, 1999.

Seeley T. *The Wisdom of the Hive.* Cambridge, MA: Harvard University Press, 1995.

Smith M, Szathmary E, Szathmary J. *The Origins of Life: From the Birth of Life to the Origin of Language.* Oxford: Oxford University Press, 1999.

Sober E, Wilson D S. *Unto Others: The Evolution and Psychology of Unselfish Behavior.* Cambridge, MA: Harvard University Press, 1998.

☰ ☷ ☷ ☰

DAVID HAIG, PHD

The Amoral Roots of Morality

David Sloan Wilson describes the biological basis of morality in lucid fashion and, although we might have minor disagreements on points of emphasis, I find myself in broad agreement with what he has to say. Natural selection is neither moral nor immoral, but amoral. Our capacity to see things in moral terms is a product of the evolutionary process, as is our capacity for treachery, selfishness and deceit. Both moral and immoral behaviors are subject to winnowing on the basis of their effects on the replication of the agent responsible for the behavior. "The ends justify the means" is almost a definition of natural selection, if "justify" is stripped of any connotations of moral approval. As it concerns morality, evolutionary biology is descriptive rather than prescriptive. It helps us to understand how morality evolved, what it is used for, and why it sometimes breaks down. It may even suggest more effective means to achieve desired ends, but it cannot suggest what these ends *should* be.

Wilson positions the evolution of morality in the context of multilevel selection theory. Immoral behaviors tend to be favored by within-group selection, with immoral individuals gaining a selfish advantage at the expense of other group members. Moral behaviors, on the other hand, tend to be favored by among-group selection, with groups of moral individuals outperforming groups of selfish individuals and thus conferring reproductive benefits on the members of the moral group.

There are two problems with the rosy view that natural selection among groups will favor ever-greater advances in moral behavior. The first is that moral groups may include, among their members, individuals who benefit from the group's moral behavior but obtain additional benefits from their own immoral behavior. Such individuals appear to have the best of both worlds. If they gain a reproductive advantage relative to their moral colleagues, moral behavior is in danger of unravelling as the proportion of immoral individuals increases, gradually converting a productive group of selfless individuals into a less productive group of selfish individuals. There are a number of theoretical routes out of this bind. For example, if groups split up sufficiently often, some of the descendant groups will by random sampling (or, better yet, by preferential association of moral individuals) receive fewer selfish individuals. Such processes, that increase the variation among groups, can sometimes keep ahead of the tendency for the proportion of selfish individuals to increase. Perhaps the most effective route, however, is to directly deny the benefits of moral behavior to the selfish members of a group, either by exclusion or by direct punishment of selfish acts. If the benefits of cooperation and the costs of being punished are large enough, selfishness no longer pays and all individuals should behave "morally," not out of conviction nor on principle, but out of pragmatic self-interest. Recent work in experimental economics (a cousin of evolutionary biology) has shown that many individuals are prepared to incur a personal cost to punish individuals who are perceived as behaving unfairly, and that such "strong reciprocity" is remarkably effective at enforcing norms of fair behavior.

Moral communities are at risk of being exploited from within. Therefore, it is no coincidence that our evolved moral sentiments include what one may call righteous anger. The individual who transgresses the moral code is its focus. He or she is cast out from the community and is no longer entitled to its benefits. Sometimes the transgressor becomes an object of moral aggression, with the aggressors no longer constrained by the dictates of morality that apply to members of the community. The evolutionary rationale of righteous anger is clear when it is directed against the selfish exploiter of others, but the emotion can also be directed against other non-conformists who abide by different moral rules. It can then be used to justify the mistreatment of the dissenter, the homosexual, the Jew, the infidel or the heretic. Osama bin Laden unleashing the World Trade Center atrocity and George W. Bush declaring preemptive war have at least this much in common: each believes his acts are justified by the immoral behavior of his adversary. Both invoke divine approval for their actions. Both are enemies of moral relativism.

Consideration of who falls inside and outside the pale of moral protection raises the second problem with the rosy view that selection among groups inexorably favors advances in morality. Within-group cooperation evolves because it provides an advantage relative to other groups, but groupishness may be even less desirable than selfishness. The capacity for genocidal warfare is an obvious candidate for a component of the human behavioral repertoire that has evolved by group-level selection. The obligations of group loyalty—and the fear of being outcast—may cause a nation to acquiesce, and many to participate, in a holocaust.

When we discuss national conflicts, we have moved into a very different world from that in which our moral sentiments evolved. Moral evolution has not ceased, but it now proceeds largely in the cultural realm. Our conception of what is right and what is wrong may have changed under the influence of philosophers, religious and political reformers, novelists, and perhaps scientists, but we are stuck with the emotional toolkit supplied by our biological heritage. Natural selection has provided us with the capacity for charity, generosity, forgiveness, courage and honesty, as well as for greed, callousness, vindictiveness, cowardice and mendacity. It has given us the ability to see things in moral terms, to put ourselves in others' shoes, and to sacrifice ourselves for a principle. But it has also given us the ability to sidestep our conscience, to practice double standards, and to sacrifice others for the same moral principle.

Our moral sentiments are powerful tools to move us to action. Moral precepts are perceived as being universal, and thus binding on all members of a group. Moral obligations are seen as overriding personal preference. If some policy can be defined as the moral course, much energy can be mobilized to advance it. If it can be defined as immoral, the forces of moral outrage can be marshalled against it. For these reasons, much of political debate is framed in moral terms, as arguments about what is right. In this world of competing interests, moral clarity is all too often a combination of a certain degree of self-deception about one's own motives and blindness to alternative points of view.

Is moral evolution progressive? There is no external standard against which to measure moral progress, at least none that would receive universal consent. But there is change. As the result of cultural evolution, we now make sacrifices to defend groups that are larger and more diverse in their membership than the groups for which our moral sentiments evolved. Moreover, moral evolution now proceeds in a marketplace of ideas, in which different moral philosophies compete for adherents. It need no longer proceed by the differential reproduction of individuals and groups.

Some might see the cultural selection of ideas as preferable to the natural selection of genes. But that, of course, is a moral judgment.

SUGGESTED READING

Fehr E, Gächter S. Altruistic punishment in humans. *Nature* 2002;415:137–40.

Paradis JG, Williams GC. *Evolution and Ethics: T. H. Huxley's Evolution and Ethics with New Essays on its Victorian and Sociobiological Context.* Princeton NJ: Princeton University Press, 1989.

REPLY BY DAVID SLOAN WILSON, PHD

David Haig and I agree on most issues. This might seem boring to the idle reader looking forward to a fight, but in fact it is a very encouraging sign that a resolution is possible on such a complicated and sensitive subject as the biological nature of morality.

Haig is especially eager to counteract the "rosy view that selection among groups inexorably favors advances in morality." Here again I agree. Not only does group selection promote a kind of morality that is primarily confined to members of the same group, but even this morality includes elements of intolerance and punishment within the group in addition to nurturing altruism.

It is important to stress that a theory should be judged by two standards. First, how well does it explain the world as it exists now and in the past? Second, can it be used to improve the world in the future? With respect to the first standard, it is clear that the moral systems of the past and present experience all of the difficulties alluded to above. They are almost always confined to an in-group, however much we might yearn for universal morality in abstract terms, and they invariably include punitive, in addition to nurturing, elements. If these are empirical facts about moral systems of the past and present, it is a strength of multilevel selection theory to be able to account for them.

With respect to the second standard, can multilevel selection (or any other) theory be used to improve the world in the future? Haig is somewhat shy about this prospect, stating, "It helps us to understand how morality evolved, what it is used for, and why it sometimes breaks down. It may even suggest more effective means to achieve desired ends, but it cannot suggest what these ends *should* be." The last part of this statement invokes something called the naturalistic fallacy, which is often used to deny that *ought* can be derived from *is*. The naturalistic fallacy is not as decisive as it is often taken to be, as I and others have discussed elsewhere.[1] Moreover, there is plenty of elbowroom in the phrase "more effective means to achieve desired ends."

Science has been spectacularly successful at achieving desired ends in some domains, such as engineering, although the unforeseen consequences are often like the man who unfortunately gets his wish in so many genie-in-a-bottle stories. We need to be careful about what we ask for, but a genuine theory of moral systems might enable us to get our wishes in the social domain more in the future than in the past or present.

NOTES

1. Wilson DS, Dietrich E, Clark AB. On the inappropriate use of the naturalistic fallacy in evolutionary psychology. *Biology and Philosophy*, 2003; 18(5): 669–681.

☰ ䷀ ䷀ ☰

LAURIE ZOLOTH, PHD

Religion and the Public Discourse of Bioethics

There is contention enough, these days, in the world of public policy and morality to last us a long time. Given this discord, what is the role for the religious voice in the discourse of bioethics? Let me make the argument here that rather than retreating from contention, the religious voice needs to be clearly and distinctively raised. Too often, theologians and religious scholars shrink from the prophetic voice out of a fear of being thought "fanatic," forgetting that a knife-edge of alarm is part of the religious imperative. Much would be lost if bioethics cannot hear the argument of religion clearly.

Medicine "works" on a collective, if not an entirely justifiable, faith that reason and science can solve any conundrum. It is a technical challenge to research and discover, but once known, the right act is inescapable and efficient, with measurable outcome data. Modern medical science trumped a religious apprehension of the world because it could be, in this important sense, proven, whereas the claims of faith could not. But the extreme uses of science and medicine in the 20th century shook the belief that rationality and objectivity were always progressive, at least in some measure because of the consequences of medicine and technology taken to the most immoral of extremes in the Holocaust. The vision of a liberating secularity that is rational, objective, and therefore truthful, was deeply shaken.

Bioethics responded with the belief that what makes one free and human are the personal, individual liberty rights that allow for choice. Then, the only structure for control left intact is the legal assertion of autonomy. This is the most desperate and most barren of the requests we honor—the right to be left alone.

There is readily apparent evidence that religion provides bioethics a missing ingredient. Americans are a very religious people, relative to many European nations, and relative to most medical staff. Americans attend church, synagogue or the mosque, and Americans believe in God. Surveys by the *New York Times* tell us that a paradigmatically typical American day includes daily prayer. We can witness this behavior at moments of national crisis, the Oklahoma City bombing, for example, when prayer becomes public and clearly genuine. And in moments of medical crisis, Americans become their most religious.

Consistently, despite the ubiquitous faith in secularity, pleasure and science, there is a persistent yearning to see a moral, meaningful trajectory in one's private life, in one's workplace and in the social goals of the state. Religion persists in asking about goals, ultimate meanings and long-term consequences. While it is not alone in this, religion insists on the question of moral meaning in the way that science insists on the question of replicable physical data. In the context of religion, humans are burdened by the obligations that are linked to this goal. This moral awareness is the mark of the person of faith.

Science and bioethics have created the illusion that we can be in disengaged, rational control of unruly processes. In fact, the notion that all of life is subject to rational control became the hallmark of early modernity, reflected in art, architecture and horticulture. This view marks the assumption that everything that trespasses on this rational control can be and ought to be progressively eliminated. This includes suffering, disease and loss. We believe that control ought to be ultimate, and that suffering is a medical failure to be medically managed. We turn over the entire problem of a fitting end to human life to unmediated medical science or yearn for physician-assisted suicide to sanction a medicalized death. But we will always live in a world where people will sicken and die. Although we cannot change this fact, we act as if we expect each encounter to be successful, that our part in it "work." This expectation affects us as ethicists. I, too, want every consultation to be successful, but living this way, without humility— which is a religious virtue—has its price.

In bioethics, we can tend to forget that medicine is about the problem of human suffering, that human loss is not a failure to be managed, but a tragedy in which we are the witnesses and the community of response. We forget this concept at our own moral peril, because forgetting one's place and confusion about one's stature is the classic problem in religion, called by the name of idolatry. But theological speculation is never far from this problem, seeking meaning in the face of suffering. For religious scholars and chaplains, attention to the existential anguish engendered by illness is imperative. The systemic theology of science is quite powerful; tantalizing not only to the clinician, but also to the ethicist. It takes the serious regard for religious faith, in part, to remind us that our faith in science and philosophy alone may leave us unfulfilled.

It is not only in the clinical arena that communities of religious meaning play a central role. Americans greet each research advance with a query toward faith commitments. When cloning or human embryonic stem cell research is on the agenda, it is apprehended as a religious-moral problem to be solved by textual recourse or the interview with the religious expert. This analysis is not a formalistic gesture. When interviewed in the popular media, Americans selected for their ordinariness speak of the problem in religious terms—unease with "playing god" or the "sanctity of life." What makes the sense of violation—or at least of controversy—in these situations, is that some boundary has been crossed, a concept that makes rational sense only if one notes a boundary. Yet it is not constraints of philosophic reason that create such a terrain. The parameters of religions, even the lost ones of childhood faith, are the ones cited when discomfiture is described.

The stance of the theologian is to be an outsider claiming possession of an unpopular truth. That this claim may seem radical is to be expected. The prophetic tradition can tell us much about the imperative of the outsider who can see an alternate vision. Challenging the "is" with the "ought" leads us to fruitful understandings about the role of the alternate claim, leads us to challenge the givenness of the relationships as presented, and leads to an ironic view of diagnostic certainty. Such language is neither safe nor endearing. That the historical place of the philosopher, as well as the theologian, was to remain the outsider easily can be forgotten. This exclusion may explain why it is uncomfortable to the discipline of bioethics to have theologians around. The first task of any theology is to remember that it is the brokenness of the world itself that calls us to the work of repair.

Even in religious communities which stress individual responsibility and individual relationships to God, the suffering stranger will not be alone. In religious discourse, the voice of the vulnerable other carries a power that is definitive. It is one that demands a rethinking of one of the most treasured concepts of bioethics: that of the privilege of the autonomous self with a set of universal and trumping rights.

Religion advocates on behalf of the most vulnerable. The theological claim is for the stranger and the powerless that dwell within our gates. The Sinaitic commands link healing with justice and the prophetic tradition scorns the society that abandons the poor. In a context where care is doled out, managed and curtailed to protect a bottom line, one might do well to invite a Jeremiah to the table of discourse, to remind us of the top line, to speak truth to power, and to persist beyond politeness. The discipline of religious studies insists that justice will be central to the matter of healthcare, admonishing us to return over and over to the need for universal access to healthcare services. Bioethics without a voice for justice cannot remain credible in a world of injustice.

Without this voice, for justice, for charity, for humility and for faith, bioethics will remain unprovoked by critical aspects of the human condition, a condition enriched by the difficult ethical questions and essential insights of theology and religious studies.

FURTHER READING

Dena D, Zoloth L (eds). *Notes From a Narrow Ridge: Religion and Bioethics.* University Publishing Group, 1999.

Hauerwas S. *The Suffering Presence: Theological Reflections on Medicine, the Mentally Handicapped and the Church.* Univ. of Notre Dame Press, 1993.

Hauerwas S. *Dispatches from the Front: Theological Engagements with the Secular.* Duke Univ. Press, 1994.

Lammers S, Verhay A (eds). *On Moral Medicine.* Erdmanns, 1998.

Marty M, Wind J (eds). *Health and Medicine and the Faith Traditions, Project 10.* Trinity Press International, 1986–95.

Shelp E (ed). *Theology and Bioethics: Exploring the Foundations and Frontiers.* D. Reidel Publishing Co., 1985.

Stout J. *Ethics after Babel: The Languages of Morals and Their Discontents.* Beacon Press, 1995.

☷ ☶ ☶ ☷

DANIEL CALLAHAN, PHD

Religion and Bioethics

I need to begin this article with a disclaimer. I am not now "religious" in any ordinary sense of that word, neither worshipping on the sabbath nor meditating alone in the woods. I left my Roman Catholic beliefs behind me 35 years ago and have never regretted that change, not for a minute. I simply ceased being a theist, rejecting the entire premise of Western religion. I consider myself an atheist, not a worried, longing agnostic.

Even so, I have tried over the years not to let myself congeal into that kind of unbeliever who is angry and rejecting of anything to do with religion. They are not an impressive crowd, the eerily mirror image of what I wanted to get away from. Moreover, I want to try to make the strongest possible case for the legitimacy, and the great value, of including religious believers as full partners in the bioethics enterprise. There are three reasons for saying this, which I will spell out as I go along: the rational legitimacy of religious belief; the valuable historical contributions of the great world religions to ethics over the centuries; and the fact that a religious perspective is able to take up problems and puzzles that a purely secular, so-called "rational," perspective simply cannot deal with in any coherent, sensitive way.

THE RATIONAL LEGITIMACY OF RELIGIOUS BELIEF

A widespread conceit of a wholly secular perspective, embodied in the secular humanism movement, is that religion is, of its essence, irrational and superstitious, based on commitments of faith that have neither reason nor science to give them credibility. By contrast, those who have put religion aside to embrace reason and science display not only greater courage in facing up to a universe and life without intrinsic meaning, but also show themselves to be more rational and mature.

The problem with that rather self-satisfied ideology is that I have never found my religious friends and acquaintances any less rational or mature than those who are not religious. They have different beliefs, that is true, but they are neither stupid nor lacking in insight or self-reflection. I came some years ago to think that those who are religious believers are mistaken in their faith and their reasoning, woefully so.

That is not, however, the same as being irrational. Rationality should be understood from two angles. There is the rationality of choosing one's ultimate premises, and the rationality of working those premises out in some logical and coherent way. I know of no secular cluster of beliefs that does not have some act of faith behind it, not provable in terms of those beliefs without begging the question (e.g., the core secular proposition that reason and science only will deliver the truth, a proposition that is not provable on rational or scientific grounds without begging the question). For me, then, believers and unbelievers start off on an equal footing, and neither has a special claim to superior reason. After that, with minimal reasonableness, both can work through logically consistent systems of values and ethics and have often done so.

THE HISTORICAL CONTRIBUTIONS OF RELIGION

It has long been remarked that the great religions of the world share many common values. They espouse the dignity of human beings, reject cruelty and oppression, deny the morality of lying, stealing, murdering and the like. The great Decalogue, the Ten Commandments, remain to this day a moral staple, difficult to reject in principle even if one can imagine exceptions, and presenting, as an ensemble, about as wise a set of moral rules as can be devised. That religious believers have hardly always lived up to those rules, even flagrantly ignored them, does not tell against them. Indeed, those very rules can be, and have been, called to judgment upon them.

Beyond that, the various religious writings and reflections over the century on such issues as abortion, truth-telling, respect for others, still have punch and pertinency. The principle of "double effect," a contribution of the Roman Catholic tradition, has been taken up into the core contemporary medical values even if there is some secular dissent. The traditional Protestant affirmation of the rights of the individual conscience, the right to make choices about one's life and faith, is surely alive and well. The Jewish halakic tradition, relying on the accumulation of cases in ethics, has been so incorporated as a method into the routine reflection on ethical dilemmas that it is hardly noticed.

BIOETHICS AND HUMAN BREADTH

As Laurie Zoloth so effectively noted in her article on "Religion and the Public Discourse of Bioethics," the very core of religious belief requires a wrestling with questions of human meaning and suffering. This is where secular ethics, of all strains, tends to fall silent. Those are not its sort of issues, which require a breadth and depth that modern ethical theories such as utilitarianism and deontology have not been devised to cope with. For scientific medicine, illness and death are simply treated as evils to be eliminated, not to be given meaning. But they have not been, and will not be, eliminated. The ancient questions are still there, never far from most people's minds.

Contemporary bioethics is prone to focus on moral dilemmas and typically those which pit some common moral rule against another rule. But historically, ethics, and particularly religious ethics, has always focused on the living of a moral life, which encompasses the shaping of ideals, the cultivation of virtues, with the fashioning of an inner life, not simply learning the right rules and how to manage them. Theological ethics has understood a point which secular ethics has never managed to quite get: the need to put ethics within the larger framework of an interpretation of life and human destiny. Secular ethics has worked with the premise that there can be ethical systems and theories not dependent upon such a framework. Perhaps so, but secular ethics is typically quite thin in that respect, resting on what reason alone can discover and develop, but which is itself only part of human nature.

Yet the religious thinkers working in bioethics have not always been helpful. There are a fair number who are simply reactionary, seeing bioethics and much of the contemporary world as simply misguided at best and corrupt at worse. Those so inclined usually stick to themselves, throwing thunderbolts from their own journals at all the evils out there—thunderbolts which have no bite because they seem oriented mainly to pleasing their own like-minded believers rather than engaging those whom they attack from afar. They usually fail, moreover, to take the bioethics problems seriously, skipping instead to the end of the chase to provide the (surely) true answers. At the other end of the spectrum are those whose religious beliefs turn out to be indistinguishable from, say, the editorial positions of the *New York Times*. But there are many in the various religious communities who fall neither within the self-certain right nor left, people who are thoughtful and have much of value to say.

Bioethics began with a strong religious bent, was quickly superseded by the advent of secular philosophers in the 1970s and then by the pressure for bioethics to speak acceptably, that is, non-religiously, in the public marketplace of courts, legislators and the media. Bioethics gained purchase and prominence when that happened. It also left behind insights and riches that cannot be supplied by an anti- or "a-religious" stance. That is a great loss. For all of its classic separation of church and state, the United States is a religious nation, in its history, its traditions and among a majority of its people. To fail to factor that reality fully into our public discourse about bioethics is to fail to take its work with sufficient seriousness.

⠿ ⠗ ⠗ ⠿

ROSEMARIE TONG, PHD

Feminist Approaches to Bioethics

In order to be "feminist," an approach to bioethics must emphasize the role gender plays in the realm of healthcare. How does one's femaleness or maleness, one's femininity or masculinity, shape the way one thinks about and behaves within the worlds of medicine and science? And, of equal significance, how does one's gender affect one's power, prestige, status and personal value within systems and structures such as the hospital, managed care organization, hospice, physician's office, medical society and research institution? In an attempt to answer these questions, feminist men and women have developed a variety of ethical approaches, most of which fall under one of two headings: care-focused or power-focused.

CARE-FOCUSED FEMINIST APPROACHES

Feminists who adopt care-focused approaches to bioethics often rely on the writings of Carol Gilligan and Nel Noddings, both of whom correlate being female with tending to cultivate such culturally associated feminine virtues as caring, and being male with tending to cultivate such culturally associated masculine virtues as justice. For example, while studying how each of 29 women decided whether it was right or wrong to have an abortion, Gilligan noted that, as a group, these women focused on how their decision would affect their relationships with those persons to whom they were already related, as well as to the future persons within their wombs. On the basis of this and several other empirical studies of women's and, more recently, men's moral reasoning patterns, Gilligan concluded that for a variety of cultural reasons, women typically utilize an ethics of care which stresses social relationships and personal responsibilities, whereas men typically employ an ethics of justice which stresses individual rights and contractual duties.[1]

In a similar vein, Nel Noddings writes that traditional ethics have emphasized theoretical, as opposed to practical, modes of reasoning, favoring things that tend to be valued by men (independence, autonomy, intellect, hierarchy, domination, asceticism and war) as opposed to things that tend to be valued by women (interdependence, community, connection, sharing, emotion, body, trust, absence of hierarchy, nature, process, joy and peace).[2]

Eschewing the interpretive style of reasoning which is characteristic of the humanities and social sciences, most traditional ethicists have instead embraced the deductive-nomological style of reasoning which is characteristic of mathematics and the natural sciences. They have favored weighing the principles of autonomy, beneficence, nonmaleficence and justice against each other, hoping to discover through their rational powers which of these principles ought to take precedence over others in a given situation. In contrast, feminists who espouse care-focused approaches to bioethics have relied on their emotional resources—on human sentiments such as empathy and on what Noddings calls "human caring and the memory of caring and being cared for . . ."[3]

Feminist care-focused approaches to bioethics are not unproblematic. The virtue of care can be distorted. People can care too much about others and not enough about themselves, they can use caring words to manipulate people to get them to do things that are not in their own best interests or they can care too much about one person and not enough about another. Before care is hailed as healthcare's quintessential moral virtue, its relationship to justice, its primary competitor, must be better understood. I, for example, believe that "care" is not some sort of principle, rule or guideline that trumps "justice," but the passion or motive that makes us want to be just in the first place.

POWER-FOCUSED FEMINIST APPROACHES

Feminists developing power-focused approaches to bioethics also value the virtue of care. However, as they see it, care cannot blossom as a moral virtue in an unjust society in which sexism, racism, ethnocentrism, classism and heterosexism thrive. Therefore, the most important task for feminist power-focused bioethicists is to expose and reform all healthcare systems, structures, institutions, principles, policies and procedures which neglect, trivialize or ignore women's and other vulnerable groups' interests, issues and identities.[4] In order to accomplish this ambitious goal, these feminists have sharpened the so-called woman question: "Why is this man's world, not woman's world?" into an analytical tool for the purpose of "identify[ing] the gender implications of rules and practices which might otherwise appear to be neutral or objective."[5]

Aided by this probing instrument, power-focused feminist bioethicists ask, for example, why women have been excluded from so many clinical research studies; why so few women are hospital presidents and chiefs of medical staffs; why such professions as nursing and social work are female dominated; and why women are far more likely than men to fall prey to eating disorders like anorexia or bulimia. The ways to raise questions about the role gender (masculine and feminine) plays in our everyday lives are many indeed—a fact that power-focused feminist bioethicists interpret as a sign of how deeply gendered our society is, and how easily most people accept as "natural" the unjust megastructure of male domination and female subordination which human beings have gradually constructed and, for the most part, successfully internalized.

AN INTEGRATED PERSPECTIVE

Both care-focused and power-focused feminist bioethicists use ways of thinking which promise to eradicate those invidious power relations that make our healthcare system less than just, and far from fully caring. For example, Dr. Joanne Lynn's remarkable essay, "Travels in the Valley of the Shadow," reveals an integrated perspective. Her story concerns an elderly man, whom she calls Mr. Phillips, who apparently was a victim of Alzheimer's type dementia and was unable to swallow. After she inserted a feeding tube and gave instructions to the home-care nurse about restraining him, Mrs. Phillips became distraught. She sobbed that she couldn't "tie" her husband down to their bed. Suddenly Dr. Lynn realized that Mr. Phillips was not her "problem of nutrition and hydration,"[6] but Mrs. Phillips' husband, lover and partner. To tie him down to his bed was not, therefore, a straightforward "mechanical solution to the problem of keeping a feeding tube in place, but a deeply offensive abuse . . ."[7]

Reflecting on Dr. Lynn's story as a feminist bioethicist, it seems to me that she initially acted like the traditional non-feminist physician. She made her decision as the physician who knows what is best for her patient. But when Mrs. Phillips broke down, Dr. Lynn recognized how little thought she had given to the effects of her decision on the relationship between Mr. and Mrs. Phillips, let alone her relationship to the Phillipses. Locked into her own world, Dr. Lynn had failed to see the world from the position of the very vulnerable couple. A securely-fastened feeding tube might be the treatment of medical choice, but it was not what the Phillipses required. Only Dr. Lynn's ability and willingness first to hear, and then to converse with Mrs. Phillips permitted her to see that the right treatment for Mr. Phillips was not artificial food and hydration but the healing ministries of his wife. By sharing her power with the Phillips family, by admitting the ultimate authority of their own fundamental good, Dr. Lynn stopped acting like an oppressor and found a treatment for Mr. Phillips with which everyone, including herself, could live. She removed the feeding tube, revoked her restraint orders, and let Mr. Phillips "live as well as he had been living as long as it lasted."[8] He died at home two months later.

Clearly, care-focused and power-focused feminist approaches to bioethics, despite their differences, can and do merge in the decisions and actions of people like Dr. Lynn. Although Dr. Lynn did not describe her decision and action in this case as feminist, it is, nonetheless, the decision a feminist would make and the action a feminist would take. In order to make the world of health care one that structures and organizes itself so as to serve men and women—and, by parity of reasoning, people of different races, ethnic backgrounds, socioeconomic classes, religions and cultures—equally well, feminist bioethicists must develop ways of thinking which permit people with differences to establish caring relationships among themselves.

Feminist bioethicists do not regard their many-faceted approaches to bioethics as consisting of self-contained bioethical theory meant to rival traditional bioethical theories, but as a series of corrective lenses that are meant to improve moral vision. Thus, feminist bioethics invite all bioethicists to reflect upon the status of women and other subordinate groups in the realm of health care. By focusing on issues related to gender, but also to class and race, for example, bioethicists will be able to play a more effective role in making the realm of health care a truly just world which fully cares about women's interests, issues, values and experiences as much as men's— indeed, a world that cares passionately about anyone who finds himself or herself deeply in need of the healing that only caring heads, hearts and hands can deliver.

NOTES

1. Gilligan C. *In a Different Voice.* Cambridge, MA: Harvard University Press, 1982:76–92.

2. Jaggar AM. Feminist ethics: projects, problems, prospects. In Card C (ed): *Feminist Ethics.* Lawrence, KN: University of Kansas Press, 1991:85–90.

3. Noddings N. *Caring: A Feminine Approach to Ethics and Moral Education.* Berkeley, CA: University of California Press, 1984:1.

4. Jaggar AM. A feminist ethics. In Becker L, Becker C (eds): *Encyclopedia of Ethics.* New York: Garland, 1992:363–364.

5. Bartlett KT. Feminist legal methods. In Weisberg DK (ed): *Feminist Legal Theory.* Philadelphia, PA: Temple University Press, 1993: 551.

6. Lynn J. Travels in the valley of the shadow. In Spiro HM, McCrea MG, Peschel E, St. James D (eds): *Empathy and the Practice of Medicine: Beyond Pills and the Scalpel.* New Haven, CT: Yale University Press, 1993:43–44.

7. Ibid, p. 44.

8. Ibid.

☶ ☷ ☷ ☶

GILBERT MEILAENDER, PHD

Feminist Approaches to Bioethics

Rosemarie Tong's "Feminist approaches to bioethics" is a clear, judicious, and I think, a fair depiction of the two most common feminist approaches to ethics generally, and, hence, bioethics in particular. Readers who come unencumbered by theory or ideology to her piece might, however, be pardoned for wondering whether, given her description, we are not all now feminists. Perhaps so. But by sharpening just a few points we may see what is at stake in her discussion.

I begin with what she calls "power-focused feminist approaches." Simply put, these approaches pay close attention to the experience and interests of women—and to the way those interests may be overlooked or denigrated in the organization and delivery of health care. More stridently put, this approach might focus on ways in which men are privileged and women oppressed in a still too patriarchally ordered world of medicine. And there are legitimate questions to be raised here, some of them noted by Tong (though the prevalence of eating disorders in women may be attributable less to patriarchy than to a world shaped, to some degree, by feminism). Important questions have been raised about, for example, the different levels of participation of men and women in medical experimentation, or about the way new reproductive technologies may alienate women from their bodies, or about the respective roles in caregiving of nurses and physicians.

Granting all this, we should still pause to reflect upon the fact that this is an approach to *moral reasoning* that places at the center the interests of women—that is, one "special interest" among others. Perhaps one might try to justify this as a temporary measure, necessary in response to a gravely unjust world. But pressing special interests and putting one's ideal of fairness on hold for a time should, at least, be worrisome. This "power-focused feminist approach" will need to explain how it differs from unjust special preference.

One way of responding to this concern—the concern that this kind of feminism seeks to justify special preference—is to broaden the range of those whose interests are favored by a feminist ethic. Thus, for example, Tong suggests that power-focused approaches are concerned about "women's and other vulnerable groups' interests, issues and identities." They are opposed to a society "in which sexism, racism, ethnocentrism, classism and heterosexism thrive." It's hard to know what to think of this move. On the one hand, large numbers of women believe quite strongly that the heterosexual bond is normative for human life. Evidently the feminism Tong describes (which brings "heterosexism" into its fold) would have to ex-communicate such women—or, perhaps, develop a theory of false consciousness, contending that such women may be oppressed even though they deny it. On the other hand, if we eliminated heterosexism from Tong's list of "isms," this broadened feminist concern for vulnerable groups would begin to sound rather like the Roman Catholic emphasis upon a preferential option for the poor—making for unusual allies, to say the least.

In short, these are not promising ways to deal with the charge of unjust special preference. It might be better to turn to what Tong calls "care-focused feminist approaches," for they argue that there is more to moral reasoning than considerations of justice alone. There is also care—an emphasis on relationships and fitting action within the bonds that tie us to others. This is, I think, a more promising approach. To be sure, it can be abused, as Tong notes (though I do not myself believe it is possible to "care too much about others").

Feminists themselves often disagree about the language of care, however. It might seem to support the notion that the sexual differentiation between male and female is of moral significance, that there are womanly and manly ways of being in the world—suggestions that will make certain feminists edgy. Others might wonder why men may not be as caring, as devoted to special relationships, as women. Tong herself seems disinclined to adopt a care-focused ethic; indeed, whatever havoc this may play with our categories, I suspect that I am more sympathetic to it than she!

Surely it is best, though, to say that somehow "care" and "justice" must be held together within any sound moral perspective. (And this must be part of what Tong means by an "integrated perspective," though I do not think it is adequate to describe care only as a passion or motive that inclines us to be just.) Joanne Lynn is simply a good physician of the sort to which anyone, male or female, might aspire. I doubt, though, whether her first instinct—to provide the feeding tube—was acting like a "traditional non-feminist physician." Rather, it was a quite proper attempt to provide useful care for her patient and to be certain that she did not treat him unjustly by deliberately hastening his death. Likewise, her second thoughts about the feeding tube were not, I think, so much the result of an imaginative breakthrough as they were a realization—perhaps possible only after trying the tube—that for this patient such a treatment was excessively burdensome and, hence, not warranted. It looks less like the insight of a feminist bioethic—or of both feminist approaches integrated in some way—than simply of good moral reasoning that is sensitive to considerations of both care and justice. And, if there is anything at all to the care-focused ethic, it may best be achieved when men listen to women and women, likewise, listen to men.

REPLY BY ROSEMARIE TONG, PHD

I am glad that Professor Meilaender thinks it possible that we are "all now feminists." What a delightful thought! Regretfully, however, I do not believe our society in general or bioethicists and health care practitioners in particular have overcome all their sexist, racist, ethnocentric, classist, heterosexist (the list goes on) ways of thinking and acting. Not everyone is a feminist, believing that gender plays an enormous role in many aspects of life; and not everyone accepts that women's views and interests have often been disregarded and should be emphasized in order to bring a balance into realms such as health care.

Meilaender's concern about power-focused feminist approaches to bioethics is a reasonable one. However, just because feminists want bioethicists to look intently at women's interests, it does not mean they want bioethics to ignore men's interests. Similarly, just because feminists stress that women's perspectives on moral issues in the realm of health care are insightful, it does not mean feminists believe that women's moral authority is incontestable. Rather, power-focused feminist approaches aim to broaden and deepen traditional ethics (which tended to neglect or trivialize the interests of women and other historically vulnerable groups) with the perspectives of those previously marginalized groups.

Admittedly, feminist approaches to bioethics are not neutral. They wear their primary interest (women) on their sleeves, opening themselves up for criticism voluntarily. However, just because an approach to bioethics emphasizes gender, it does not mean it is sexist. An approach to bioethics becomes sexist only when it systematically excludes the interests, identities, issues and values of one sex in favor of another.

That feminists are concerned about vulnerable groups, including gay men and lesbian women, does not mean they disregard the interests of other groups. Most humans oscillate between roles of oppressor and oppressed and positions of power and vulnerability. However, some groups of humans—according to race, gender or class, for example—are oppressed more frequently and severely. The fact that I oppose heterosexism does not mean that I think all heterosexual women (or men, for that matter) should renounce the values they associate with being heterosexual (e.g., beliefs about what constitutes a proper family, a meaningful sexual liaison or marriage). However, it does mean I think it is wrong for heterosexual persons to discriminate against gay men and lesbian women in the public realm (including employment, insurance, housing and so forth).

Feminists who espouse care-focused or power-focused approaches to bioethics are not advocating women's perspectives *über alles*. Far from it. It's just that by focusing on how gender shapes and misshapes one's power to care and be cared for in the world of medicine and science, they are identifying ways for everyone to improve bioethical reasoning.

⌗ ⦀ ⦀ ⌗

LEIGH TURNER, PHD

Bioethics in Culturally Diverse Societies

Anyone examining the last three decades in the history of medicine, healthcare and biotechnology can identify both longstanding zones of ethical conflict and areas of relatively stable social norms. Morality is neither fully stable and ordered or dominated by conflict.[1] With some topics, individuals from many different cultural, religious, philosophical and political traditions are able to reach shared understandings. In other instances, cultural and religious differences play an important role in generating and perpetuating moral disputes. Serious moral conflicts occur in Canada, the United States, New Zealand and Australia, but they rarely threaten to destroy the entire social order.

Contemporary liberal democracies are multicultural, multifaith, pluralistic societies. Globalization is dispersing individuals, families and larger social networks from small geographic niches to cities and towns around the world.[2] Most democratic societies contain multiple political traditions with very different understandings of social justice, individual liberty and conceptions of the common good. Similarly, the religious landscape in many societies is remarkably variegated. In Chicago, Miami, New York and Los Angeles, it is possible to visit mosques, temples, churches, synagogues and other religious institutions serving as gathering places for innumerable religious communities. These communities often have very different understandings of health, illness, suffering, death, dying, aging, medicine and healing. Most of us live in multifaith societies.[3]

Despite the multifaith, multicultural nature of contemporary societies, the most well-known and widely used methods and theories in bioethics make some very large assumptions about the existence of shared, common moral norms or intuitions held by all "reasonable" or "moral" individuals. For example, the principlist ethical framework of Beauchamp and Childress assumes the existence of a "common morality" that can be found throughout history and across different cultural settings. The "common morality," they argue, "contains moral norms that bind all persons in all places; no norms are more basic in the moral life."[4] Describing the contents of the common morality, Beauchamp and Childress write: "Since virtually everyone grows up with a basic understanding of the institution of morality, its norms are readily understood. All persons who are serious about living a moral life already grasp the core dimensions of morality. They know not to lie, not to steal property, to keep promises, to respect the rights of others, not to kill or cause harm to innocent persons, and the like."[4]

Without engaging in comparative, crosscultural analysis or detailed historical research, Beauchamp and Childress make empirical claims about the universality of the common morality. Acknowledging that "amoral, immoral or selectively moral persons" do not recognize the common morality, Beauchamp and Childress insist "we believe that all persons in all cultures who are *serious about moral conduct* do accept the demands of the common morality." Developing this claim, they state, "we think it is an institutional fact about morality, not merely our view of it, that it contains fundamental precepts. These fundamental precepts alone make it possible for persons to make cross-temporal and crosscultural judgments and to assert firmly that not all practices in all cultural groups are morally acceptable."[4] Individuals persuaded by common morality approaches rarely pause to consider whether the empirical claims of proponents of the common morality approach are accurate. However, there is a crucial difference between making normative claims about how humans ought to act and making transhistorical, cross-cultural claims about the empirical status of particular moral practices. Beauchamp and Childress assume that "virtually everyone" is raised with a basic understanding of various moral norms. While these claims might coincide with what we would like to think about human nature and human conduct, they ignore historical and anthropological research challenging such broad generalizations about moral practices. Notions of property and private possessions are culturally shaped. Lying, deception and nondisclosure can be sanctioned in particular social contexts. Deliberately inflicted violence against the innocent is a staple of human history.

Beauchamp and Childress, along with other proponents of common morality approaches, provide a very sunny view of human nature and a common moral sense operating across societies and throughout time, but rarely provide anthropological, historical or sociological evidence in support of these claims. Let me emphasize that I am not taking issue with the substance of morality typically described by common morality theorists. Clearly, I am not making an argument for lying or harming the innocent. Rather, I am challenging the common and unsubstantiated assertions that we can find broad empirical support for the common morality through time and across different cultural settings.[5,6,7,8,9]

The problem with the "common morality" framework of Beauchamp and Childress is that it ignores the powerful role of culture and religion in shaping very different understandings of morality, family life, illness, suffering, healing and death. They make numerous assumptions about what individuals find "intuitive." Principlist bioethics has yet to grapple in a serious manner with the scholarship on "local knowledge" and the cultural shaping of "common sense." Principlist bioethics largely overlooks the challenges posed by the work of such anthropologists as Clifford Geertz and Richard Shweder.[10,11]

Though I am critical of the empirical claims made by Beauchamp and Childress, I can sympathize with their effort to develop a cross-cultural, universal core of moral norms that can be used to judge cultural practices around the world. What critic of the common morality approach would want to defend many of the practices Beauchamp and Childress oppose? Still, the substance of the common morality is vaguely described and the challenges posed by plural moral traditions are underestimated. The ethical framework of Beauchamp and Childress offers limited insight into how the principles of biomedical ethics are supposed to resolve conflicts where fundamental differences exist concerning what it means to be a thoughtful, moral individual and member of a particular community.

Much like principlists, case-based proponents of practical moral reasoning, also known as "casuists," similarly assume that humans share a common morality providing cross-cultural moral intuitions and maxims about ethical and unethical practices.[12] Casuists, like principlists, minimize the powerful role of cultural and religious norms in shaping different understandings of what constitutes "common sense" approaches to ethical issues. Proponents of case-based "clinical" moral reasoning have yet to fully grapple with the challenges of case-analysis and policy formation in multicultural, multifaith societies. Case-based moral reasoning relies upon the existence of widely shared tacit moral knowledge. However, with many subjects, the moral intuitions of some citizens can be quite at variance with what other interlocutors find ethical and reasonable.

Just as cultural and religious pluralism raises challenges for principlists and casuists, more "emotivist" modes of reflecting upon ethical issues underestimate the significance of different cultural models of "commonsense" moral reflection. Leon Kass, chair of the President's Council on Bioethics, makes a detailed case for "the wisdom of repugnance."[13] Much like the work of principlists and casuists, Kass's discussion of the intuitive wisdom of repugnance insufficiently attends to the cultural and historical variability of reactions of "disgust" and "revulsion." The wisdom of "repugnance" can have only limited usefulness as an effective guide for moral deliberations or the creation of social policy when individuals have markedly divergent responses to whether a particular practice or phenomenon is "repugnant."

Having briefly noted how different approaches in bioethics pay little attention to the role of culture and religion in shaping understandings of moral practice, I would like to consider just one example of an issue where religious and cultural norms often play a role in generating different understandings of what constitutes "ethical" conduct.

While many moral norms have broad public support, substantial backing in courts and legislatures, and endorsement in hospital policies and professional codes of ethics, there are other topics where substantial disagreement exists. In Canada, the United States and many other countries, for example, ethical disputes persist concerning "medical futility" or questions about what constitutes "appropriate" forms of end-of-life care when patients or family members demand medical care deemed "nonbeneficial" by healthcare providers. Within North America, the debate concerning how to craft policies and respond to individual cases reveals very different understandings of how best to care for seriously ill patients. Some disputants insist upon the importance of respecting religious and cultural norms concerning doing everything possible to keep a patient alive. Other commentators emphasize the significance of the quality of life of patients and the ethical obligation to treat patients with dignity. They argue that there are moral limits to demonstrating respect for cultural and religious differences.

Debates over medical futility are not reducible to religious and cultural conflicts. However, cultural and religious norms sometimes lead family members to request further medical interventions to preserve life regardless of quality-of-life considerations, provide an occasion for a "miracle," or meet obligations imposed by religious doctrines and texts.[14,15] Bioethicists are free to contest the religion-based moral claims of family members. Still, bioethicists need to recognize that these family members have very clear moral intuitions of their own about what it means to act responsibly when a family member is ill. Reference to "moral intuitions" or "common sense" does not provide much help in such situations.

Long-standing debates are not limited to disputes concerning end-of-life care. Such topics as the ethics of embryonic stem cell research and stem cell therapies, germline gene therapy and physician-assisted suicide reveal tremendous public controversy. Citizens from different cultural, religious, political and philosophical traditions differ over how various biomedical technologies are best regulated. While I dwell upon the topic of medical futility, many other examples could be provided of ethical disputes where cultural and religious norms play important roles in shaping diverse understandings of what constitutes ethical, responsible conduct.

Too often, bioethicists exaggerate their capacity to bring long-standing ethical debates to ultimate closure. They mistakenly claim that morality is settled, orderly, and in state of reflective equilibrium when this account tells only one part of a very complex story. In pluralistic societies, we find both relatively stable social norms as well as conflicting understandings of how we should live and die. Several of the dominant approaches in bioethics rely upon the notion of shared, common, intuitively obvious moral norms. However, many of the issues addressed by bioethicists reveal the existence of disagreements over what constitutes "common sense" moral reasoning. Disputes about ethical issues in medicine, health care, and biotechnology often occur along cultural and religious fault lines. Such conflicts emerge in clinical settings, the deliberations of advisory bodies and professional organizations, and in legislative arenas.

We need to better recognize limits to bioethics and acknowledge that finding common modes of addressing ethical issues is very difficult in multicultural, multifaith, heterogeneous societies. There are some ethical issues that simply do not seem to be near "closure" or "resolution." Canonical methods, theories and other tools of ethical deliberation in bioethics glide over deep social and moral conflicts rather than acknowledging the depth of ethical controversies found in pluralistic societies. Bioethics has its limits. Perhaps it is better to recognize these limits than to claim that some method, theory or technique of reasoning is available that will magically resolve longstanding moral conflicts.

NOTES

1. Turner L. Zones of consensus and zones of conflict: Questioning the "Common Morality" presumption in bioethics. *Kennedy Inst Ethics J* 2003;13(3):193–218.

2. Giddens A. *Runaway World: How Globalization Is Reshaping Our Lives.* New York: Routledge, 2000.

3. Sowell T. *A Conflict of Visions: Ideological Origins of Political Struggles.* New York: Basic Books, 2002.

4. Beauchamp TL, Childress JF. *Principles of Biomedical Ethics.* New York: Oxford University Press, 2001;3–5.

5. Carrithers M, Collins S, Lukes S (eds). *The Category of the Person: Anthropology, Philosophy, History.* Cambridge: Cambridge University Press, 1985.

6. MacPherson CB. *Political Theory of Possessive Individualism: Hobbes to Locke.* Oxford: Oxford University Press, 1964.

7. Nisbett RE. *The Geography of Thought: How Asians and Westerners Think Differently . . . and Why.* New York: The Free Press, 2003.

8. Nisbett RE, Cohen D. *Culture of Honor: The Psychology of Violence in the South.* Boulder, Colorado: Westview Press, 1996.

9. Schmidt B, Schroder I (eds). *Anthropology of Violence and Conflict.* London: Routledge, 2001.

10. Geertz C. *The Interpretation of Cultures.* USA: BasicBooks, 1973 and *Available Light: Anthropological Reflections on Philosophical Topics.* Princeton, NJ: Princeton University Press, 2000.

11. Shweder R. *Why Do Men Barbecue? Recipes for Cultural Psychology.* Cambridge, MA: Harvard University Press, 2003,

12. Jonsen AR, Toulmin SE. *The Abuse of Casuistry: A History of Moral Reasoning.* Berkeley: University of California Press, 1988.

13. Kass L. The wisdom of repugnance. *The New Republic* 1997; June 2:17–26.

14. Orr RD, Genesen LB. Requests for "inappropriate" treatment based on religious beliefs. *J Med Ethics* 1997;23(3):142–7.

15. Brett AS, Jersild P. "Inappropriate" treatment near the end of life: conflict between religious convictions and clinical judgment. *Arch Intern Med* 2003;163(14):1645–9.

≡ ‖‖ ‖‖ ≡

BERNARD GERT, PHD

Bioethics in Culturally Diverse Societies

The last two sentences of Leigh Turner's article, "Bioethics in culturally diverse societies" are "Bioethics has its limits" and "Perhaps it is better to recognize these limits than to claim that some method, theory or technique of reasoning, is available that will magically resolve longstanding moral conflicts." I am in complete agreement. Furthermore, it is not merely bioethics that has its limits; there is no method, theory or technique of reasoning available that will resolve long-standing moral conflicts in any area of morality.

However, Leigh Turner takes himself to be providing an attack on the notion of a common morality and I am a leading defender of the view; something is quite puzzling.[1-4] Part of the puzzle is due to the fact that the view that Leigh Turner is attacking is the principlist version of common morality, a view that Beauchamp and Childress adopted in later editions of their book, *Principles of Biomedical Ethics.* This principlist version of common morality has only a distant relationship to the account of common morality that we put forward in *Bioethics: A Return to Fundamentals.*[5]

Common morality cannot and should not be used to settle long-standing moral conflicts in bioethics. Rather, common morality explains why, although there is agreement about the vast majority of moral decisions and judgments, there are some unresolvable moral disagreements.

The agreement about the overwhelming majority of moral decisions and judgments, e.g., it is morally wrong to subject a patient to a serious risk of death simply to make money, is overlooked because these kinds of cases are rarely if ever discussed. The relatively few controversial issues, e.g., the moral acceptability of abortion or the use of "medical futility" to discontinue treatment, are widely discussed, and thus are mistakenly taken as constituting the vast majority of moral decisions and judgments. But although the number of unresolvable moral issues is small relative to the number about which there is complete agreement, it is a mistake to think that any moral theory will resolve these long-standing moral conflicts.

Common morality is not a theory; it is the system that people use, usually not consciously, when they make their moral decisions and judgments based on a thoughtful consideration of the facts involved in a specific situation. The correct account of common morality is similar to the correct account of grammar provided by grammarians. These grammarians simply describe the grammatical system that is used, usually not consciously, by speakers of the language when they speak and when they interpret the speech of others. People are speakers of a language if they can understand and can be understood by other speakers of the language. If a grammarian puts forward a description of the grammatical system of a language that is in conflict with the way in which any significant number of speakers use it, that grammarian has put forward a mistaken account.

Philosophers who put forward moral theories that conflict with the moral judgments of any significant number of moral agents, are similarly mistaken. People are moral agents if they can understand what morality prohibits, requires, discourages, encourages, and allows and can guide their conduct by it. That is why any accurate account of common morality must allow for unresolvable moral disputes concerning issues about which a significant number of moral agents disagree.

However, although I agree with Leigh Turner about the limits of common morality, we have a significant disagreement about what counts as morality. He says "there is a crucial difference between making normative claims about how humans ought to act and making transhistorical and crosscultural claims about the empirical status of particular moral practices." He seems to hold that any claim about how humans ought to act is a moral judgment. This is a common mistake of philosophers. Turner seems to offer the following in support of his view that moral practices differ: "Deliberately inflicted violence against the innocent is a staple of human history." That he thinks that inflicting violence against the innocent is a moral practice can only be explained by his acceptance of the view that however any society claims that people ought to act is a moral practice.

When philosophers talk about morality, they are not talking about all of the diverse practices that different societies put forward as guides to conduct. Morality has certain features that they rightly take to be essential. Among these features is that it is inappropriate to make a moral judgment about the actions of a person if he is legitimately ignorant that what he is doing is morally discouraged or prohibited. This distinguishes morality from law and religion, for it is appropriate to make a legal or religious judgment about the actions of a person even if he is legitimately ignorant that what he is doing is legally or religiously discouraged or prohibited. Together with the fact that, unless they are legitimately ignorant of the facts of the situation, it is appropriate to make moral judgments about the actions of all normal adult human beings, this feature of morality has a somewhat surprising implication. The conclusion is that morality cannot be based on religion, for no religion is known to all normal adult human beings. Thomas Aquinas's acceptance of this conclusion explains why he tries to show that the moral views put forward in the Christian scriptures are the same as those known by natural reason. Neither Aquinas nor I deny that a particular religion may put forward correct moral views, but both of us deny that what makes them correct moral views is that they are put forward by that religion.

Genuine unresolvable moral disagreements are the result of a number of factors, of which two are the most important. The first is a difference in the rankings of the various benefits (goods) and harms (evils). Everyone agrees that death, pain, disability, loss of freedom, and loss of pleasure are evils or harms. Everyone also agrees that abilities, freedom, and pleasure are goods or benefits. However, within fairly wide limits, rational persons differ in their rankings of these goods and evils. For example, two people suffering from the same painful terminal illness may make different choices, both rational. One may choose to stop life-prolonging treatment in order to avoid the continuing pain, whereas the other may choose to continue life-prolonging treatment despite the pain. Turner is correct that these differences are often the result of different cultural and religious backgrounds, but it is the rationally allowed differences in the rankings of the evils that are directly responsible for the unresolvable moral disagreement.

A second important source of unresolvable moral disagreement is differences about who is included in the group that is impartially protected or protected at all by morality. The group must include all moral agents, those about whom it is appropriate to make moral judgments. If a person denies that any group of moral agents is impartially protected by morality, e.g., women or blacks, he is a sexist or a racist, he is not putting forward a rationally allowed way of being moral. But there is considerable disagreement about who else in addition to moral agents should be included in the impartially protected group. Almost everyone in western societies wants to include infants, but there is considerable disagreement about whether fetuses should be included. Some people want to include non-human animals, especially highly intelligent mammals such as chimpanzees and dolphins, but others disagree. Like the differences in the rankings of the harms and benefits, this difference about who is included in the group impartially protected by morality is often decisively influenced by cultural and religious factors. However, these cultural and religious factors are only indirectly responsible for the unresolvable moral disagreement; the differences in deciding who besides moral agents should be included in the impartially protected group are what is directly responsible for the unresolvable moral disagreement.

Leigh Turner is correct in claiming that common morality cannot resolve long-standing moral conflicts, but because he equates moral practices with any practices that a society puts forward to guide behavior, he offers mistaken arguments for his claim. Were he to have recognized the distinction between morality and other guides to conduct such as legal or religious guides, he would have been able to support his claim that common morality cannot resolve long-standing moral conflicts without lapsing into what seems like ethical relativism.

NOTES

1. Gert B. Common morality and computing. *Ethics and Information Technology.* 1999;1(1): 53–60. Reprinted in *Readings in CyberEthics,* 2nd ed. Sudbury, MA: Jones and Bartlett, 2004;308–322.

2. Gert B, Culver CM, Clouser KD. Common morality versus specified principlism: reply to Richardson. *J Med Philos* 2000;25(3):308–22.

3. Clouser KD, Gert B. Common Morality. In *Bioethics: A Philosophical Overview.* Kushf G (ed). Norwell, MA: Kluwer Academic Publishers, 2004.

4. Gert B. *Common Morality: Deciding What To Do.* New York: Oxford University Press, 2004.

5. Gert B, Culver CM, Clouser KD. *Bioethics: A Return to Fundamentals.* New York: Oxford University Press, 1997.

REPLY BY LEIGH TURNER, PHD

OUBLIER AQUINAS (IT'S TIME TO FORGET AQUINAS)

Once again, let me review two problems with common morality approaches in bioethics. First, the common morality is often described as being in "reflective equilibrium." Gert suggests that the common morality provides a "system." The language of reflective equilibrium emphasizes orderliness and stability. One point of my commentary was to suggest that in contemporary social orders we can identify both zones of moral conflict and zones of moral stability. Postmodern theorists typically emphasize the existence of conflict. Principlists and casuists tend to emphasize order and stability. If postmodernists overemphasize conflict, philosophers of the common morality exaggerate the degree of stability and order in contemporary societies. Gert argues that there is agreement about the "vast majority of moral decisions and judgments." I'm not convinced there is agreement on "the overwhelming majority" of moral issues and decisions. Gert suggests there are "relatively few" controversial moral issues. However, any newspaper reader knows that moral controversy surrounds many different topics. Furthermore, these issues are not just of interest to a small cadre of academic specialists. Should the U.S. have invaded Iraq? Is it both legal and moral for the U.S. to detain "enemy combatants" without trial in Guantanamo Bay? Should same sex marriage be both legalized and celebrated? Should governments provide substantial funding for embryonic stem cell research or should research involving embryonic stem cells be prohibited or highly restricted? Should governments fund "faith-based" social institutions? These issues have a moral dimension and "we" do not all agree upon what constitutes appropriate moral decisions and judgments. Caution must be exercised when offering judgments about whether there are "relatively few" or "many" controversial moral issues. This is one area where scholarship by sociologists, anthropologists, and other interpreters of societies might make a useful contribution to bioethics. To what extent is there a broadly shared "common morality" in such countries as Australia, Canada, and the United States? It is not possible to address such questions simply by offering question-begging claims about what "everyone" thinks.

Second, as I indicate in my commentary, I do not challenge the substance of what many scholars characterize as the common morality. When I note that humans often seem to take pleasure in inflicting harm, violence, and suffering, I am not presenting a brief for warfare, genocide, or organized famine. Rather, I am suggesting that we need to be skeptical of sunny notions about human nature and the fundamental moral decency of all thinking humans. The last century alone ought to make us skeptical of the notion that humans are generally guided by a beacon of natural reason that prompts them to be honest, trustworthy, and respectful of property rights. In short, I am noting problems with empirical claims made by proponents of common morality approaches to moral reasoning. Too often, they make wholly unsupported assertions about the widespread prevalence of common moral intuitions. I wish they would provide some evidence to buttress their claims concerning what "everyone" thinks about pain, death, and loss of pleasure. Such experiences might seem like bedrock dimensions of human existence. However, is it accurate to claim that death, pain, loss of freedom, and loss of pleasure are always and everywhere experienced as evils or harms? If this claim is inaccurate, proponents of the common morality draw upon a great many mistaken assumptions when they describe what "everyone" thinks.

Claiming that "right-thinking" people know the "essential features" of morality seems to offer a tautology rather than an argument.

If I am prepared to suggest that conflict is a part of moral existence and many moral "intuitions" appear to be local, culturally and historically shaped phenomena, am I properly labeled "an ethical relativist"? I nowhere suggest that all social practices are equally morally defensible. I might take issue with aspects of the substance of the common morality if philosophers ever clarified in fine detail just what this concept is supposed to include. It is hard to criticize the substance of a concept more often assumed than defended or even described in depth.

Contemporary inhabitants of societies such as Canada and the United States are socially and historically shaped beings. We live at a particular moment in human history. We are enculturated into particular social and cultural traditions. Some of "our" moral norms have long-standing roots and can be found in many different social settings around the world. Other moral norms are of more recent vintage and local provenance. Richard Rorty, Jeffrey Stout, and other philosophers with pragmatist leanings think it possible to defend particular social practices and institutions even if the moral norms these practices and institutions embody are not hardwired for all eternity into the human mind. We can say good-bye to Aquinas and his account of natural reason because in the 21st century we inhabit multicultural, multifaith, pluralistic democratic societies where moral agreement is often difficult or impossible to achieve. We should think of the common morality creed in bioethics as more an article of faith than a detailed framework for normative deliberation.

⁝ ⫴ ⫴ ⁝

DAVID STEINBERG, MD

Introduction: The Power of Language

The expression of thought requires words and concepts that in turn demand definition. Language is the indispensable medium through which reasoning in ethics is communicated. We must be scrupulous in our use of language and carefully scrutinize its use by others because it can be manipulated to unduly affect reason. This section is devoted to the importance and influence of language.

Wolf, an anthropologist, considers whether a woman who is using a donated egg for in vitro fertilization but still wants a genetic connection to her child, can request her father be the sperm donor. The question is whether the use of her father's sperm would constitute incest. Wolf notes this would not be biological incest, but worries that the word *incest* is so emotionally charged that its mere mention might stigmatize a child conceived in this manner. The use of the term *Frankenfoods* in the discussion of genetically modified organisms is another example of damning by the employment of emotionally charged language.

Words often are used to generate emotional reverberations that support or undermine an argument. Veatch contemplates the future widespread availability of a total artificial heart and asks whether its removal and the associated cessation of the heartbeats that define life would constitute murder. He recognizes "killing" and "murder" are words with a dubious reputation and that their use could damn an action of which he approves. To avoid the implication of direct intended killing, he proposes changing the definition of death to the loss of brain function, not heart function.

Steinberg, in response, maintains that removal of an artificial heart, though justified in some cases, should, nonetheless, be called killing; however, he advocates a nuanced concept that recognizes the complexity of killing. Veatch and Steinberg agree that removal of a total artificial heart may be justified; the substance of their disagreement is the most appropriate use of language to explain and support their position. In a similar discussion Taylor suggests "terminal sedation" should more properly be called "palliative sedation" because the term *terminal sedation* suggests a form of euthanasia.

Couples who use in vitro fertilization to have children may create excess embryos that are frozen indefinitely or may be given to other infertile couples. Brakman notes that the name given to the donation process has significant conceptual implications. She lists several candidate terms: *embryo transfer, embryo donation, embryo rescue,* and *embryo adoption.* Because children are adopted it is claimed the term *embryo adoption* implies, by the manipulative use of language, that embryos are children and therefore warrant protection. Majumder is ambivalent about using the word *adoption* and notes those who use adoption language in this context have been accused of mounting a deceptive "rear-guard attack" against human embryonic stem cell research.

Chervenak and McCullough in their discussion of an ethical framework for considering fetal research explicitly acknowledge the power of language. They caution against using the words *mother, father,* and *baby* because those words suggest moral relationships that they believe do not exist; instead, they advise the words *pregnant woman, husband, fetus,* and *fetal patient.* Callahan calls their suggestion that only neutral language be used unrealistic because pregnant women considering fetal surgery do not think of themselves as carrying a "fetal patient"; they believe they are carrying a "baby" with a problem. Words have persuasive and manipulative power and we must be wary of their ability to subtly influence without resort to argument and reason.

Philosophers have long understood that language is problematic because conceptual definitions which purport to describe reality are human constructs and vulnerable to subjective interpretation. A 339-page book, *The Definition of Death,*[1] offers numerous opinions of the meaning of death. Skeptics can be forgiven their doubts about the value of a bioethics enterprise that cannot find unanimity on the nature of a state—being dead—that for centuries has been intuitively obvious. In defense of bioethics, the circumstances of modern medicine ask it not only to define established death but also—and here is the difficulty—the first moment of death.

In voluntary postmortem organ donation, organs are recovered from patients who have been removed from life supports and allowed to die; only after their heart has stopped beating for a defined period are these patients declared dead and their organs taken.[2] The longer the time interval after the heart has stopped beating, the longer organs are deprived of oxygen and the less likely they will be useful for transplantation.[3] Because of the "dead donor rule" organs are not taken from people who have not first been declared dead.[4] Tension exists between an early declaration of death to obtain viable organs and the fear of being accused of killing people for their organs by taking them from people not yet dead.

In contrast to patients declared dead using neurological criteria (brain death), the heart has stopped beating in patients removed from life supports. When first adopted this type of organ donation was called "non-heart-beating organ donation." The transplant community did not feel comfortable with the emotions evoked by this term and provided another example of the power of language when they scuttled the words *non-heart-beating* in favor of the less visceral death by cardiac determination ("DCD" organ donation).

Bernat defends the concept of whole brain death, "an unfortunate and misleading term" that refers to the use of neurological criteria to determine death. He rejects as a "contrived redefinition of death" a higher brain criterion that would declare death when consciousness and cognition were permanently lost. Bernat argues that failure to agree on a uniform criterion of death and allowing the removal of organs for transplantation as a justified form of killing would be bad public policy. In response, DeVita and Arnold claim the criteria for death are not simply matters of biologic fact but "value-laden propositions." They regret the term *non-heart-beating organ donation,* initially attached to their policy of declaring death using cardiopulmonary criteria prior to organ retrieval. In their discussions Bernat, DeVita, and Arnold confront the distinction between language as a reflection of objective reality and language distorted by value-laden propositions. Their debate concerns language, but the consequences are not trivial.[5]

The use of language has been important in discussions of human cloning. Brock acknowledges a strong right to "reproductive freedom" but questions whether the term *reproductive freedom* includes the right to clone humans. Brock concludes that in some limited cases it does; however, opponents of human cloning have said cloning is not reproduction and claim it is a manufacturing process. Macklin notes that many official bodies have declared human cloning a violation of "human dignity," then questions the precise meaning of "human dignity" and what constitutes its violation.

Spack describes illness as susceptible to mislabeling when he argues that "gender dysphoria" has erroneously been called a psychiatric condition. The Soviets were guilty of mislabeling language when political dissidents were locked up under the pretext of a psychiatric diagnosis. Hughes criticizes the medical model used to classify individuals with gender dysphoria and advocates "morphological liberationism." He objects to "passé binary assumptions" that linguistically divide gender into male and female and argues for recognition of various intermediate "ambiguous gender positions." The concept of gender dysphoria can therefore be defined as a psychiatric condition, a medical condition that merits treatment or the reflection of a sexual preference that merits respect. In this exchange much of the debate is about what words ought to mean. The influence of language on the perception of illness has been described by Sontag in her classic work, *Illness as Metaphor.*[6]

Ethics cannot exist without reasoned linguistic expression. The articles in this section highlight the important role of language in ethical debate. Language has power and its use warrants careful scrutiny; it should reveal the world objectively and facilitate impartial reason. But, as these discussions illustrate, that is much easier said than done.

NOTES

1. Youngner Stuart J; Arnold Robert M; Schapiro Renie. *The Definition of Death.* The Johns Hopkins University Press, 1999.

2. *Non-Heart Beating Organ Transplantation Medical and Ethical Issues in Procurement.* Institute of Medicine National Academy Press, Washington, D.C., 1997; *Non-Heart-Beating Organ Transplantation Practice and Protocols.* Institute of Medicine National Academy Press, Washington, D.C., 1999. Full text available online at www.nap.edu/readingroom

3. A flat electrocariogram and the cessation of breathing for 5 minutes is a commonly used standard for the declaration of death.

4. Under very different circumstances organs or parts of organs may be recovered from "live organ donors."

5. Bioethics confronts similar disagreement in the definition of when life first begins.

6. Sontag Susan. *Illness as Metaphor* (Paperback) Picador USA, 2001.

☰ ☷ ☶ ☴

ROBERT M. VEATCH, PHD

The Total Artificial Heart: Is Paying for It Immoral and Stopping It Murder?

Slowly, but surely, we are developing the ultimate replacement part for the human body. The idea of a total artificial heart (TAH) has been with us for decades.[1] A range of devices to totally replace the heart are in clinical trials. Some are envisioned as a bridge to transplant while others are seen as permanent replacements for the human's biological pump.[2–9] As long as these devices are used as temporary support while a patient awaits transplant, most of the moral issues raised by them will not be too novel or too challenging. The issues of consent,[10] government approval,[11] and the use of humans as subjects[12,13] have arisen with the artificial heart from the beginning and will continue.

MURDER VS. FORGOING TREATMENT

The development of a permanent replacement device, especially the TAH, will, by contrast, create some truly new problems. One of these involves terminal care ethics. Over the past two or three decades a mainstream consensus has emerged that relies on some conceptual distinctions: between actions and omissions, as well as between directly intended killing and death that results as a side effect of actions that are in themselves good.[14] It is now commonplace to accept the forgoing of life support even though active interventions to kill are illegal and many consider them unethical. Patients may withhold or withdraw consent, as long as doing so does not intentionally, directly cause their death. The death is thought of as a side effect of forgoing a burdensome or useless intervention.

The TAH may change all of that. How should we think about patients who demand that their TAHs be stopped? When dealing with life-supporting technologies not directly related to the heart, many concluded that we could forgo a technology that was maintaining life even if the end result was that death could proceed unabated. We accepted, for example, a patient's decision to forgo hemodialysis even though everyone knew that the patient would die without it. The common wisdom was that the purpose of forgoing the treatment was to remove an intervention that failed to offer more benefit than harm. As long as the death of the patient was merely a foreseen, but unintended outcome and it was the consequence rather than part of the patient's action, even traditional Roman Catholics opposed to all euthanasia have found the forgoing of life-supporting technologies morally acceptable.

Now, however, we anticipate the case in which the life-supporting technology does not merely make continued life possible, but whose functioning actually is the basis for saying that life continues. In the old world of 20th century medical ethics, clinicians could choose to believe that, when the patient refused dialysis or a ventilator and the physician removed the technology deemed disproportionately burdensome, the physician didn't cause the patient's death; some intervening disease process did.

Some have always found this distinction between direct and indirect killing problematic. The new TAH technology, however, presents a new twist. If one stops a TAH or removes the machine, one does not merely permit the dying process to continue. The very act of stopping the machine is the event that, by traditional cardiac-based definition of death standards, we call "death." A person dies, according to that definition, when cardiac function ceases irreversibly. Turning off the TAH is the direct and immediate cause of death just as certainly as injecting potassium into the ventricle.

We have some options: One would appeal to "liberals" who never accepted the doctrine of double effect. They have tended to be consequentialists. They have long believed that it makes no difference whether one forgoes life support or actively, intentionally kills a patient. According to them, it is not the action/omission distinction or the direct/indirect distinction that is critical; it is whether the patient is better off dead. For them, even if turning off the TAH is an act of direct killing it may be morally justified.

Another option might appeal more to conservatives. They might insist that stopping the TAH is somehow different from stopping any other technology necessary for life and insist it is both unethical and illegal.

There is a third option, however. The conclusion that stopping the TAH is a direct killing rests on the use of the traditional cardiac definition of death. One dies according to current law when *either* the heart or the brain function ceases irreversibly. A patient is legally dead when the heart stops permanently (even if, hypothetically, the brain continued to function).

Some of us are now convinced that can't really be correct. If we believe in brain death, it is because we accept the notion that the essence of a living human being has something to do with the functioning of the brain. Imagine the hypothetical case of someone whose cardiac function had irreversibly stopped, but whose brain continued to function—who continued to think, feel, reason, and emote. Surely, that person is not dead just because the cardiac function is gone.

If so, then stopping the TAH is no more the immediate cause of death than stopping a ventilator or a dialysis machine. The patient would continue to live for the few seconds or minutes when the heart was not beating, but the brain was still alive and functioning. Stopping the TAH would turn out to be no different from stopping any other life-supporting treatment.

It could turn out that the TAH will force us to fix our now naive and implausible two-pronged definition of death that permits death to be pronounced when either heart or brain function is lost and replace it with one relying only on brain function loss. We could, of course, continue to use loss of heart function as a sign that the brain function is irreversibly gone just as we always have, but it would now be merely an indicator of brain function. Moreover, the first few minutes of heart function loss would not imply brain death; only loss long enough to conclude that brain cells could not survive would signal death.

The TAH will raise an additional problem. Until now, we have generally assumed that the right to refuse treatment implies the duty of the clinician to stop whatever life support is currently functioning. The removal of treatment has generally been noninvasive or only minimally so. But removing a TAH would involve significant surgery. It may be we will have to develop an entirely new set of moral standards for the duty of clinicians in such cases. It may be, for example, that the clinician would have a duty to turn the TAH off, but not a duty to remove it. Some clinicians may object to stopping the TAH, which they perceive as direct killing, but they plausibly would nevertheless have such an obligation.

We may also have to contemplate the reverse case: the one in which the clinician sees no point in continuing, but the patient insists that the TAH be maintained. The clinician may come to see the TAH as "futile" in the case of someone whose life cannot otherwise be maintained. Some commentators have claimed that physicians should not be forced to provide support for a TAH once they conclude it is serving no purpose,[15] but they usually don't address the interesting case of when the patient still sees value in the treatment. One thing seems clear: when the physician and patient disagree about the value of a treatment that could continue to maintain life, there is no reason to assume that the physician's view must prevail.

THE ULTIMATE RESOURCE ALLOCATION PROBLEM

The transplant of human hearts is one of the most expensive medical technologies. It currently comes, however, with a natural constraint. In the United States, fewer than 2,500 human hearts are available in a given year. Because of that limit, the cost of heart transplants in the United States is in the range of $350–700 million a year.[16]

If that natural limit were overcome through the use of artificial organs, present heart transplant costs would dwarf in comparison. Estimates are that as many as 100,000 patients a year could be candidates for these devices. For the first implantable heart attempts, the devices alone would cost $75,000. Although they expect costs could be reduced to about a third with mass production, that would amount to $2.5 billion a year—just for the pump. Evans estimates that the total direct annual costs for cardiac assistance and replacement would be in the range of $5–24 billion.[16]

When the technical problems are solved, the scarcity of transplantable hearts will be replaced by financial scarcity. Providing them for all Americans would tax the system significantly. The TAH may be the device that pushes the inevitability of rationing into the open. If the TAH arrives before universal health insurance, money will determine which patients are covered for the TAH. Otherwise the society will have to decide which factors justifiably limit access—medical hopelessness, low expected benefit, patient age, or an element of voluntary lifestyle risk that was the cause of the cardiac disease. They would all be better than ability to pay or judging the social usefulness of the recipients.

They would probably all be better than blindly attempting to pay for all artificial organs and leaving other important projects underfunded. When the TAH arrives, we should be ready to figure out whether giving the machine to everyone who could benefit will break the bank as well as be ready to figure out whether stopping it would be murder or merely forgoing disproportionally burdensome treatment.

NOTES

1. Report by Artificial Heart Assessment Panel. The totally implantable artificial heart. *National Heart and Lung Institute* June 1973.

2. Goldstein DJ. Worldwide experience with the MicroMed DeBakey Ventricular Assist Device as a bridge to transplantation. *Circulation* 2003;108 Suppl 1:II272–7.

3. Dowling RD, Gray LA Jr, Etoch SW, Laks H, Marelli D, Samuels L, et al. The AbioCor implantable replacement heart. *Ann Thorac Surg* 2003;75(6 Suppl):S93–9.

4. Jeevanandam V, Jayakar D, Anderson AS, Martin S, Piccione W Jr, Heroux AL, et al. Circulatory assistance with a permanent implantable IABP: initial human experience. *Circulation* 2002;106(12 Suppl 1):I183–8.

5. Copeland JG, Arabia FA, Smith RG, Sethi GK, Nolan PE, Banchy ME. Arizona experience with CardioWest Total Artificial Heart bridge to transplantation. *Ann Thorac Surg* 1999;68(2):756–60.

6. Catanese KA, Goldstein DJ, Williams DL, Foray AT, Illick CD, Gardocki MT, et al. Outpatient left ventricular assist device support: a destination rather than a bridge. *Ann Thorac Surg* 96;62(3):646–52.

7. Pierce WS, Sapirstein JS, Pae WE Jr. Total artificial heart: from bridge to transplantation to permanent use. *Ann Thorac Surg* 1996;61(1): 342–6.

8. Frazier OH, Myers TJ, Westaby S, Gregoric ID. Use of the Jarvik 2000 left ventricular assist system as a bridge to heart transplantation or as destination therapy for patients with chronic heart failure. *Ann Surg* 2003;237(5): 631–6; discussion 636–7.

9. Dowling RD, Etoch SW, Stevens KA, Johnson AC, Gray LA Jr. Current status of the Abio-Cor implantable replacement heart. *Ann Thorac Surg* 2001;71(3 Suppl): S147–9.

10. Goldberg D. Artificial heart implant leads to suit over consent process: recipient's widow says she and her husband were misinformed and misled on risks, benefits. *Washington Post* 2002;Nov 30:A3.

11. Altman LK. Unsanctioned artificial heart implanted in Arizona patient. *NY Times* 1985: Mar 7: A1, A25.

12. Eichwald EJ, Woolley FR, Cole B, Beamer V. Insertion of the total artificial heart. *IRB* 1981;Aug./Sep.; 3(7): 4–5.

13. Morreim H. AbioCor: an experiment in research. *Hastings Cent Rep* 2001;31(6):7.

14. Meisel A. The legal consensus about forgoing life-sustaining treatment: its status and its prospects. *Kennedy Inst of Ethics J* 1992(4):309–45.

15. Bramstedt KA. Replying to Veatch's concerns: special moral problems with total artificial heart inactivation. *Death Stud* 2003;27(4):317–20.

16. Evans RW. Economic impact of mechanical cardiac assistance. *Prog Cardiovasc Dis* 2000;43(1):81–94.

☷ ☳ ☳ ☷

DAVID STEINBERG, MD

The Total Artificial Heart and the Morality of Killing

The words and concepts we use make intellectual discourse possible; but language is not simply an inert enabler; it can resonate emotionally charged implications, and not only facilitate discourse, but also influence it. In his discussion of the total artificial heart (TAH), Veatch engages two high-voltage concepts, "killing" and "death." He would alter the definition of death to avoid the direct "killing" that would follow stopping or removing the TAH and seems more comfortable if those acts could be conceptualized as merely permitting "the dying process to continue." These linguistic maneuvers raise interesting questions.

According to Veatch, stopping mechanical ventilation or dialysis may allow death to "proceed unabated" but these maneuvers do not directly cause death. However, the functioning of the artificial heart "actually is the basis for saying life continues." According to the cardiac definition of death, one dies when heart function ceases irreversibly; therefore, terminating an artificial heart kills directly and immediately, "as certainly as injecting potassium into the ventricle."

Veatch proposes changing the definition of death to "one relying only on brain function loss." Stopping the TAH would then no longer be the immediate cause of death and would "turn out to be no different from stopping any other life-supporting treatment." Veatch, it seems, would agree with stopping or removing a TAH if that intervention was "deemed disproportionately burdensome" but he is intent on avoiding the accusation of direct intended killing.

Before consigning "killing" to the trash can of immoral acts, the concept warrants further exploration. Although Veatch mentions "liberals" for whom direct killing may under certain circumstances be morally justified, he has done a disservice by implying in his title that killing is equivalent to "murder." "Killing" is a more complex phenomenon with a spectrum that includes genocide, mass murder, first-degree murder, second-degree murder, manslaughter, second-degree manslaughter, the execution of criminals, euthanasia, and killing in battle and self-defense. Could the termination of life supports be more honestly construed as yet another form of "killing" but one that under appropriate circumstances might be justified?

The removal of a mechanical ventilator, stopping dialysis, and stopping an artificial heart all lead to death. There is a cause and effect relationship. When you remove a mechanical ventilator from a person with terminal cancer, they don't die of cancer, they die because they stop breathing. When you stop dialysis in a demented man, he doesn't die of dementia, he dies of renal failure. Cancer and dementia may be the initiating factors, the root problems that ultimately lead to death, but they are not the immediate mechanism of death.

Veatch's desire to avoid direct killing also warrants examination. Whether an act causes instantaneous direct death, as when stopping a TAH, or delayed death, as after removing a ventilator or stopping dialysis, may not be morally significant. If a man is pushed off the roof of a high-rise building he doesn't die directly and instantaneously; nonetheless, we don't allow that the push merely enabled him to die of gravity.

It is not uncommon for surrogate decision makers to express the feeling that removing life supports is tantamount to killing their relative. We use convoluted language to convince them of the importance of their good intentions and that they are simply allowing the patient to die of some underlying disease. Perhaps we should acknowledge the truth in their intuitions. If the removal of burdensome therapy is construed as a justified form of killing, it should not meet automatic public disapproval precisely because the absolute rejection of killing is not a widespread belief.

Intention is important, but the use of intention to exculpate a bad effect that can be foreseen is problematic. In double effect whether an act is moral or immoral can depend on the psychological predisposition of the actor. The same act may be judged differently depending on the actor's state of mind. Intentions can be murky, complex, and difficult to decipher. Should the intention to relieve pain become suspect if it briefly crosses the actor's mind that the patient might be better off dead?

If the heir to his uncle's fortune surreptitiously disconnected his uncle from a mechanical ventilator, most people would consider that killing; but if the ventilator is disconnected by a nurse or physician, Veatch might call it enabling death from another cause. That the identical act can be considered both killing and not killing is a troubling inconsistency. Let's for the moment confront reality bluntly and label the removal of life-sustaining treatment "killing" and see where that leads us.

I first propose a new category of life, "medically contingent life." This concept defines people who are alive only because of an active medical intervention. The removal of that intervention will directly and in a short time lead to death. This would place people dependent on ventilators, on dialysis and on a TAH in the same category. The concept might require further elaboration, but by defining life differently among a specific group of people, the boundary of any permissible killing is drawn and restricted. A form of "killing"—let's tentatively call it "termanasia"—would be defined as that which consisted of the removal of life-supporting treatment from people whose lives are "medically contingent." Just as killing in self-defense may be justified, killing by the removal of life supports from people living "medically contingent lives" might also be justified as long as defined appropriate rules are followed.

Veatch and I seem to have reached the same conclusion; we both agree a TAH can be stopped or removed when that is appropriate. Veatch would arrive at that conclusion by altering the definition of death so that removal cannot be considered intended direct killing. I would arrive at the same conclusion by allowing that removal is a specific form of killing, albeit justified killing. I have also downplayed the moral significance of direct versus indirect killing and expressed some reservations concerning the exculpatory power of intention.

It might be argued, in another testament to the power of language, that to justify killing in one sphere facilitates its justification under other circumstances. It's important to refrain from drawing conclusions that go beyond what is actually stated in an argument. If the removal of life supports under appropriate conditions from people leading "medically contingent lives" is acknowledged as justified killing, it does not follow that killing under other circumstances is also being justified.

At this point readers might legitimately ask whether I believe what I have written. Have I concocted this discussion merely to illustrate that the legitimacy of an act can be a function of how we use language? As a physician who struggles against death, do I want to endorse a form of killing? And do I want to be in a position where I have to tell a woman whose husband is hopelessly ill with metastatic cancer that she ought to kill him by allowing the removal of his ventilator? My answer to both of these questions is no. I feel conflicted because I believe we have an obligation to use language as precisely and accurately as possible. When we alter and distort language to facilitate an ulterior motive, the line that separates honest discussion from manipulation and propaganda begins to blur; but honesty can be brutal.

I think we more closely approximate moral reality when we consider the removal of burdensome life-sustaining medical interventions as its own category. We can call it a category of killing but should judge it on its own terms rather than describing it as analogous to something else, such as other forms of killing or enabling the dying process. The interventions that sustain medically contingent life should from their initiation themselves be considered to be morally contingent on their benefits outweighing their burdens. Veatch has argued elsewhere in favor of a higher brain definition of death.[1] I have bypassed that argument and only mean to say that justification for stopping or removing a TAH should not be the reason to alter the definition of death.

NOTES

1. Veatch RM. *Transplantation Ethics.* Georgetown University Press, 2000:70.

REPLY BY ROBERT M. VEATCH, PHD

David Steinberg has challenged my approach to stopping an implanted total artificial heart (TAH). Since death is traditionally understood as irreversible heart stoppage, deactivating TAHs could plausibly be understood as direct, active killing. I pointed out that, with a proper understanding of the definition of death, stopping TAHs could still be classified as only an indirect killing.

Steinberg points out that there is an alternative: confronting the traditional active killing forgoing distinction directly. We could simply accept that some patients might actively end their own lives *by authorizing* TAH stoppage and that some surrogates might instruct physicians to actively kill their loved ones. If active killing were potentially morally acceptable, we could admit these patients were killed when their machines were turned off, but deny this was wrong.

My analysis was not as antithetical to Steinberg's position as he thought. I stated that there were three options: We could follow the "liberals" accepting that direct, active killing can be justified. We could follow the "conservatives" and acknowledge that turning off TAHs is morally unacceptable active killing. I proposed a third option: limiting death to brain death so that stopping the TAH becomes indirect killing, a forgoing of life support that would indirectly lead to death when (and only when) brain function ceases irreversibly. This does not require adopting a higher-brain definition; merely acknowledging that heart-stoppage alone doesn't count as death. Our multiple-option definition has always been wrong. Now we have a reason to acknowledge it.

Steinberg assumes I reject options one and two in favor of option three. But I didn't quite say that. It is true that option three is only needed in the TAH context if one wants to retain the possibility of stopping the TAH without directly causing death, but I have for the last decade been perplexed over the question of whether the traditional active-killing/ forgoing distinction can be sustained. I put forward the third option for those who end up supporting the traditional formulations, but still believe stopping the TAH can be moral.

While I am open to Steinberg's liberal alternative of legitimizing active, direct killings, for both practical and theoretical reasons I remain skeptical. First, as a practical matter, the active-killing/forgoing distinction is remarkably robust. It has withstood political attacks for at least a century and in the US no jurisdiction has yet overturned it. While Oregon has legalized active self-killing, no other state has followed suit and Oregon militantly retains a prohibition on merciful homicides. Even the Netherlands continues to prohibit merciful homicides of those who do not persistently and voluntarily request to be killed. Hence, in the case of an incompetent patient, in no place in the world would stopping a TAH be legal if it is conceptualized as an active, direct killing.

Of course, Steinberg can argue that this does not make the distinction valid. In order to make his case, Steinberg needs to defend more than merely active, direct killing by TAH stoppage. Imagine someone with a TAH who has made a competent, adequately informed decision to stop the machine and has authorized a physician to do what is necessary to get it stopped.

There is another problem with Steinberg's solution. Physicians can be forced by patients or valid surrogates to stop life support, but surely cannot be forced to kill their patients. My proposal serves the interests of a patient whose physician was unwilling to kill, but would be obliged to withdraw life support by turning off a TAH.

The underlying problem is that something remains very troublesome about killing another human being. Some of us have even gone to the extreme of rejecting (at least *prima facie*) all human killing and have become pacifists. Of course, if killings by omission are conceptualized as being included in this prohibition, the norm would be impossible to follow. (We all omit life support for starving people throughout the world every day.) Hence, we have trumped up an active-killing/forgoing distinction that provides a more-or-less bright line that sorts into two group behaviors leading to death.

For those who have not chosen pacifism, the active killing of unjust aggressors is sometimes added as another qualification, but the prohibition on the active, direct killing of the innocent is remarkably stable, in spite of its logical ambiguities.

In claiming that stopping TAHs is forgoing rather than active, direct killing, I speak to the substantial majority who retain these bright lines, but still see stopping a TAH as acceptable. I am willing to continue conversing with the minority preferring my first option, but the evidence is that that position is not selling. Even if it does sell, it opens the door to a much broader range of active killings than I was addressing. I am yet to be convinced that legalizing active merciful homicide is the way to go.

⚎ ䷀ ䷀ ⚎

ARTHUR P. WOLF, PHD

Is This Incest?

QUESTION: Janet M. is a 42-year-old single mother with two sons who are 4 and 6 years old. Both boys were conceived using anonymous donor sperm from different donors. A few months ago, Janet, a successful advertising executive, moved from Los Angeles to San Francisco to take a new and more exciting job and to be closer her widowed father, a healthy 70-year-old retired high school English teacher. Janet's father, who now lives with her, has been helpful in caring for her sons while she works full time. Janet comes to a fertility clinic for a third child, again using donor sperm. After one in vitro fertilization (IVF) cycle using donor sperm, Janet learns that she has poor quality eggs. To become pregnant, she would need a donated egg. Because she badly wants genetic connection to her child, she requests that her father be the sperm donor. She would use an anonymous egg donor. In this manner she would be able to maintain a genetic link through her father and still experience pregnancy. Her father has agreed to this arrangement.

This request generated alarming and uncomfortable feelings for the IVF staff. While this would not be genetic or carnal incest, they felt that in some manner they might be violating the incest taboo because Janet would be giving birth to her father's child. Should the IVF staff honor Janet's request?

REPLY: Anthropologists are generally agreed that incest is sexual intercourse between individuals related in certain prohibited degrees of kinship. Some would add "and/or affinity," but the core of the matter is proscribed sexual relations between kin. Strictly speaking, a woman's having a donated ovum impregnated with her father's sperm is not incest because it does not involve sexual relations with her father. But why then, does anyone object to the procedure? Why do some people insist that it is like incest? Does their reaction indicate there is something about it that ought not to be allowed? One possibility is that the consequences are similar to those produced by incest. Obviously, there is no reason to fear that the biological consequences will be similar, but what about the social consequences? Accepting Freud's view that "an incestuous love choice" is in fact the first and regular one[1] many anthropologists have argued that the incest taboo exists to protect society from the deleterious consequences of these choices. One argument is that in its absence, families would become isolated "self-perpetuating units, over-ridden by their fears, hatreds, and ignorances."[2] Another is that if it were not for the taboo, sexual rivalry between parents and children and between siblings would "subvert the most fundamental bonds of kinship on which the further development of all social relations is based."[3]

For reasons I will note below, I do not accept these arguments. But even if they were valid, they do not account for the unease people feel about the proposed procedure. The woman's family would not be isolated or its functioning subverted by her bearing a child carrying her father's genes. There is no more reason to predict dire social consequences than dire biological consequences. Yet the question remains: Why does the proposal make people uneasy? Why does it elicit what amounts to moral disapproval?

I think the answer is to be found in the work of the Finnish sociologist and philosopher Edward Westermarck.[4] Westermarck argued that the dangers of inbreeding have selected for something that causes us to develop an aversion to sexual relations with people by whom or with whom we are reared. In the normal course of affairs, the aversion is experienced as a comfortable indifference. It only manifests itself as an aversion when incestuous behavior forces us to entertain the possibility of sexual relations with a parent or sibling. This is painful and prompts us to condemn the cause of our pain. Thus, in Westermarck's view, the moral disapproval at the core of the incest taboo is rooted in our reaction to what he characterized as "living closely together from childhood."[5]

For the greater part of the 20th century Westermarck's argument was condemned to oblivion by Freud's claim that psychoanalytic investigations show "beyond the possibility of doubt" that incest is our first choice. The evidence that finally turned the tide of anthropological opinion against Freud came from two natural experiments—one in Israel and the other in Taiwan. The evidence from Israel says that when children are reared together in communal nurseries and allowed to choose their own sexual partners they never choose a childhood associate.[6] The evidence from Taiwan says that when children are reared together and forced to marry the result is abnormally low fertility and an abnormally high divorce rate.[7]

Thus, following Westermarck, I think the reason some people are reluctant to allow the proposed procedure is because it arouses their aversion to sexual relations with their relatives. The procedure does not involve the woman's having sexual relations with her father, but it does involve allowing her father's sperm to pass through her body. It is not incest, but it brings to mind the possibility of incest. It arouses an image of sexual relations between father and daughter, and, for many people, this is enough to transform a comfortable indifference into a painful aversion.

Should the requested procedure be disallowed because it arouses an aversion that prompts disapproval? In my view, no, if the only persons affected are the medical personnel who perform the procedure. The woman's request is not frivolous. A wealth of evidence says that we are so constituted as to act to perpetuate our genes. The only reason I can see for refusing the request is the possibility that the child will suffer if it becomes known that he or she is the product of an incestuous-like procedure. The reaction to the request is sufficient reason to fear that the child may be stigmatized. My recommendation is to allow the procedure but warn the woman that she may cause her child harm if she reveals the source of the sperm.

OUTCOME: The fertility clinic decided not to go through with the procedure because of the complex psychological relationship between Janet and her father. Janet decided not to pursue IVF and use donated sperm from another source.

NOTES

1. Freud S. Riviere J (trans). *A General Introduction to Psychoanalysis*. New York: Pocket Books, 1920:221.

2. Levi-Strauss C. The family. In Shapiro HL (ed): *Man, Culture, and Society*. New York: Oxford University Press, 1960:278.

3. Malinowski B. Culture. In *Encyclopedia of the Social Sciences*. New York: Macmillan, 1930, vol. 4:630.

4. For a detailed account see: Wolf AP. *Sexual Attraction and Childhood Association: A Chinese Brief for Edward Westermarck*. Stanford, CA: Stanford University Press, 1995.

5. Westermarck E. *The History of Human Marriage.* 5th ed., rev., 3 vols. New York: Allerton, 1922, vol. 2:192.

6. Shepher J. Mate selection among second generation kibbutz adolescents and adults: incest avoidance and negative imprinting. *Arch Sex Behav* 1971:1(4);293–307.

7. The most recent evidence is summarized and discussed in: Wolf AP, Durham W (eds): *Inbreeding, Incest and the Incest Taboo: The State of Knowledge at the Turn of the Century.* Stanford, CA: Stanford University Press, 2004.

☱ ☲ ☲ ☱

SARAH-VAUGHAN BRAKMAN, PHD

Embryo Adoption

Couples who have used in vitro fertilization (IVF) may choose to give their no longer needed (frozen) embryos to other couples wishing to bear and raise children. The name given to this process (based on one's frame of reference and/or ideological commitments) is embryo donation, embryo adoption, embryo rescue, or human embryo transfer. This practice has been around for over 20 years[1] but has only gained widespread attention recently. Why is this?

Four reasons may account in part for the current interest in embryo adoption. First, with estimates of over 400,000 embryos currently frozen in the United States and significant numbers in other countries, the question of what to do with them has become urgent.[2] Storage is an issue in terms of space and cost as well as the "shelf life" of frozen embryos, which will become nonviable over time. Interestingly, one option, relinquishing the embryos for research, is not chosen by significant numbers of couples for psychological and moral reasons.[3] Embryo adoption offers those couples an alternative that they may find morally more palatable than donating their embryos to research.

Second, proponents of human embryonic stem cell research (which entails the destruction of embryos) argue for the moral permissibility of stem cell research on the grounds that only "excess" embryos from reproductive medicine will be used (i.e., no new embryos will be created for research purposes). Furthermore, since frozen embryos will expire eventually, using them for stem cell research is not depriving them of a better fate. Consequently, many believe the growing interest in embryo adoption is largely politically motivated by the stem cell debate.

As evidence for this claim, some bioethicists point to the Department of Health and Human Services 2001 announcement of close to one million dollars in grants for "Public Awareness Campaigns for embryo adoption."[4] These bioethicists claim that even calling the practice embryo adoption instead of donation implies that embryos are children. Elsewhere, I have argued the error of this claim.[5] Data show that couples "considering the embryo as a child choose destruction as frequently as donation but refuse experimentation on the embryo."[6]

Third, a significant number of couples with fertility problems or hereditary disorders are seeking embryo adoption.[1,3] Some couples are attracted by the lower costs of embryo adoption in relation to traditional IVF.[7] For example, embryo adoption programs currently list costs of $3,600 to $10,000 per cycle, regardless of outcome and not including the expenses of pregnancy and delivery. These expenses include: the identification of a match; the cost of thawing; screening and testing of donors, embryos, and possibly recipients; the hormonal preparation of the prospective mother; and the embryo transfer. Costs per cycle for IVF, using fresh embryos, range from $12,000 to $20,000, also exclusive of outcome. Costs are lower for embryo adoption, because the original couple has paid for the harvesting of gametes and fertilization of the ovums. The success rate using embryo adoption is slightly less than that of IVF using fresh embryos; however, it currently appears comparable to IVF with one's own frozen embryos.[8]

Finally, embryo adoption is also on average less expensive than traditional newborn adoption (for example, in the US, domestic adoption fees vary from $9,000 to more than $35,000). However, each cycle of embryo adoption, just like traditional IVF, includes a greater than 60 percent chance of failure; whereas, traditional adoption fees are paid in relation to the placement of a child. Even so, embryo adoption may appeal to people in this country who have been waiting (sometimes years) to adopt newborns and has the added advantage of prospective parental control of the prenatal environment and the chance to experience the birth of the child.[9] Embryo adoption may also afford older women, who are often not chosen by birth mothers in domestic adoptions, a chance to become mothers—a practice that raises ethical considerations in itself.

Yet despite long waiting lists for embryo adoption, it is rarely done, because people with frozen embryos are reluctant to donate. The most common reasons given are: having unknown children, the possibility of sibling marriage, and legal ramifications.[10] Some studies identified willingness to donate "was associated with greater comfort about disclosing personal information, a desire to know the outcome of donation and willingness to have future contact with a child, but not with current family size."[11] Seventy-six percent of fertility clinics do not allow donors any control over who receives their embryos and further stipulate anonymous donation with no knowledge of outcome.[12]

In my view, embryo adoption is conceptually different than gamete donation, with which it is often compared. With embryo adoption, couples
view the embryos as their once possible and perhaps future children. Decisions about giving the embryos to others more closely resemble adoption
decisions than decisions about "donating" sperm or egg.[13] Fertility centers
ought to change their policies concerning donating couples' choices to better respect the reality of this activity, to respect couples' views and finally to
increase the supply of embryos available for embryo adoption. Some agencies, like Snowflakes, and clinics, like the National Embryo Donation Center, in fact, have policies that allow for greater choice of involvement for
couples with embryos.

Other ethical issues raised by embryo adoption have been raised by other
forms of assisted reproductive technology and by traditional infant adoption. These include: permissibility of the practice; payment for the embryos;
who decides which embryos are given to which couples and on what basis;
screening of donors, embryos, and recipients; genetic disclosure to recipient couples; privacy and disclosure to children; anonymous recordkeeping,
and future relationships between genetic and rearing families.

Consensus seems to exist for one of these issues—the impermissibility of
paying the donor couple for the embryo itself (though reimbursement for
some specific expenses is permissible).[14] This is based on views about gift
giving, solidarity, and the risk of commodification of human life. The policy
is consonant with other practices in medicine, such as forbidding payment
for organs and for babies.

Some major religious traditions have difficulties with the permissibility
of embryo adoption, even those most associated with pro-life positions. For
example, controversy regarding embryo adoption exists among scholars
who accept Roman Catholic official teachings. Arguments in favor of it include the appeal to rescuing innocent human lives, for embryos are viewed
as persons with inherent dignity. Arguments against embryo adoption hold
that condoning embryo adoption is not acceptable, because it is too closely
associated with practices considered inherently immoral, such as IVF and
the freezing of embryos. Reasons of this type do not seem particularly persuasive since traditional adoption is not denounced as condoning acts (i.e.,
extramarital intercourse) that have, in most cases, led to the availability of
children for adoption.

A second type of argument against embryo adoption from Catholic
scholars is that the ends do not justify the means. It is wrong for a woman to
intentionally become pregnant with a child that is not the fruit of marital
intercourse. Just as surrogacy and the use of donor gametes is impermissible, so is embryo adoption, despite the seemingly "good" intentions in this
case. This set of arguments is currently at the heart of the debate among
Catholic scholars.[15]

A separate set of ethical issues arises once embryo adoption successfully has been accomplished. I will discuss just one of these here—parental privacy. With embryo adoption, no one, including the child, will know that a baby born into a family is not genetically related to that family, unless the couple chooses to share that information. I hold that children's best interests are served by knowing about their origins as early as possible. Counterarguments about the privacy of the couples, the liberty of parents to decide for children, and the privacy of the genetic parents are weaker claims. Moreover, secrets of this magnitude, if discovered, are usually very damaging to the parent-child relationship and will be more difficult to keep as genetic testing becomes more comprehensive and routine.[16] The obligation of parents to inform their children about the use of embryo adoption is founded on philosophical views about the rights of individuals and the obligations of the parents. It is also based, in part, on outcome data from the literature on traditional adoption concerning disclosure to children. Telling those other than their children entails different considerations, including that of the children's privacy. Centers and agencies offering embryo adoption should counsel, if not require, couples to agree to disclose the use of embryo adoption to their future children.

NOTES

1. Eisenberg VH, Schenker JG. Pre-embryo donation: ethical and legal aspects. *Int J Gynaecol Obstet.* 1998;60:51–57.

2. Eydoux P, et. al. How can the genetic risks of embryo donation be minimized? *Hum Reprod.* 2004;19(8):1685–1688.

3. Lee J, Yap C. Embryo donation: a review. *Acta Obstet Gynecol Scand.* 2003;82:991–996.

4. Caplan A. "The problem with 'embryo adoption': why is the government giving money to 'Snowflakes?'" http://www.msnbc.com/id/3076556/print/1/displaymode/1098/

5. Brakman S-V. "Ethics and 'Embryo Adoption': a rose by any other name . . ." Presentation at the annual meeting of the American Society of Bioethics and Humanities; October 2004.

6. Laruelle C, Englert Y. Psychological study of in vitro fertilization-embryo transfer participants' attitudes toward the destiny of their supernumerary embryos. *Fertil Steril.* 1995;63(5):1047–1050.

7. Robertson JA. Ethical and legal issues in human embryo donation. *Fertil Steril.* 1995;64(5):885–894; Van Voorhis BJ, et al. Establishment of a successful donor embryo program: medical, ethical, and policy issues. *Fertil Steril.* 1999;71(4):604–608.

8. Kovas GT, Breheny SA, Dear MJ. Embryo donation at an Australian university in-vitro fertilization clinic: issues and outcomes. *Med J Aust.* 2003;178(3):127–129.

9. Robertson, 1995; Lee, Yap, 2003.

10. Burton PJ, Sanders K. Patient attitudes to donation of embryos for research in Western Australia. *Med J Aust.* 2004;180(11):559–561.

11. Newton CR, et al. Embryo donation: attitudes toward donation procedures and factors predicting willingness to donate. *Hum Reprod.* 2003;18(4):878–884.

12. Kingsberg, et al. 2003.

13. Brakman, 2004.

14. The American Society for Reproductive Medicine. Guidelines for cryopreserved embryo donation. *Fertil Steril.* 2004;82(supplement 1):S16–S17.

15. For more, see *Natl Cathol Bioeth Q,* Spring 2005 issue.

16. McGee G, Brakman S-V, Gurmankin A. Debate: disclosure to children conceived with donor gametes. *Hum Reprod.* 2001;16(10):2033–6.

☷ ☶ ☵ ☴

MARY ANDERLIK MAJUMDER, JD, PHD

The Politics of Embryo Transfer

I will examine aspects of the current embryo "adoption" controversy introduced by Sarah-Vaughan Brakman through the lens of law and policy. I will begin by looking at possible legal and policy responses to the concerns of those who regard an embryo as morally equivalent, or nearly morally equivalent, to a child.

LEGAL AND POLICY RESPONSES

Our society is sharply divided over the moral status of a human embryo. If the segment of society committed to full(er) moral status for embryos is given some policy space, at least three options are possible: (1) avoid any public expenditure that supports or promotes embryo destruction, (2) expend public funds to promote the use of embryos for purposes of reproduction or (3) require implantation of all viable embryos and/or prohibit embryo destruction.

The first option is the compromise enshrined in federal law since 1995 through a rider to an appropriations act and known as the "Dickey Amendment." This legislation prohibits the use of appropriated funds for the creation of a human embryo or embryos for research purposes or research in which a human embryo or embryos are destroyed, discarded, or knowingly subjected to risk of injury or death above the threshold set for research with fetuses in utero.[1]

Using the second option, the Bush administration has spent over $1 million of public money to promote embryo "adoption." Although this outrages some commentators, it is, in general, considered legitimate for the majority to use public resources to advance its agenda, even if others believe a particular expenditure is wrongheaded or foolish.

Bioethicist Arthur Caplan does not share the view that a human embryo is the moral equivalent of a human infant. He also makes the argument that paying for the promotion of embryo adoption is a relatively ineffective way of helping infertile couples have babies. Caplan writes that "most frozen embryos are not healthy enough to ever become babies," because the highest quality embryos are usually used first by the generating couple, and because over time frozen embryos degrade.[2] But if the goal of President Bush and his supporters is to help save embryos with the potential for becoming children from destruction as well as to help the infertile, this objection is unlikely to change minds or policy.

The third option is the most draconian. A number of countries have laws that limit the creation and destruction of embryos in ways that impinge quite significantly on the use of assisted reproductive technologies. For example, Italy limits fertilization to three eggs at a time and requires implantation of all resulting embryos. An Italian judge ordered a couple to transfer all the embryos produced with their eggs and sperm to the woman's womb, despite the fact that both the man and the woman carried the recessive gene for beta thalassemia, wanted preimplantation genetic diagnosis, and would not keep a child born with the condition.[3] Of course, this is an unlikely scenario in the US given the current state of constitutional law. Yet Louisiana law declares a viable in vitro fertilized human ovum to be a juridical person "which shall not be intentionally destroyed."[4] While the goal of reducing the number of excess embryos is arguably a worthy one, such laws seem at odds with recognition of moral pluralism and with respect for privacy and the intimate nature of procreation.

TERMINOLOGY

Brakman notes that debate exists over the terminology that should be used to describe the transfer of an embryo from the progenitors to others and states her own position in support of the use of the word "adoption." My ambivalence is reflected in my repeated placement of that word within quotation marks. Brakman links her position to information on how participants feel about or regard what is going on. Others accept or reject the use of the word "adoption" according to how they stand on the question of moral status. Nightlight Christian Adoptions, which runs the Snowflakes Embryo Adoption Program, describes embryos as "pre-born children" of the "genetic parents" and uses the word *adoption* to describe the transfer to another couple, because it reinforces the view that an embryo is just like a baby in all important respects.[5] Caplan sees the use of adoption language as a rearguard attack on human embryonic stem cell research.

Caplan also believes that the rhetoric of adoption is deceptive given the low odds that a frozen embryo will become a baby even where every effort is made to realize that end. The National Embryo Donation Center notes that "only about two-thirds of embryos survive the thawing process" (other *advocates* say only half), and the "chance of pregnancy after transfer of frozen embryos is currently 20–25%."[6] The statistic that likely matters most to prospective recipients is the chance of bringing home a baby, often referred to as the "take-home baby" rate, which tends to be considerably lower.

Does use of the word "adoption" imply that prospective parents should be subjected to background checks to assure that the gestational couple will be good parents? In unassisted reproduction, restraints based on evidence of unsuitability to parent are rare and controversial. In assisted reproduction, assessment is much less systematic than in the case of adoption, though clinics appear to do some screening.[7,8] While I believe that professionals involved in aiding conception have a responsibility to attend to the welfare of future children, the challenge in assisted reproduction is distinguishing between standards based on reasonable evidence-based consensus about characteristics likely to be inconsistent with good parenting and standards based on unreflective prejudice.

Finally, as even the National Embryo Donation Center acknowledges, "[b]ased on current law, adoption only refers to the placement of a child after birth."[6] "Regardless of what terminology is used to explain the procedure, adoption law does not and cannot apply to donating embryos because many state statutes specifically invalidate biological parents' consent to adoption that is given prior to childbirth."[9] In short, state adoption laws are not currently being applied to embryo donation. If embryo transfer were to be subsumed under the law of adoption, donors would retain the power to assert parentage throughout the pregnancy, and if a donated embryo results in a child, the gestational mother might have to return the baby to the genetic parents.

The Uniform Parentage Act, a model act offered as a guide to state lawmakers, creates certainty about assignment of parentage in the context of assisted reproduction. The Act states: "A donor is not a parent of a child conceived by means of assisted reproduction."[10] (The definition of assisted reproduction expressly includes donation of embryos.) Rather, a birth mother who intends to parent the child is the legal mother, and if she is married, her husband becomes the legal father. The Uniform Parentage Act approach is commendable for its clarity, but it has been adopted by only six states to date, however, more states have laws that declare that embryo donors do not have parental rights and responsibilities.

A pragmatic resolution of the terminology debate might consist of allowing Nightlight/Snowflakes and others who prefer the language of adoption for a variety of reasons to use it in peace and to make contracts that accord embryo donors some of the choices now offered to parents surrendering a child for adoption (such as playing a role in the selection of the adoptive parents), while favoring the intent-based approach that makes no distinction between gamete and embryo donation for purposes of determining legal parentage.

NOTES

1. The original version, introduced by Representative Jay Dickey, was in § 128 of the Balanced Budget Downpayment Act, I, Pub. L, No. 104–99, 110 Stat. 26 (1996). The most current version (identical in substance to the rest) is in § 509 of H.R. 3010, the appropriations bill that, as of the writing of the commentary, has passed the House and is pending in the Senate in the 109th Congress.

2. Caplan A. "The problem with 'embryo adoption': why is the government giving money to 'Snowflakes?'" http://www.msnbc.msn.com/id/3076556.

3. Turone F. New law forces Italian couple with genetic disease to implant all their IVF embryos. *BMJ* 2004;328:1334.

4. Louisiana Revised Statues (2005), §§ 9:121, 9:124, 9.129.

5. Nightlight Christian Adoptions, "Message to Genetic Parents," www.nightlight.org/message_genetic.asp.

6. National Embryo Donation Center, "Embryo Adoption Information," http://www.embryo donation.org/adoptions.php.

7. Gurmankin AD, Caplan AL, Braverman AM. Screening practices and beliefs of assisted reproductive technology programs. *Fertil Steril* 2005;83:61–67.

8. Stern JE, Cramer CP, Green RM, Garrod A, DeVries KO. Determining access to assisted reproductive technology: reactions of clinic directors to ethically complex case scenarios. *Hum Reprod* 2003;18:1343–1352. .

9. Kindregan CP, McBrien M. Embryo donation: unresolved legal issues in the transfer of surplus cryopreserved embryos. *Vill L. Rev* 2004;49:169–206, at 175.

10. National conference of commissioners on Uniform State Laws, Uniform Parentage Act (2002), §§ 102, 702. For information on state legislative action with regard to the Uniform Parentage Act, see http://www.nccusl.org/Update/uniformact_factsheets/uniformacts -fs-upa.asp.

REPLY BY SARAH-VAUGHAN BRAKMAN, PHD

Professor Majumder's reply enriches our appreciation of the political and legal difficulties regarding embryo adoption. Those like Caplan who assume "adoption" terminology necessarily implies a moral status claim about embryos, however, are mistaken. Pets are adopted, so are laws and highways. I readily agree that some may in fact use the term to draw the connection between infants and embryos, but logically there is no direct implication from one to the other.

I do not argue for the use of the word *adoption,* but rather for the use of the *adoption paradigm.* Though some law at present equates gamete donors and embryo donors for the purposes of determining parentage, there is a distinction of note here. Gamete donors never intended to actively parent.

Embryo "donors" originally intended to be parents. To equate couples' interests in the disposition of their embryos to those of gamete donors (as most fertility centers do when denying couples the ability to choose the gestational couple or to know the outcome of the "donation") is to gravely mistake the reality of these families' lives and to inappropriately conflate the two practices.

Professor Majumder asks if "adoption" implies screening for the gestational couple. The answer is yes. While legally pre-adoption screening may represent the state's interests in ensuring the welfare of its most vulnerable citizens, birth parents who place their infants with adoptive parents expect, indeed demand, that adoptive couples have undergone such screening. From the data I found, screening would increase the availability of embryos for adoption. Perhaps what is troubling is that it seems like these "fertility patients" would be treated unequally compared to other patients at the clinics who are not subject to any screening. While this may be, they would not be treated unfairly, because the situation by definition would be different than all others; the "gestational" couple would be choosing to bear and rear children from another couple's once valued embryos. No such prior interest in genetic material exists for any other assisted reproductive technology alternative.

Finally, Professor Majumber correctly worries that applying current adoption laws to embryo adoption would have disadvantages making the practice unattractive. Surely laws may be amended, or new regulations proposed specific to embryo adoption that acknowledge its unique place in the spectrum between the donation of genetic material and the gift of a born child.

☰ ☷ ☷ ☰

JAMES L. BERNAT, MD

Defending Challenges to the Concept of "Brain Death"

The concept known colloquially as "brain death" holds that a human organism is dead if and only if all the clinical functions of the entire brain have irreversibly ceased functioning. Over the past 30 years, "brain death" has become accepted so uniformly by Western society that every state in the United States and the legislatures of many other countries have codified it into statutes of death. These statutes provide two tests of death: (1) if the patient is not on mechanical ventilation, death can be determined by the prolonged absence of circulation and ventilation; or (2) if the patient is on mechanical ventilation, death can be determined by the irreversible cessation of clinical functions of the whole brain.

Brain death is an unfortunate and misleading term, erroneously connoting that there are two types of death, rather than simply two methods for determining human death. But because the more precise term, *the determination of human death using a neurological criterion and tests* is cumbersome, the term *brain death* has become popularized. However, the term has led to misunderstanding and must be used and understood precisely.

When the concept of "brain death" first evolved in the 1960s, it was a prerequisite for stopping physiological support of the patient. However, now that there are accepted guidelines for stopping life-sustaining treatment on living patients, the only act for which "brain death" remains a prerequisite is multiorgan procurement for transplantation. This fact has established a clear causal linkage between "brain death" and organ transplantation. A secondary application may be to permit physicians to terminate medical treatment over the objection of the patient's family.

Despite the widespread public acceptance of "brain death," several scholars recently have called for its abandonment on three grounds: (1) that it is an anachronism because it is no longer a necessary condition for discontinuing life-sustaining therapy; (2) that it is an incoherent concept that does not accurately represent biological death, principally because most of the patient's other organs continue to function; and (3) that multiorgan donation can be uncoupled from "brain death," permitting organ procurement from living patients who are beyond harm, with their consent or that of their proxy decision makers.[1-3]

Concerns about these questions are one reason the Vatican Pontifical Academy for Life has decided to re-examine the Roman Catholic doctrinal acceptance of "brain death" as human death. Because the Roman Catholic Church cannot condone killing, even in the case of an imminently dying person who has consented for organ donation, determining whether "brain dead" patients are truly dead is of paramount ecclesiastical importance.

At first glance, the determination of death seems like a straightforward task, a purely medical diagnosis. Indeed, it was fairly simple in the era before the invention of the mechanical ventilator. At that time, all vital functions (breathing, heartbeat, brain functions) stopped within minutes of each other so it was unnecessary to consider whether a human organism was alive who had lost some but not all vital functions. But this simple matter changed forever with the advent of the mechanical ventilator. Cases then were reported of patients who had permanently lost all brain functions and breathing capacity but were kept supported by a mechanical ventilator. Were these tragic victims dead or alive?

Unfortunately, this question could not be answered solely by physicians because it was no longer clear what their examination was supposed to measure. As my colleagues, Charles M. Culver and Bernard Gert, and I pointed out 17 years ago,[4] and I restated in another article,[5] an optimal analysis of the concept of death should proceed in three sequential phases: (1) identifying the definition of death to make explicit the traditional meaning of the concept of death; (2) choosing a criterion of death, a measurable general standard, that shows that the definition has been fulfilled by being both necessary and sufficient conditions for death; and (3) devising tests to show that the criterion has been satisfied with no false-positive determinations. Even many scholars who disagree with our conclusions concur with this method of analysis.

The most reasonable definition of death is "the permanent cessation of the critical functions of the organism as a whole." Critical functions are those that are necessary for the continued health and unity of the organism, such as breathing, functional integration, homeostasis, and consciousness. The criterion that is necessary and sufficient for death by this definition is "the permanent cessation of all clinical functions of the whole brain." Because the brain stem, hypothalamus, thalamus and cerebral hemispheres subserve the functioning of the organism as a whole, critical functions of all these areas must be lost. The tests of death are those outlined in the statute in the first paragraph of this article. The specific brain tests were enumerated by the American Academy of Neurology[6] and comprise the quartet of utter unresponsiveness, absence of the capacity to breathe (apnea), loss of brain stem reflexes, and irreversibility.

Some proponents of "brain death" oppose a whole-brain criterion and instead favor a higher-brain criterion of death. They claim that because consciousness and cognition are the unique features of human life, only their absence, and not the absence of vegetative functions such as breathing, should be necessary for death.[7] I oppose such a formulation because it is a contrived redefinition of death. The higher-brain formulation would declare as dead patients in a persistent vegetative state who are considered alive in every country. It would also create the disquieting situation of burying, cremating, or removing organs from individuals who remain spontaneously breathing and moving. Indeed, no jurisdiction anywhere in the world is even considering such a radical change.

Most opponents to "brain death" propose a circulation formulation in its place: the human organism is not dead until its circulation ceases irreversibly. They regard "brain dead" patients as alive, though hopelessly ill. However, circulation proponents do not necessarily insist on mandatory treatment of "brain dead" patients; they merely assert that such patients are not yet dead.[2,3]

Of the several arguments refuting this position, the most powerful is that the brain is the central generating, regulating, and integrating organ of the body and it is responsible for the unity of the organism. The brain is the critical system of the organism without which the remaining organs may continue to function independently but cannot together comprise an organism as a whole. As the critical system of the organism, the brain can neither be transplanted nor replaced with a mechanical device. When the brain is destroyed, the entropy of the organism increases inexorably because the critical system opposing entropy and subserving the functional unity of the organism as a whole is gone forever.[8]

There are pragmatic reasons not to abandon the dead donor rule—the axiom of multiorgan transplantation, which requires that the multiorgan donor first must be dead. Loss of public confidence in physician death determination has followed several highly publicized cases in which the press alleged that physicians were prematurely determining death merely to procure organs for transplantation.

One proposed solution is to use non-heart-beating organ donors. For example, the "Pittsburgh" protocol allows dying patients or their surrogate decision makers to authorize organ donation immediately after life-sustaining treatment has been removed and the heart has stopped beating for a few minutes. However, I question whether non-heart-beating donors are truly dead at the moment of donation because their hearts potentially could be restarted before all brain function had been lost. Some have suggested that instead of struggling to agree upon a uniform definition of death, organ removal could be permitted in certain situations as a form of justified killing. Irrespective of the moral issues, procuring organs from people who are not yet dead constitutes poor public policy. Public confidence in death determination is precarious and can be shaken easily. As a conceptual issue and a matter of public policy, continuing to use the concept of "brain death" as the basis of human death determination, particularly to qualify as a donor for multiorgan procurement, remains both coherent conceptually and prudent pragmatically.

NOTES

1. Truog RD. Is it time to abandon brain death? *Hastings Cent Rep* 1997;27(1):29–37.

2. Taylor RM. Re-examining the definition and criterion of death. *Semin Neurol* 1997;17: 265–270.

3. Shewmon DA. Recovery from 'brain death': a neurologist's apologia. *Linacre Q* 1997;64(1):30–96.

4. Bernat JL, Culver CM, Gert B. On the definition and criterion of death. *Ann Intern Med* 1981;94:389–94.

5. Bernat JL. A defense of the whole-brain concept of death. *Hastings Cent Rep* 1998;28(2): 14–23.

6. American Academy of Neurology Quality Standards Subcommittee. Practice parameters for determining brain death in adults (summary statement). *Neurology* 1995;45:1012–1014.

7. Veatch RM. The impending collapse of the whole-brain definition of death. *Hastings Cent Rep* 1993;23(4):18–24.

8. Korein J. Ontogenesis of the brain in the human organism: definitions of life and death of the human being and person. *Adv Bioethics* 1997;2:1–74.

☷ ☶ ☵ ☳

MICHAEL A. DEVITA, MD AND ROBERT M. ARNOLD, MD

The Concept of Brain Death

In his article on the concept of brain death, James Bernat makes several claims. First, he argues *brain death* is misleading as a descriptive term. Second, he believes *death* is a term that refers to a specific biologic event, and the most reasonable definition of death is "permanent cessation of the critical functions of the organism as a whole." He asserts that the only criterion that meets this definition is "the permanent cessation of all clinical functions of the whole brain." Bernat supports the "dead donor rule"—that organ procurement can neither be the cause of death nor proceed before the patient dies—because he feels it is necessary to maintain public confidence in organ procurement. He is concerned that non-heart-beating organ donors might be alive because "hearts could be restarted before all brain function had been lost." Following this line of reasoning, we assume—given his belief that permitting pre-death donation will undermine confidence in organ donation— he must believe non-heart-beating organ donation is poor public policy.

Each of these assertions is extremely controversial and has been extensively discussed in the literature.[1] While we focus our attention on his concern about non-heart-beating organ donors, we do have several questions regarding Bernat's position.

First, how can Bernat be so confident that there must be a single unifying criterion for death? Our society has been unable to define when life begins, not due to disputed facts, but because of differing values. Are questions about the criteria for death matters of biologic fact or are they value-laden questions about which reasonable persons may disagree?

Second, Bernat suggests that death requires cessation of the critical functions of the organism as a whole, but shouldn't the definition require cessation of *all* critical functions of the organism as a whole? If the brain is the critical integrating organ, how does he explain individuals who have been declared dead using neurologic criteria surviving for years; some of whom have gone through complex hormonal and growth changes such as puberty and pregnancy.[2]

Third, how do we decide what constitutes the brain's critical functions? Bernat equates the "critical" with the "clinical" functions of the whole brain. Why? While he includes hypothalamus in the critical functioning of the brain, he does not require testing its neuroendocrine function.

Finally, given that with time, we have permitted withdrawal of life-sustaining treatment before "brain death," why is Bernat so convinced that our society will not tolerate organ procurement from nearly dead individuals? Because both death and organ donation are value-laden propositions, might not such viewpoints change?

Regarding *non-heart-beating organ donation,* first let us say that if we had to do it over again, we would not use this term. While descriptively accurate, the term has engendered as much confusion as has the term *brain death.* Today, most organs are procured from individuals who are declared dead using neurological criteria and whose hearts are still beating at the time of procurement. Recently there has been renewed interest in procuring organs from individuals who are declared dead using cardiopulmonary criteria. Their hearts are not beating at the time of procurement (thus the name, non-heart-beating organ donors). We are concerned that this term has increased the confusion over whether these individuals are "really dead" and wish we had insisted on a different terminology, for example, *organ procurement from dead individuals certified dead using cardiopulmonary criteria.*

Second, non-heart-beating organ donation is not new. Prior to the acceptance of "brain death," non-heart-beating organ donors were a common source of organs for transplantation.[3] Interestingly, at that time, there was no controversy regarding the death of those donors. Instead, the controversy questioned whether "brain-dead" individuals were really dead. Non-heart-beating organ donation was largely abandoned because the organs did not perform as well as those procured from brain-dead donors. Not every center stopped non-heart-beating organ donations. For example, in Wisconsin it has always been a source of kidneys.

There are two approaches to limiting ischemia, or lack of blood supply, to an organ and thus ensuring that viable organs are procured from non-heart-beating organ donors.[4] First, ischemia can be limited by controlling the time and place of death. So called "controlled non-heart-beating organ donors" was developed in response to families' requests to donate their loved one's organs after a decision to withdraw life-sustaining treatment. The Pittsburgh Protocol was the first published policy detailing and justifying the procurement of organs in such situations. Second, quickly infusing cold preservatives after death decreases warm ischemia. This method must be used in uncontrolled circumstances when death is unexpected, but can be utilized in controlled situations as well.

The most controversial issue in non-heart-beating organ donation is when death can be declared. The University of Pittsburgh Medical Center's policy for non-heart-beating organ donors requires two minutes of absent circulation, apnea, and unresponsiveness. There is scientific support for this position. First, there is no brain function within 15 seconds after the heart stops beating in normothermic patients. Second, the little data available demonstrate that auto-resuscitation—the heart restarting on its own—is very rare and never occurs after more than two minutes.[5] Tomlinson argues that because these individuals refuse resuscitation, it is unethical to attempt to restart the heart. Therefore they are dead.[6]

Critics have objected to this formulation in a number of ways. The Institute of Medicine questions the power of the data regarding the potential for auto-resuscitation and recommends a longer waiting time.[7] Bernat argues that the Pittsburgh policy relies on a faulty definition of irreversible. Just because one chooses to not try to restart the heart does not mean it cannot be restarted. Until the heart (or the brain) loses the potential for resuming function, the loss is not irreversible and the patient should not be declared dead. Finally, because of the dichotomous certifying criteria, one may argue that a patient can be dead using cardiopulmonary criteria, but if such an individual was immediately placed on a cardiopulmonary bypass machine, some brain function may resume. This possibility led individuals at the First International Conference on non-heart-beating organ donation to call for requiring ten minutes of pulselessness prior to declaring death.

We agree with the critics that non-heart-beating organ donor policies raise important questions regarding the definition of irreversibility, highlight the tension between brain and cardiopulmonary-based criteria for death, and force re-examination of the data regarding auto-resuscitation. While we believe the Pittsburgh Protocol offers a conceptually and pragmatically defensible answer to these questions, we understand the controversy is unlikely to go away. Like the debate regarding the definition of death and criterion for "brain death," they reflect the socially and philosophically ambiguous nature of death. Finally, it seems that the current growth in non-heart-beating organ donation may render moot Bernat's concern about its public policy implications.

NOTES

1. Youngner SJ, Arnold RM, Schapiro R (eds): *The Definition of Death: Contemporary Controversies.* Baltimore, MD: Johns Hopkins University Press, 1999.

2. Shewmon DA. Chronic "brain death" meta-analysis and conceptual consequences. *Neurology* 1998;51:1538–45.

3. DeVita M, Snyder J, Grenvik A. History of organ donation by patients with cardiac death. *Kennedy Inst Ethics J* 1993;3(2):113–29.

4. Youngner SJ, Arnold R. Ethical, psychosocial, and public policy implications of procuring organs from non-heart-beating cadaver donors. *JAMA* 1993;269:2769–74.

5. DeVita M. *The Death Watch.* Unpublished.

6. Tomlinson T. The irreversibility of death: reply to Cole. *Kennedy Inst Ethics J* 1993; 3(2):157–65.

7. *Institute of Medicine: Non-heart-beating Organ Transplantation: Medical and Ethical Issues in Procurement.* Washington, DC: National Academy Press, 1998.

REPLY BY JAMES L. BERNAT, MD

Drs. DeVita and Arnold highlight several areas of current controversy that the brevity of my article permitted me to address only tangentially. I have considered them in greater detail elsewhere.[1] I will respond briefly to two of their questions.

Their claim that the definition and criterion of death are "value-laden propositions" underscores that any analysis of a biosocial issue must carefully distinguish between those elements contingent on the science of biology and those related to the creation of social policy on the biological issue. We can only study, describe, and try to understand the scientific facts of biology; we cannot change or contrive their objective reality to fit social agendas or for other purposes.[2] However, we remain free to design and continuously alter our public policy about biological issues as a result of societal debate on both consensually held values and pragmatic issues of what works best for society. The analysis of the definition and determination of death contains both scientific and social policy elements but, unlike in the question posed by Drs. DeVita and Arnold, they must be clearly separated for adequate analysis.

Because death, like life, fundamentally is a biological phenomenon, determining the definition and criterion of death are biophilosophical tasks that can be studied and modeled but cannot be assigned arbitrarily. Much of the current scientific debate on the coherence of the concept of "whole brain death" as a formulation of death results from our incomplete understanding of the theoretical biology of complex organisms and their emergent functions. Our current models of complex living systems remain primitive, regrettably including the concept that I endorse of the "organism as a whole." But it is from this biological perspective that I hold that my account of the definition and criterion of death best captures the objective reality of the demise of the human organism. Recently, Julius Korein has further consolidated this view using the thermodynamic concept of the brain as the critical system of the organism.[3] Nevertheless, we need greater sophistication in our understanding of the theoretical biology of complex systems to finally settle this scientific debate.

Whether "whole brain death" or an alternative concept of death conforms to our consensually held values or works best for our society, however, remains an active but entirely separate point of public policy debate. This choice may evolve over time based upon changing public opinion, and may vary among societies. Here, unlike in the biological question, values and pragmatism become relevant. In this regard, I believe that Drs. DeVita and Arnold would concur that the current widespread acceptance of the "whole brain" concept of death by every jurisdiction in the US and most Western nations is *prima facie* evidence that it represents a workable and coherent public policy. Similarly, the dead donor rule represents a successful public policy because it has been accepted around the world as an axiom for determining candidacy for multiorgan procurement for transplantation.

The non-heart-beating organ donor protocols are an innovative and creative solution for increasing the supply of scarce organs available for transplantation. When I pointed out that the donors of such organs may not be unequivocally dead at the point of donation (because of the potential reversibility of their illness and the fact that death, by definition, is irreversible) this was merely acknowledging a biological fact. Whether we as a society are willing to overlook this fact, because of the obvious social benefits gained by endorsing the practice of non-heart-beating organ donors, is a question of policy. As Drs. DeVita and Arnold predict, the consensus may well turn out that because these patients will neither be actively resuscitated nor will auto-resuscitate, they are "as good as dead" for the purposes of organ transplantation. It is entirely possible that our society may decide that incipient death is close enough to actual death for us to construct a workable and acceptable public policy on multiorgan procurement. But, as I noted in the article, despite many years of successful operation, public confidence in our current system of organ procurement remains precarious and I fear that altering the dead donor rule could backfire.

NOTES

1. Bernat JL. A defense of the whole-brain concept of death. *Hastings Cent Rep* 1998;28(2): 14–23.

2. Wilson EO. *Consilience: The Unity of Knowledge.* New York: Alfred A. Knopf, 1998:45–65.

3. Korein J. Ontogenesis of the brain in the human organism: definitions of life and death of the human being and person. *Adv Bioethics* 1997;2:1–74.

☰ ☷ ☷ ☰

FRANK A. CHERVENAK, MD AND LAURENCE B. MCCULLOUGH, PHD

An Ethical Framework for Fetal Research

Fetal surgery involves the repair of a fetal anomaly either through a hysterotomy or endoscopy. Such procedures carry risks of harm and potential benefit to both the pregnant woman and the fetal patient. For the pregnant woman, these risks include morbidity and, rarely, mortality associated with major surgery and anesthesia, the psychosocial risks of losing a pregnancy or living with the burden of iatrogenic injury to a future child, and risks to future pregnancies from uterine rupture. Risks to the fetal patient include iatrogenic prematurity, injury, and, rarely, death. The potential benefits of fetal surgery are reduction of mortality and improvement in functional status for the fetal patient with consequent psychosocial benefit to the pregnant woman and her family. Although fetal surgery has been attempted to correct a variety of fetal anomalies, including meningomyelocele, diaphragmatic hernia, cystic adenomatoid malformation of the lung, and sacrococcygeal teratoma, at this time fetal surgery is not considered standard treatment. Increasingly, investigation in that area is being conducted under research protocols.[1,2]

A randomized, controlled clinical trial of surgical repair of spina bifida is being sponsored by the National Institutes of Health. These and other trials that are sure to follow underscore the need for an ethical framework for experimental fetal surgery.

The purpose of this article is to outline such a framework, which the authors have presented in greater detail elsewhere.[3] We will address ethical criteria for the initiation and assessment of clinical trials, the informed consent process, selection criteria based on abortion preference, and cooperation of physicians in the clinical investigation.

ETHICAL CRITERIA FOR INITIATION & ASSESSMENT OF CLINICAL TRIALS

Innovation in fetal surgery usually begins with a single case and then case series, preceded by work on appropriate animal models. These steps are necessary to determine the feasibility, safety, and efficacy of innovations.

We have defended three criteria that must be satisfied in order to conduct such preliminary investigations in an ethically responsible fashion that takes into account beneficence-based obligations to both the fetal patient and the pregnant woman.[3] The previable fetus is a patient in these cases because the woman has made a decision to continue her pregnancy[4] to have the opportunity to gain the potential benefits of the innovation. She remains free to withdraw that status before viability.[4] The viable fetus is a patient in these cases in virtue of viability.[4]

Our criteria include: (1) the proposed fetal intervention is reliably expected (on the basis of previous animal studies) either to be life-saving or to prevent serious and irreversible disease, injury, or handicap for the fetus; (2) among possible alternative designs, the intervention is designed in such a way as to involve the least risk of mortality and morbidity to the fetal patient; and (3) on the basis of animal studies and analysis of theoretical risks, both for the current and future pregnancies, the mortality risk to the pregnant woman is reliably expected to be low and the risk of disease, injury, or handicap to the pregnant woman is reliably expected to be low or manageable.

The third criterion is important because fetal surgery is also maternal surgery. Investigators have an independent beneficence-based obligation to protect human subjects from unreasonably risky research and should use beneficence-based, risk-benefit analyses. The phrase *maternal-fetal surgery* is useful when it reminds investigators of the need for such comprehensive analysis. If it is used to subordinate fetal interests to the pregnant woman's interest and rights, it undermines the concept of the fetus as a patient in favor of the concept that the fetus is merely a part of the pregnant woman.

Preliminary innovation should cease and randomized clinical trials begin when there is clinical equipoise. Clinical equipoise means that there is "a remaining disagreement in the expert clinical community, despite the available evidence, about the merits of the intervention to be tested."[5] Brody notes that one challenge here is identifying how much disagreement can remain for there still to be equipoise.[5] Lilford has suggested that when two-thirds of the expert community, measured reliably, no longer disagrees, equipoise is not satisfied.[6] When the experimental intervention is more harmful than non-intervention, equipoise cannot be achieved. We propose that the satisfaction of the previous three criteria with slight modifications should count as equipoise in the expert community.[3]

The above three criteria can be used in a straightforward manner to define stopping rules for such clinical trials. When the data support a rigorous clinical judgment that the first or third criterion is not satisfied, the trial should be stopped. When the clinical trial is completed, its outcome can be assessed to determine whether the innovative fetal surgery should be regarded as standard of care. The trial results should meet the three criteria in order to establish the innovation as standard of care.[3]

Brody has underscored the value of data safety and monitoring boards to prevent investigator bias and to protect subjects.[5] Such boards should be used in fetal research, especially to ensure adherence of the above-mentioned ethical criteria as a basis for monitoring such research.

THE INFORMED CONSENT PROCESS

The informed consent process should always be led by a physician competent to explain any intervention, its alternatives and their benefits and risks. This requirement means that the physician-investigator should lead the consent process.

Like all consent processes for human subject research, counseling the pregnant woman about initial innovation or clinical trials should be rigorously non-directive. Investigators should emphasize the distinction between research and treatment to prevent the therapeutic misconception. This is the belief of patients that research, like treatment, will be beneficial and not involve disadvantages that do not occur in the therapeutic setting.[7] Words such as *mother, father,* and *baby* should not be used, because these suggest moral relationships and moral status that do not apply.[8] Words such as *pregnant woman, husband, fetus,* and *fetal patient* should be used instead. The pregnant woman should be clearly informed that she is under no obligation to the fetal patient to enroll it in a clinical research project.

To protect a woman from potential coercion, her husband or partner and other family members should be reminded that while they may have strong views for or against her participation, their role should be to support and respect the woman's decision-making process and its outcome.

SELECTION CRITERIA BASED ON ABORTION PREFERENCE

There should be no exclusion criteria in research on fetal surgery based on willingness to countenance elective abortion. Study designs would therefore have to include elective abortion and birth of adversely affected infants as endpoints.[3]

COOPERATION OF PRACTICING PHYSICIANS WITH CLINICAL INVESTIGATION

It is widely accepted that practicing physicians are justified in informing their patients about relevant clinical investigations, and, with the patient's consent, referring them to the investigators. In our view, there is also an obligation to do so. The justification for this obligation cannot appeal to the benefit to the pregnant woman or fetal patient, because by definition, the existence of clinical investigation does not establish clinical benefit. However, there is an obligation to future patients, pregnant and fetal alike, to establish whether fetal intervention improves the current standard of care or not. All physicians should take seriously their obligation to future patients to assure that innovation has the opportunity to be validated scientifically and ethically, rather than introduced in an unmanaged fashion or simply ignored.[3]

NOTES

1. Bruner JP, Tulipan N, Paschall RL, et al. Fetal surgery for myelomeningocele and the incidence of shunt-dependent hydrocephalus. *JAMA* 1999;282:1819–25.

2. Sutton LN, Adzick NS, Bilanivic LT, et al. Improvement in hindbrain herniation demonstrated by serial fetal magnetic resonance imaging following fetal surgery for myelomeningocele. *JAMA* 1999;282:1826–31.

3. Chervenak FA, McCullough LB. A comprehensive ethical framework for fetal research and its application to fetal surgery for spina bifida. *Am J Obstet Gynecol* 2002;187:10–4.

4. McCullough LB, Chervenak FA. *Ethics in Obstetrics and Gynecology.* New York: Oxford University Press, 1994.

5. Brody BA. *The Ethics of Biomedical Research: An International Perspective.* New York: Oxford University Press, 1998.

6. Lilford RJ. The substantive ethics of clinical trials. *Clin Obstet Gynecol* 1992;35:837–45.

7. Appelbaum PS, Roth LH, Lidz CW, Benson P, Winslade W. False hopes and best data: consent to research and the therapeutic misconception. *Hastings Cent Rep* 1987;17(2):20–4.

8. DeCrespigny L, Chervenak F, McCullough L. Mothers and babies, pregnant women and fetuses. *Br J Obstet Gynaecol* 1999;106:1235–7.

☲ ☷ ☷ ☲

SIDNEY CALLAHAN, PHD

Ethics and Fetal Research

The news that something has gone wrong in one's pregnancy will be devastating to a woman. Experts may refer to "a fetal anomaly," "a fetal patient," and discuss the possibility of experimental "maternal-fetal surgery," but these words cannot begin to capture the anguish and anxiety of the situation. Nor can the dreadful choices presented to a pregnant woman with a damaged fetus be fully conveyed by the term of *informed consent.* Decisions to be made in such cases are emotionally charged and present excruciating moral dilemmas.

Such dilemmas have appeared in the developed world as part of the modernization and medical control of reproduction. The possibility of innovative, sophisticated technologies of maternal-fetal surgery have only emerged in the wake of the reduction of infant mortality, the development of the medical specialty of obstetrics, and new technologies of fetal monitoring and ultrasonography. The ready availability of contraception and legal access to elective abortion has further complicated childbearing decisions. The landscape of family formation has been forever changed.

At the same time a new awareness of the maternal-fetus relationship has emerged in many fields from feminist theory, psychosocial research, and evolutionary biology. Today it is clear that there can exist female ambivalence toward childbearing and the potential for different kinds of maternal-fetal conflict. Yet epidemics of infertility and other cultural developments that newly enhance the value of children have raised the stakes in women's reproductive decisions. Maternal satisfactions are newly appreciated and parental altruism can be seen as the mainstay of social and biological flourishing.

For both biological and cultural reasons women will invest enormous effort and energy in childbearing and child rearing. They have a strong drive to protect their offspring and can identify with the fetus as their own flesh and blood. Maternal bonding with a fetus can begin early and be strengthened by ultrasound images. Women's emancipation and freedom to choose can make their desires for children more intense. Fortunately, new respect for women's rights has been part of a general human rights movement that has also benefited other vulnerable groups such as infants, children, patients, prisoners, and experimental subjects.

In this complex new cultural context Laurence B. McCullough, PhD, and Frank A. Chervenak, MD, have proposed an admirable ethical framework for dealing with the challenges presented by innovative fetal research. The authors attempt to give proper moral weight to the claims of the pregnant woman, the "fetal patient," and to the physician-investigators who want to further medical progress. The authors set forth ethical criteria for the initiation and assessment of clinical trials, selective criteria for inclusion of subjects, guidelines for the informed consent process, and justifications of the obligation of treating physicians to support clinical investigations that will benefit future patients.

In undertakings of innovative medical experiments, risks, and benefits remain uncertain. The uncertainty along with the promise of benefits produces the need for clinical trials accompanied by thorny problems of informed consent. Constructing ethical criteria for experimental maternal-fetal surgery is a particularly complex challenge because two lives are involved and the stakes for a woman and her family are enormously high.

Looming in the background of the authors' proposed framework are continuing ethical conflicts over abortion and the moral status of the fetus at different stages of development. Other complicating debates exist concerning the medical and moral indications for starting and stopping experimental clinical trials. Fundamental difficulties in acquiring truly informed consent also have to be confronted. Without delving into the ongoing arguments and conflicts of bioethics, the general criteria proposed in McCullough and Chervenak's ethical framework seem sensible.

They propose that clinical trials can begin when (1) there exist reliable expectations that fetal interventions may be life-saving or prevent serious and irreversible disease, injury, or handicap for the fetus; (2) the pregnant woman's risks of disease or injury for the present and future pregnancy are reliably expected to be low; and (3) among alternative designs for intervention, those with the least risk for the fetal patient will be chosen. In other words neither the welfare of the woman nor the fetus can be disregarded or sacrificed for the other.

Of course there is always the problem remaining of who decides whether ethical criteria to initiate or stop clinical trials have been met. Who will measure the disagreement or agreement in the expert clinical community and by what methods? The authors recommend outside monitoring boards to prevent investigator bias and to protect subjects. Unfortunately, medical research enthusiasm and a desire to recruit subjects can produce subtle pressures upon subjects to agree to interventions. False hopes or therapeutic misconceptions have to be avoided. Potential coercion of women from all—investigators, treating physicians, husbands, and families—must be guarded against by rigorous non-directed procedures for obtaining consent.

In order to further protect the autonomy of a woman's decision, the authors recommend (somewhat unrealistically?) that only neutral language be used. Thus no loaded words such as *father* or *mother* should be allowed. And in this approach the very worst four letter-word to be avoided is b--y. Of course pregnant women do not usually think of themselves as carrying a fetal patient, but as having something wrong with the baby. Still the authors insist that the woman must be clearly informed that "she is under no obligation to the fetal patient to enroll it in a clinical research project."

In the same neutral spirit, there should be no exclusion criteria regarding a woman's countenancing of elective abortion or the choice to produce an affected infant. Throughout the process the individual woman must be granted the power to give, or withdraw, the status of patient to the fetus. This acceptance of the individual woman's power to unilaterally confer or deny the status of patient to the fetus will disturb those who judge that human life has moral claims beginning with conception. But this aspect of the proposed ethical framework, along with the use of neutral language, can be seen as an effort to protect a woman from external pressures while making her decision.

Yet, even if external pressures are minimized, a woman will still confront inner moral struggles. In such a crisis women will have to make an incredibly difficult moral decision. Both positive and negative responses may be aroused in the process. Intense hopes can be invested in a pregnancy as well as anxiety and fear over future consequences. Morally socialized persons desire to do good and avoid evil; women will feel the ethical pull and pressure of conscience to do the right thing. In the case of a pregnant woman, there can be further strong desires to become a good mother and not harm her offspring. The prospect of regret and guilt over a decision can be sobering. The risk of unknown outcomes produces anxiety, even in normal pregnancies. Ironically, women's new freedom to determine their own maternal obligations produces its own burdens.

A woman's choice may be determined in great part by her perception or estimate of the probabilities that the experimental procedure can be of possible benefit for her fetus. If there is minimal or little benefit to be expected, then it seems too much to ask that a woman should volunteer herself and her fetus to risks of harm in order to further the good of future patients and medical progress. The primary moral obligation of parenthood is to protect one's own specific offspring. To offer one's fetus for a risky experimental procedure seems morally callous, even if abortion is ultimately to be elected. A personal sacrifice is one thing; sacrificing one's offspring another.

However, if there is some chance of actual benefit to the fetus, then the situation is different—involving a more tortuous decision. The risks to be taken may be more acceptable if both one's own fetus and future fetal patients may benefit. After all, the human species has only survived this far by continuing acts of maternal altruism. Consenting to innovative experimental fetal surgery may be one more gift that women can give to the next generation.

SUGGESTED READING

Brody BA. *The Ethics of Biomedical Research: An International Perspective.* New York: Oxford University Press, 1998.

Chervenak FA, McCullough LB. *Ethical issues in obstetric ultrasonography. Clin Obstet Gynecol* 1992;4:758–62.

Chervenak FA, McCullough LB. What is obstetric ethics? *Clin Obstet Gynecol* 1992;4:709–19.

Hardy SB. *Mother Nature: A History of Mothers, Infants, and Natural Selection.* New York: Pantheon Books, 1999.

Levine RJ. *Ethics and Regulation of Clinical Research,* 2nd ed. Baltimore-Munich: Urban & Schwarzenberg, 1986.

Rothman BK. *Recreating Motherhood: Ideology and Technology in a Patriarchal Society.* New York: W.W. Norton & Company, 1989.

REPLY BY FRANK A. CHERVENAK, MD, AND LAURENCE B. MCCULLOUGH, PHD

Sidney Callahan rightly points out that the abortion controversy is "looming in the background" of our proposed framework. Current "debates" about the morality of abortion have hit a dead end, because they have focused on whether or not the fetus has independent moral status, is a person, or has rights. There is no way to resolve these disputes, because there is no single, intellectually and morally authoritative perspective from which to resolve them. As a serious intellectual discipline, ethics in general and bioethics in particular should be willing to recognize conceptual failure when it repeatedly occurs. A distinct advantage of our framework is that it liberates the ethics of maternal-fetal research and medicine from intractable disputes about fetal rights. Indeed, our framework explicitly rejects the concept and language of fetal rights, in favor of the clinically applicable concept and language of the fetus as a patient.

Callahan correctly underscores the difficulty of reaching a reliable judgment that equipoise exists or should exist in the expert clinical community. It is certainly clear that new forms of surgical management—as distinct from innovative changes to existing techniques—should never be presumed to be clinically beneficial, despite the sometimes understandable enthusiasm of investigators who have developed them. Before they are tested, such expectations of benefit must properly be understood to be only theoretical. Moreover, as we pointed out, new forms of surgical management should always be tested in animal models as the first step toward establishing more than theoretical benefit. If animal models are promising, small, well-designed, and thoroughly evaluated experimental case series should be undertaken. These steps will ensure the collection of data that can then discipline enthusiasm and result in considered judgments about whether equipoise exists.

We agree with, and want to emphasize strongly, Callahan's point that a pregnant woman's decision to enroll herself and her fetal patient in maternal-fetal research involves serious "inner moral struggles," especially when there are nontrivial risks of fetal loss. Investigators and others involved in the consent process can help potential subjects think through their decision with care and thus manage their moral struggles. Pregnant women should—after they have developed a reliable understanding that the intervention involves research and what the research involves—be asked what is important to them in their decision about whether to enroll in the trial. They should also be encouraged to draw fully on their social supports, including spouse or partner, family, spiritual or religious advisers, and others whose judgment and wisdom they trust. Leaving pregnant women without an opportunity to reflect on their values and leaving them on their own to make a complex decision could result in such struggles becoming more difficult than they would be in the context of a compassionate and supportive informed consent process.

☷ ䷀䷀ ☶

NORMAN SPACK, MD

Transgenderism

Transgendered individuals are people who, by all known biologic measures, are male or female, yet feel like a member of the opposite sex. The discomfort they suffer is called gender dysphoria. Theirs is a relatively rare condition and cannot be explained by factors such as chromosomes, prenatal hormones or toxin exposure, genital variability, postnatal circulating hormone levels, gender of rearing, birth order, or the presence or absence of same-sex siblings.

Is it possible that the brains of the transgendered are uniquely "wired"? Subtle differences between female and male brains have been reported for decades in research studies that identify gender-related size differences between specific brain nuclei by staining slices of post-mortem specimens.[1] One recent study showed that the nuclei of transgendered male-to-females (MTFs) are the size of the nuclei of genetic females.[2] An earlier study revealed that males dying of prostate cancer who had been treated for years with female hormones, and females dying of virilizing adrenal tumors, had nuclei consistent with their genetic sex.[3] Their hormonal exposure did not affect the gender-specific nuclei of their brains.

Gender dysphoria is listed as a psychiatric condition in the psychiatric diagnostic coding manual DSM-IV. I believe that the psychiatric manifestations are a reaction to the situation, not the underlying condition. A transgendered individual who has not had hormonal therapy or surgery may require psychopharmacologic medications, but after a patient receives medical and/or surgical treatment, psychotropic medicines are often unnecessary.

Nearly all transgendered adults recall feelings of being in the wrong body early in childhood. Patient histories resonate with the common theme of dressing secretly in the clothes of the opposite gender during childhood. However, the age at which a transgendered individual fully acknowledges his or her gender identity varies from mid-childhood to middle age. Delayed acknowledgment can usually be traced to a fear of stigmatization and rejection by family, friends, and employers.

The majority of children who express recurrent interest in being the opposite sex are not transgendered, although many become homosexual.[4] A small percentage of children who are emphatic and consistent in their desire to be the opposite gender (less than 20% of the above) prefer to be called by a pronoun and name consistent with their gender identity. Their friends, dress, and activities correspond with that identity. Their greatest fear is puberty because of the irreversible changes that threaten how they are perceived (their "gender attribution"). During adolescence, when unwanted and permanent secondary sexual characteristics transform the patient's body into an adult form that is asynchronous with the brain, depression and anxiety are typical reactions. When menses become a monthly reminder of femaleness in a teenager with a male identity, self-abusive behavior is common. The incidence of suicide among transgendered youth is high.[5] Adult transgendered individuals who find it threatening to acknowledge their gender identity publicly may adopt a lifestyle of marriage and parenthood that matches their genetic sex. Inevitably, maintaining this charade takes its psychic toll.

Who is qualified to assess a patient's condition for referral for endocrine treatment and ultimate surgery? "Standards of care" have been created by the Harry Benjamin International Gender Dysphoria Association, a professional society that includes mental health professionals, endocrinologists, internists, and surgeons (www.hbigda.org). The standards define stages of treatment, beginning with "extensive exploration of psychological, family and social issues" by a mental health professional who has abundant experience working with this population, and only then moving to physical intervention, which should take place in stages, from reversible to irreversible interventions.

Physicians may be uncertain how to address transgendered patients who have not legally changed their name and gender but have transitioned to a gender role consistent with their gender identity. Some states require reconstructive surgery—genitoplasty or mastectomy—before allowing name and gender changes on documents such as driver's licenses and health insurance cards. Whether or not patients have made legal changes or undergone surgery, they are entitled to the dignity of being referred to by the name and pronoun of choice. Male-to-female patients should be offered a gown in the exam room, and female-to-male (FTM) patients should be asked what they prefer to wear during the exam. No assumption should be made about the patient's sexual orientation. Like anyone else, a transgendered individual may be straight, gay, or bisexual. Sexual orientation reflects physical attraction, not gender identity.

The labeling of transgenderism as a psychiatric condition has the ironic effect of inducing psychological problems in transgendered individuals. This fuels the notion that a psychiatric disorder is at the heart of the condition, which influences the diagnostic coding and billing structure. Under the DSM-IV code, few health insurers in the United States cover the cost of hormonal replacement therapy. Mastectomies in FTMs, which cost $6,000 to $10,000, and genitoplasties (sex reconstructive surgery) in MTFs, which cost $15,000 to $25,000, are considered by almost all health insurers to be cosmetic surgeries on patients with a mental illness.

To enable patients to transition physically, endogenous gonadal sex steroid output must be lowered to levels consistent with the gender of choice, which may not be easy. Both MTFs and FTMs require supraphysiologic doses of "cross-hormones": estrogen for MTFs, testosterone for FTMs. High dose estrogen poses a risk of blood clots, which can be fatal if they travel to the lungs (pulmonary embolism) and doses of testosterone sufficient to prevent menses can induce hypertension, cystic acne, and excess red blood cell production with the risk of blood flow "sludging." Alternatively, endogenous sex steroids can easily be suppressed by GnRH analogues, which block pituitary gonadotrophin (LH and FSH) release, enabling cross-hormone treatment to be accomplished with safer physiologic doses of estrogen or testosterone. Unfortunately, GnRH analogues are prohibitively expensive in the US, and patients are forced to take the higher doses of sex steroids until they have their gonads removed. Genitoplasty in MTFs and reduction mammoplasty in FTMs are not covered by most health insurers, and patients may have to wait years saving for it.

In the Netherlands and Belgium, national health insurance covers all costs related to evaluation and treatment of transgendered individuals, including children.[6] Interdisciplinary gender teams evaluate patients psychologically, and patients become potential candidates for sex reconstructive surgery at government expense after living for at least a year in the gender of choice (the "real-life experience") while taking corresponding sex steroid hormones. This discrepancy in coverage across nations raises questions about US health insurance policy decisions.

Because treatment with cross-gender hormones has irreversible effects, challenging choices inevitably arise. For the MTF, estrogen produces breast enlargement and diminished sperm production. Some MTFs request sperm banking before estrogen treatment or gonadectomy just to maintain their reproductive capacity, regardless of who will receive that sperm. For the FTM, testosterone produces a deeper voice, facial hair, temporal balding. Loss of ovulation and menses ensue, and the ovaries become polycystic while retaining retrievable ova. When cryopreservation of ova becomes technically routine and successful, some FTMs will request the procedure to serve as egg donors for their partner or surrogate.

A significant ethical question in transgender care concerns potential intervention with children. Should transgendered children who have had a careful and protracted evaluation by a skilled gender specialist be compelled to complete puberty before being offered the same therapy used for adults? No national or international protocol exists, and there are opposing views on how to proceed. One side argues that physical intervention should be delayed until the completion of puberty because teenagers are more likely than adults to change their minds about their gender identity. The opposing view, with which I concur, argues for early endocrinologic intervention to prevent the severe depression that accompanies the onset of an unwanted puberty and to avoid the physically and psychologically painful procedures required to reverse puberty's physical manifestations.

A model protocol currently employed in the Netherlands begins with a lengthy screening process in gender-variant pubescent teens at the "Tanner 2" stage of pubertal development: breast budding in girls and testicular volumes of 8 cc, preceding phallic enlargement in boys. At this stage the pubertal manifestations are reversible. GnRH analogues are given for at least two years, potentially until age 16, when adolescents in the Netherlands are capable of giving informed consent to receive cross-hormones. By blocking puberty, GnRH treatment buys time for FTMs to achieve a height more typical of males and for continued assessment of all patients' desire to transition. If the Dutch clinical trial proves medically and psychologically safe, it will become the standard of care in the Netherlands, and treatment will be covered by the government health insurance.

Adoption of such therapy in the US, except by a research protocol, is unlikely to be reimbursed by most health insurers as long as transgenderism continues to be coded and billed as a psychiatric condition. The only alternative drug capable of achieving comparable gonadotrophic suppression is high dose progesterone, which has effects similar to high dose prednisone or cortisone and can produce ACTH suppression, fluid retention, "moon face," central obesity, and insulin resistance.

"Precocious puberty" is the only approved indication for pediatric use of GnRH analogue therapy in the US. For a patient's insurance to pay for this drug a physician would have to use this diagnosis for an 11-year-old FTM or 12-year-old MTF, even though the patient hardly meets the age criteria of sexual precocity. If the Dutch protocol is approved by the Harry Benjamin Society, would it be right for US health insurers to withhold payment for GnRH in properly screened transgendered teens?

Transgendered individuals have long faced discrimination in medical institutions, including physicians' offices and hospitals.[7] Reminiscent of the medical/psychiatric approach to homosexuality not so long ago, some physicians and psychologists maintain that the goal of psychiatric treatment is to convince transgendered individuals to remain in the gender role of their genetic sex, which is an impossibility for most patients. Everyone involved in patient care should have some awareness of gender identity disorders, however rare they may be. Primary care physicians interested in providing hormonal replacement therapy for transgendered patients should consult the Harry Benjamin Society Standards of Care. Physicians and mental health professionals who are neither comfortable nor sufficiently knowledgeable to treat transgendered patients should refer them to more experienced colleagues.

NOTES

1. Woodson JC and Gorski RA. Structural differences in the mammalian brain: reconsidering the male/female dichotomy. In Matsumoto A (ed.) *Sexual Differentiation of the Brain.* New York and London: CRC Press, 2000.

2. Kruijver FP et al. Male-to-female transsexuals have female neuron numbers in a limbic nucleus. *J Clinical Endocrinology & Metabolism.* 85(5):2034–41, 2005.

3. Zhou JN et al. A sex difference in the human brain and its relation to transsexuality. *Nature.* 378(6552):15–16, 1995.

4. Zucker KJ and Bradley SJ. *Gender Identity Disorder and Psychosexual Problems in Children and Adolescents.* New York and London: The Guilford Press, 1995.

5. Kreiss JL and Patterson DL. Psychological issues in primary care of lesbian, gay, bisexual, and transgendered youth. *Journal of Pediatric Health Care.* 11(6):266–74, 1997.

6. Cohen-Kettenis PT and Pfafflin F. *Transgenderism and Intersexuality in Childhood and Adolescence. Making choices.* Thousand Oaks and London: Sage Publications, 2003.

7. Feinberg L. *Transgender Warriors.* Boston: Beacon Press, 1996.

ADDITIONAL READINGS

Boylan JF. *She's Not There.* New York: Broadway, 2003.

Brown ML and Rounsley CA. *True Selves: Understanding Transsexualism—for Families, Friends, Coworkers, and Helping Professionals.* San Francisco: Jossey Bass, 1996.

Israel GE and Tarver DE. *Transgender Care.* Philadelphia: Temple U. Press, 1997.

▓ ▐▌ ▐▌ ▓

JAMES J. HUGHES, PHD

Beyond the Medical Model of Gender Dysphoria to Morphological Self-determination

The psychiatric diagnosis of gender dysphoria and its more recent medical treatment, as admirably summarized by Dr. Spack, is contested and eroding. Although "medicalization" has helped transgendered people to acquire therapy and social acceptance, transgenderism is part of a larger social struggle between defenders of the "natural" and "God-given" and the right of individuals to control their own bodies and define their own lives.

In 2003, psychologist Michael Bailey stepped into this volatile debate with his book *The Man Who Would Be Queen: The Science of Gender Bending and Transsexualism.*[1] Based on observations of transsexuals and transvestites, the book purported to confirm an out-of-favor psychosexual etiology of transsexualism rather than the dominant medicalized diagnosis of gender dysphoria. For Bailey, male transsexuals can be parsed into two broad groups, neither appropriately understood as a "woman trapped in a man's body": (1) effeminate homosexual men who want to have sex with men and believe that as women they can better attract straight men, and (2) straight men fixated on having sex involving female genitals, but who get confused and turned on by the idea of having their own female genitalia, i.e., "autogynephiles."

Not surprisingly, the book created a firestorm of protest among transgender activists, who condemned Bailey's unscientific methodology. Transgender activists also saw that Bailey's psychosexual etiology would be ammunition for the opponents of transgender therapies. The Christian Right embraced Bailey's book as evidence that transsexuals should be denied surgery and hormones, and directed to psychotherapy instead.

For instance, writing in the conservative Christian journal First Things in 2004, Dr. Paul McHugh, psychiatrist-in-chief of Johns Hopkins Hospital, said "I have witnessed a great deal of damage from sex-reassignment . . . We psychiatrists have been distracted from studying the causes and natures of their mental misdirections by preparing them for surgery and for a life in the other sex. We have wasted scientific and technical resources and damaged our professional credibility by collaborating with madness rather than trying to study, cure, and ultimately prevent it."[2]

In 2002 Dr. McHugh was appointed to the President's Council on Bioethics (PCB) and participated in the deliberations that led to the PCB's critique of human enhancement therapies, *Beyond Therapy*.[3] In his 2004 critique of sex reassignment, Dr. McHugh pointed to the larger philosophical issue swirling around the contested diagnosis of gender dysphoria. "There is a deep prejudice in favor of the idea that nature is totally malleable," he said. "Without any fixed position on what is given in human nature, any manipulation of it can be defended as legitimate."

The emerging attack on the diagnosis of gender dysphoria and the malleability of "human nature" does not come only from cultural conservatives, however, but also from some on the Left. For bioethicist Carl Elliot, author of *Better Than Well,* gender dysphoria is one of many forms of self-mutilation sold to Americans by a profit-driven medical-industrial complex.[4] To underline his point, Elliot compares sex reassignment surgery to the psychiatric condition "apotemnophilia," the obsession that one should be an amputee. Like gender dysphorics, apotemnophilics are chronically depressed, because they see their "true selves" without the offending appendages. Unlike gender dysphorics, apotemnophilics are almost universally seen as needing psychiatric treatment, rather than medical help to transition to their desired body. For Elliot, like the conservative critics, sex reassignment is a sign that we are using technology inappropriately to cure spiritual and psychiatric ailments.

Advances in global access to sex reassignment surgery, our understanding of the diversity of biological sex, and our technologies of body modification all promise to make the battles over sex reassignment even more intense in the near future, and to further polarize bioconservatives from advocates of morphological self-determination.

As transgender attorney Dean Spade points out, we don't make women suffering from "rhino-identity disorder" live as small-nosed people for a year before their surgery. But the protocols of the Harry Benjamin International Gender Dysphoria Association (HBIGDA) call for the "patient" to spend a year attempting to live as the opposite sex before they receive surgery. While an understandable attempt to prevent postsurgical regret (which is extremely rare among transsexuals), many transgender people find the HBIGDA protocols patronizing and, in a world in which crossdressers can be the victims of violence, potentially dangerous. Thai surgeons, who perform some of the highest volume sex reassignments in the world, for an order of magnitude lower cost than North American surgeons, do not follow the HBIGDA protocols, but instead make a case-by-case assessment of psychological appropriateness. As medical tourism to Latin America and Asia becomes more common and attractive, the rigid HBIGDA protocols will become irrelevant.

The idea of passing as the "opposite" gender is also based on passé binary assumptions about gender. Just as transgendered people are no longer expected to manifest "appropriate" sexual preferences, there is a growing acceptance of transgendered people who decide to only partially transition, or consciously adopt a neither-male-nor-female gender identity.[5] Female-to-male patients may decide to take testosterone, but forego phalloplasty and traditional male dress. Male-to-female patients may get breast implants, take hormones, and cross-dress, but see no need for genital reconstruction. "Gender-queer" theorists such as Kate Bornstein and Martine Rothblatt argue that such ambiguous gender positions are a political statement against binary "gender apartheid."[6,7]

The evolution of gender dysphoria from a male/female gender correction, to an experimental, analog form of self-expression is also in line with recent thought on the non-binary nature of biological sex.[8] Anne Fausto-Sterling has popularized the fact that about 1% of all births are "intersexed," from classical hermaphrodites and people with a mismatch of body genitalia and DNA to genital malformations such as hypospadias, a congenital deformation of the penis.[9,10] If easily observable morphological differences are as prevalent as 1%, brains that are neither completely male nor female must presumably be at least as common, to the extent that there is a "gendered brain."[11] The Intersex Society of North America[12] has emerged to campaign for the right of intersex children to define their own gender identity and not be surgically "fixed" at birth.

Emerging medical technologies promise to make the modification of physiological gender even easier, cheaper, and safer. Tissue engineering is rapidly advancing, growing breast tissue for breast implants and penile erectile tissue that could be used for phalloplasties. Within decades we will likely have gene therapy to modify the endocrine system, making exogenous hormones unnecessary. Surgeons are perfecting the shaving down of Adam's apples and reshaping of the chin, buttocks, and knees. Whatever neurochemistry and neurophysiology may characterize the gendered brain, if any, they will also become malleable, allowing more complete gender transitions.

Insofar as we discover genetic, hormonal, and neurophysiological determinants of gender identity and sexual preference, future neurotechnology (gene therapy, pharmaceuticals, or neurocybernetics) will permit the transgendered to not only adjust their desires and gender identity into alignment with their identity, but also with their born sex. Some gender dysphorics may follow the path of least resistance. But as the medical risks and social sanctions of gender transgression decline, and our lifespans and the efficacy of body modification technologies increase, a growing proportion of us will want to try on features of the other gender from metro-sexual cross-gender dress, to hormone supplementation to modify personality, to topical gene therapy to change skin and hair, to designer genitalia.

As the medical model of gender dysphoria is challenged by morphological liberationism on the one hand, and bioconservativism on the other, it will be difficult to make the case for covering the therapies with public or private insurance. But instead of reifying the medical model, transgender therapy should be used to challenge the illusory therapy/enhancement distinction, and establish that facilitating full self-expression is as legitimate a use of biotechnology as the fixing of diseases and disorders. There is little difference in the utility produced in someone's life from plastic surgery after an accident or burn, and plastic surgery to adjust a feature that has caused lifelong dissatisfaction. There is no reason for insurance to discriminate against the latter in favor of the former. Why is breast reconstruction for the woman recovering from breast cancer surgery politically privileged over breast construction for the trans-woman? Neither are "medically necessary" and both done to give psychological relief.

The bioconservatives are correct that we might all be happier if we were enlightened enough to be content with whatever we were dealt by fate. But that is also a formula for personal and social stasis. Transgendered individuals are entitled to access to medical technology not because, as the advocates of the medical model such as Dr. Spack assert, they have a medical condition that demands correction, but because we should respect the right to morphological self-determination. I pin my hopes with John Stuart Mill that we all will be enriched when society helps each of us find our own personal self-expression.

NOTES

1. Bailey JM. *The Man Who Would Be Queen: The Science of Gender Bending and Transsexualism.* Washington, DC: Joseph Henry Press; 2003.

2. McHugh P. Surgical sex. *First Things.* November 2004;147:34–38.

3. The President's Council On Bioethics. *Beyond Therapy: Biotechnology and the Pursuit of Happiness.* Washington, DC: October 2003.

4. Elliot C. *Better Than Well.* New York, NY: W.W. Norton & Co.; 2003.

5. Israel GE.Transgenderists: when self-identification challenges transgender stereotypes. 1996. http://www.firelily.com/gender/gianna/transgenderists.html.

6. Bornstein K. *Gender Outlaw: On Men, Women and the Rest of Us.* New York, NY: Vintage; 1995.

7. Rothblatt, M. *The Apartheid of Sex: A Manifesto of the Freedom of Gender.* New York, NY: Crown; 1995.

8. Dreger, AD. *Hermaphrodites and the Medical Invention of Sex.* Cambridge, Mass: Harvard University Press; 2000.

9. Fausto-Sterling A. *Myths of Gender: Biological Theories About Women and Men.* New York, NY: Basic Books; 1992.

10. Fausto-Sterling A. *Sexing the Body: Gender Politics and the Construction of Sexuality.* New York, NY: Basic Books; 2000.

11. Moir A, Jessel D. *Brain Sex: The Real Difference Between Men and Women.* New York, NY: Delta; 1989.

12. http://isna.org

☷ ☶ ☶ ☷

DAVID STEINBERG, MD

Introduction: Novel Technologies

Advances in biomedical science and technology have given man unprecedented power to influence human destiny and perhaps human evolution. While its potential benefits for human health and flourishing have been acknowledged as powerful, progress in biomedicine also has evoked a "certain vague disquiet,"[1] fear of a dehumanizing "post human future"[2] and concern that if human hubris tempts man to play God "things will go where no one intended."[3]

Leon Kass, former chairman of the President's Council on Bioethics, noted that the dangers of technology are seductive because "the evils we face are intertwined with the goods we so keenly seek" and "distinguishing good and bad thus intermixed is often extremely difficult."[4] Paul Lauritzen puts it more bluntly, "The road to hell is still paved with good intentions."

Scientific and technological advances have an inherent momentum that is independent of our ability to understand how these advances may best be employed. Science can outpace ethics because, as Callahan, notes "a glaring deficiency of bioethics is it has few if any good methods for dealing with new and novel technologies." An attempt to separate what's permissible from what's suspect by distinguishing therapy from enhancement, though a problematic conceptual distinction, served as the title for a cautionary book, *Beyond Therapy,* from the President's Council on Bioethics.[5]

Another publication from the council, *Being Human,* begins with the nineteenth century Hawthorne story, *The Birth-mark*.[6] In it Georgiana, wife of an alchemist named Aylmer, would be a creature of perfect beauty were it not for a hand-shaped birthmark on her left cheek that penetrates "as deep as life itself," a "visible mark of earthly imperfection." Aylmer concocts a potion to repair "what nature left imperfect"; unfortunately, his pretensions result in Georgiana's death. The selection of this nineteenth century tale of overconfidence in science was protested as ideologically motivated and irrelevant to modern science.

In this section our authors note the impressive powers the biological sciences and technology have bestowed on man. Humans use "technology to create human life" and transform how "new members are admitted to the human race." We can prenatally identify and then eliminate those with future disabilities and decide "which characteristics in a fetus are acceptable." Some predict that with "the selection of human traits" and "made to order children" we will "create novel meanings of the self" and alter "our understanding of what it means to be human." Biological enhancement technologies will make us more beautiful, more intelligent, more athletic, and vastly expand our memory capacities. Part human and part material "cyborgs" will roam the earth. Today's normal will become tomorrow's subnormal. By "playing God" we will make today's science fiction tomorrow's reality. Man will control human evolution and change the earth. Crops will grow luxuriously in poor soil, food will have greater nutritional value, and our frivolous impulses may germinate "Brussels sprouts that taste like chocolate."

These current and future powers have for many of our authors evoked fear of a deadly human hubris that will misappropriate science and technology, lead to a collection of horrors, and "threaten deep and fundamental values." The faint-hearted should read no further. We are warned of the loss of personal satisfactions, possible dehumanization, threats to individuality, the creation of "new disadvantaged groups," a Nazi-like "eugenic resurgence," reduced respect for human life, a denial of the worth of the disabled and their elimination, "sinister invasions of liberty and privacy," and the "totalitarian control of humans" by the state. If this were not sufficiently frightening, these disasters will occur on terrain that has lost its biodiversity and is inhabited by "superweeds" and "deadly pathogens."

How many of these fears are realistic? Should progress in science and technology be held hostage to a lack of faith in human judgment? Should technology and public policy intended for a legitimate purpose be condemned because of a speculated potential for misapplication down a dangerous slippery slope? Does experience with a policy or technology over time create a sense of familiarity and comfort that makes it easier to move to the next, perhaps more dangerous, step? Or is the slippery slope argument itself a slippery slope because it can be used to damn any reasonable technology or policy as being unable to remain within its intended confines?

A nasty political schism over the use of novel technologies has developed between conservative and traditional bioethicists. Macklin accuses conservatives of replacing reasoned arguments with a mean-spirited rhetoric of emotional metaphors and slogans such as "human dignity," "the wisdom of repugnance," "people without souls," "a true bioethics," and "children as a gift." Conservatives also have been accused of thinking they have a handle on the "one true bioethics," "akin to religious believers who assert that theirs is the one true religion." Macklin also claims conservatives are "yearning for a more activist government that regulates or bans whole technologies."[7]

In response, bioethicist Eric Cohen[8] has outlined the foundations of conservative bioethics and its relation to novel technologies. He notes that from the moment of conception a human embryo is "innocent life" that must be protected. Any endeavor that involves the destruction of a human embryo "exploits some lives to help others" and is therefore immoral. Technology is acknowledged as "a great blessing" before being damned for seducing us into using "morally illegitimate means" in a quest for the "illusion of man-made immortality."

The conservative notion of family requires parents to "accept off-spring unconditionally" including ill or disabled children. Cohen writes, "Selective abortion is a form of eugenics antithetical to the spirit of parenthood." Parents should not "exert novel control over the genetic make-up of new life." Many conservatives oppose in vitro fertilization because "it turns the mysterious birth of new life into a technological project." Enhancement of any particular set of human attributes merits moral caution because it "risks undermining the human whole" and creates similarity between humans and thoroughbred animals. Neuroscience should not develop drugs that erase painful memories because a "trouble free life" lacks "the defining marks of our humanity."

Madison Powers has ascribed these types of fundamental disagreements to differences in "background assumptions" and to our inability to compare qualitatively distinct parameters.[9] He notes it is incoherent to imagine "that there exists a quantitative way to assess the qualitatively incommensurable." There is no generally accepted method for performing the calculus that weighs the destruction of potential (for many, actual though embryonic) human life against the benefits of having a child free of disease or disability. We don't know how to calculate the net benefit (or harm) of creating a child for an infertile couple after factoring the perceived degradation of abandoning sexual reproduction for a manufacturing process. Powers concludes there is a "limit to moral expertise because multiple morally acceptable options" exist and "below the surface of bioethical debate is an inherently political contest."

The unknown can be frightening especially when it is difficult to distinguish future promise from peril. I suspect dramatic change, even in basic human nature, is not quite as novel as some philosophers imply. The nature of modern man who lives in a house, drives a car, buys food in a supermarket, reads books and newspapers, and watches television and movies surely is different from early man who roamed the plains barefoot in search of food, had primitive clothing and shelter, and had to fear the jaws of poisonous snakes and marauding tigers.

Callahan warns us to "watch out for the blatant bias of a Luddite or progressive-enthusiast" as "we think about novel technologies with no clear historical precedents." The greatest ethical challenge posed by advances in biomedical science and technology will be to define "how human beings can best flourish." As the readings in this section make clear, that will not be an easy task.

NOTES

1. *Beyond Therapy: Biotechnology and the Pursuit of Happiness.* A Report of The President's Council on Bioethics. 2003; 5

2. Fukuyama, Francis. *Our Post Human Future: Consequences of the Biotechnology Revolution.* Picador New York NY 2002

3. *Beyond Therapy: Biotechnology and the Pursuit of Happiness.* A Report of The President's Council on Bioethics. 2003; 13

4. Kass Leon. Opening Remarks to The President's Council on Bioethics. May 17, 2002 available at http://www.bioethics.gov/transcripts/jan02/opening01.html. Accessed March 21, 2006.

5. *Beyond Therapy: Biotechnology and the Pursuit of Happiness.* A Report of The President's Council on Bioethics. 2003.

6. The Birth-mark by Nathaniel Hawthorne in *Being Human* pages 5–20. The President's Council on Bioethics. Washington D.C. 2003.

7. Macklin Ruth. The new conservatives in bioethics: Who are they and what do they seek? *Hastings Center Report* 2006; 36 (1): 34–43

8. Cohen Eric. Conservative bioethics and the search for wisdom. *Hastings Center Report* 2006; 36 (1) 44–56

9. Powers Madison. Bioethics as politics: The limits of moral expertise. *Kennedy Institute of Ethics Journal* 2005; 15(3):305–322

☲ ☶ ☶ ☲

DAN W. BROCK, PHD

Cloning Human Beings

Ian Wilmut shocked the world by announcing the successful cloning of Dolly from a single cell of an adult sheep. The possibility of cloning a human being could no longer be dismissed as science fantasy. Around the world, public officials, scientific and medical spokespersons, and, indeed, even Wilmut himself, joined in the condemnation of human cloning. President Clinton called for a moratorium on all human cloning and asked his newly formed National Bioethics Advisory Commission (NBAC) to report in 90 days on the ethical and legal issues raised by it. NBAC issued a 110-page report calling for continuing the moratorium, based largely on the unacceptable risks that human cloning would pose at the present time to the fetus.[1] But it argued as well that federal legislation enforcing such a moratorium should have a sunset clause of three to five years, thereby forcing a revisiting of the issues after a period of more extended public and professional debate. This temporary moratorium is reasonable because, although there is no denying that many people react to the prospect of human cloning with deep unease and even repugnance, compelling reasons for a permanent ban have, in my view, not yet been persuasively articulated by the opponents of cloning.

In this article, I shall briefly state a few of the principal ethical arguments for and against human cloning; although none can be fully explored here, my hope is to help point the debate in the right direction. Both proponents and opponents have appealed to moral rights, as well as to the good and bad consequences to which the practice likely would lead.

REPRODUCTIVE FREEDOM

Proponents of human cloning, if and when the issues about its safety are resolved, have argued that access to it should be protected by individuals' moral and legal right to reproductive freedom.[2] A strong right to reproductive freedom has a deep place both in common morality and the law, and many have argued that this right includes preventing reproduction by contraception or abortion, as well as access to new assisted reproductive technologies (ARTs) such as in vitro fertilization (IVF) or oocyte donation. One issue about human cloning is whether it is also a means of reproduction properly subsumed by this right. Opponents argue that current ARTs are remedies for inabilities to reproduce sexually, whereas cloning is an entirely new means of creating persons, more a means of manufacturing a person than reproducing. Yet for some, cloning might be their only or best means of successfully having genetically related children. My own view is that, in some limited uses, cloning is a reasonable means for satisfying some individuals' reproductive interests and is properly a part of reproductive freedom.

BENEFITS FROM CLONING

At the same time, it is hard to see human cloning as promising widespread benefits. It could enable some otherwise infertile individuals or couples to reproduce in a way that maintains a biological link with their offspring. It might also allow a couple, in which one party risks transmitting a serious hereditary disease, to reproduce without doing so. Cloning a later twin could enable a person to obtain needed organs or tissues for transplantation, so long as taking them would not violate the rights of the later twin. And finally, human cloning, or research on human cloning, might make possible important advances in scientific knowledge, for example about human development. But these benefits appear to be limited and speculative. Some other benefits that have been claimed for human cloning, such as enabling the duplication of individuals of great talent or genius, are illusory and based on confusions; they presuppose a crude and false genetic determinism according to which persons' genes alone determine their identity, character, and properties.

RIGHT TO A UNIQUE IDENTITY

Opponents of human cloning argue that cloning would violate the right to a unique identity. There are two important issues here—is there such a moral or human right and, if so, would human cloning violate it? Skeptics note that this right does not appear in typical theories of moral or human rights. They also argue that if cloning would violate this right, then so apparently would genetically identical twins occurring naturally. No one claims rights' violations there; however, this might be because only the deliberate or negligent actions of another person, not "nature," can violate rights.

Accepting, for the sake of argument, that there is a moral or human right to a unique identity, human cloning would not violate it. This argument assumes the same crude and false genetic determinism that undermined the last putatively beneficial use of human cloning considered previously. For cloning to violate individuals' rights to a unique identity, their identity would have to consist of nothing more than their genes. But we know that this is not so because it ignores the impact of the environment on individuals' identity, and we confront its falsity in the case of genetically identical twins who differ from each other in myriad ways. Our uniqueness comes not just from our genes, but as well from our environment, personal history, human relationships, and choices through which we each create our own biographies. Cloning would not deny anyone a unique human identity. There are other possible moral rights that human cloning might violate which I have explored elsewhere, such as a right to an open future or to ignorance about one's future, but they cannot be pursued here.[3] Instead, I shall look briefly at the harms opponents of human cloning fear.

PSYCHOLOGICAL DISTRESS

As noted, NBAC rested its central recommendation for continuing the moratorium on human cloning on the unacceptable risks that it would pose at this time to the clone, and in that they were surely correct. But this risk of harm may only be temporary. There is no reason to believe that further research on animal cloning, as well as on human cloning, might not at some point establish that appropriate standards of safety and efficacy are met. Opponents have argued that even a perfected process of human cloning would produce serious psychological distress and harm in the later twin. For example, the later twin may feel, even if mistakenly, that his or her fate has already been laid out, and so experience a diminished sense of autonomy and individuality. While psychological harms of this sort are certainly possible, they remain at this point only speculative since we have no experience with human cloning and the creation of later twins.

It is also feared that human cloning could diminish the worth of individuals and lessen society's respect for human life. It could also undermine important parental and societal attitudes of acceptance of difference and disability. These social harms are inevitably even more speculative, but they make clear how human cloning, in the eyes of some, threatens deep and fundamental values. The issue for public policy is whether these possible harms are sufficiently serious and likely to justify a prohibition of human cloning, including a restriction on people's reproductive freedom.

CONCLUSION

Even in this compressed account, there are serious moral rights, as well as potential harms and benefits, on both sides of the human cloning debate, and reasonable people can and do disagree about whether the balance of these reasons could ever support permitting it. I have tried only to articulate a few of the moral issues that should have an important place in the public deliberation about human cloning for which NBAC rightly called in its report.

NOTES

1. *Cloning human beings: report and recommendations of the National Bioethics Advisory Commission.* Rockville, MD, June 1997.

2. Robertson JA. *Children of choice: freedom and the new reproductive technologies.* Princeton, NJ: Princeton University Press, 1994.

3. Brock DW. Cloning human beings: an assessment of the ethical issues pro and con. Prepared for the National Bioethic Advisory Commission, April 1997.

☰ ☷ ☷ ☰

RUTH MACKLIN, PHD

Commentary on Human Cloning

In "Cloning Human Beings," Dan Brock describes some responses to the news that the first mammal had successfully been cloned, and summarizes the main arguments for and against human cloning. I concur with Brock's view that once appropriate standards of safety and efficacy are met, at least in some limited uses, cloning may be a reasonable means of satisfying some individuals' reproductive interests and can be justified by the principle of reproductive freedom. Brock provides a balanced account of human cloning, noting that there are serious moral rights, as well as potential harms and benefits on both sides of the debate. What has puzzled me since the news from Scotland was first announced is the strength of the visceral reactions of people opposed to cloning, and the swift calls for prohibition by governments and international bodies. In this brief commentary I will focus on those responses to human cloning.

One of the most vigorous opponents of cloning in the United States has been Leon R. Kass, a professor at the University of Chicago. Kass testified in March 1997 before the National Bioethics Advisory Commission and later expanded his testimony into an article published in *The New Republic* (June 2, 1997). Kass' position is remarkable for the intensity of its emotional tenor. Like some others fearful of cloning, Kass employs an array of adjectives—revolting, repugnant, repulsive—that represents an extreme emotional reaction. Kass acknowledges that "revulsion is not an argument," yet he contends that "repugnance is the emotional expression of deep wisdom, beyond reason's power fully to articulate it."

Unfortunately, however, Kass makes the move of so many commentators on cloning when he cites the main source of that repugnance: the "mass production of human beings, with large clones of look-alikes . . ." But this is hardly a realistic worry. Even if it might be contemplated by some hypothetical dictator in an evil authoritarian government, policy makers in a democracy could insist on a perfectly sensible restriction: prohibition on the use of cloning to produce more live births than would ordinarily occur in nature (probably five). This and other appropriate restrictions could be embodied in regulations that would govern cloning, just as regulations exist to protect human subjects of biomedical and behavioral research.

National governments and international groups issued statements, declarations, and resolutions in the months following the cloning of Dolly, the sheep. As Brock noted, the National Bioethics Advisory Commission called for continuing the moratorium initially proposed by President Clinton. In the United Kingdom, The House of Commons Scientific and Technology Committee issued a report in March 1997 urging that an existing law be tightened to ensure that human cloning does not occur. President Jacques Chirac of France called on the French National Committee for advice and subsequently ordered a ban on cloning in his country.

The European Parliament issued a resolution confirming its opposition to the cloning of human embryos and calling for an explicit worldwide ban on the cloning of human beings. The European Commission's bioethics advisory panel called human cloning "ethically unacceptable" and said it should be prohibited by law.[1] The Steering Committee on Bioethics of the Council of Europe drafted an additional protocol to an existing Convention, which asserted that "Any intervention seeking to create a human being genetically identical to another human being, whether living or dead, is prohibited."[2] The Fiftieth World Health Assembly met in Geneva in May and issued a statement affirming that "the use of cloning for the replication of human individuals is ethically unacceptable and contrary to human integrity and morality."[3]

We are left to wonder why so many official bodies throughout the world acted so swiftly and with such certainty in declaring human cloning to be a violation of human dignity or human rights, and, therefore, unethical. Vague references to human dignity are no substitute for reason and argument. The many commentators who contend that it is important to respect and preserve human dignity need to provide a more precise account of just what constitutes a violation of human dignity in the case of human cloning. Of course, safeguards would have to be erected and regulations put in place to ensure that no one's rights are violated and no one's interests are harmed if cloning does become a reality. But beyond the considerations of safety and efficacy that justify calling for a moratorium, it is hard to see what moral arguments can justify a permanent, worldwide prohibition. It is surely worth considering such arguments if they are forthcoming, but so far the policy statements issued throughout the world have simply been assertions, devoid of empirical evidence or rational justification.

NOTES

1. *Opinion of the Group of Advisors on the Ethical Implications of Biotechnology to the European Commission: Ethical Aspects of Cloning Techniques.* 28 May 1997.

2. Steering Committee on Bioethics of the Council of Europe. *Draft Additional Protocol to the Convention for the Protection of Human Rights and Dignity with Regards to the Application of Biology and Medicine.* Strasbourg: Directorate of Legal Affairs: July 1997.

3. World Health Assembly 50.37, *Cloning in Human Reproduction.* 14 May 1997.

REPLY BY DAN W. BROCK, PHD

I did not explore the content or grounds of a moral right to reproductive freedom, though I and others have done so elsewhere.[1,2] For human cloning, the important point about the content or scope of reproductive freedom is that it does not just include the use of means to avoid reproduction, but also access to available assisted reproductive technologies—potentially including human cloning—that can be used by many otherwise infertile couples to have children.

What are the moral grounds of women's control over their reproduction that a moral and legal right to reproductive freedom secures? I believe they are mainly three: first, people's interest in controlling their reproduction is one component of their broader interest in self-determination—roughly their interest in making important decisions about their lives for themselves and according to their own values; second, satisfying people's desires to have and raise children typically has a fundamental impact on their well-being or happiness; and third, for women in particular, having control over their reproduction is important in preventing or mitigating unjust gender inequalities they would otherwise suffer. This still leaves more questions about reproductive freedom than it answers, but it should make clear that the notion of "reproductive freedom" is not just a partisan political slogan, but instead refers to deeply personal and important interests in having and raising children, interests that are grounded in the familiar, more fundamental moral values of individual self-determination, well-being and happiness, and equality.

I am in full agreement with Ruth Macklin's points, in particular, regarding the striking contrast between the intense emotional nature of many condemnations of human cloning—both from political and health-policy leaders but also from academics like Leon Kass—and the lack of clear and convincing arguments pointing to demonstrable harms, individual or social, or serious threats to important values that might warrant such strong condemnation. No doubt public policy will be affected by these intense reactions of repugnance and revulsion, but the responsibility of bioethicists is to insist instead on clear and persuasive arguments from those who support human cloning's permanent prohibition.

NOTES

1. Brock DW. Reproductive freedom: Its nature, bases and limits. *Health Care Ethics: Critical Issues for Professionals.* Thomasma D, Monagle J (eds): Gaithersburg, MD: Aspen Publishers, 1994.

2. Robertson JA. *Children of choice: freedom and the New Reproductive Technologies.* Princeton, NJ: Princeton University Press, 1994.

☳ ☶ ☶ ☳

DANIEL CALLAHAN, PHD

Cloning Human Beings

The debate on human cloning has brought to the surface a glaring deficiency of bioethics. It has few if any good methods for dealing with new and novel technologies. By that I mean those technologies where there seem to be no relevant historical precedents and where the potential benefits and harms are speculative only, not yet available for empirical testing. How might we best try to assess such technologies, and what counts as a good or bad argument for ethics and for public policy?

Macklin and Brock, for instance, both want "clear and persuasive" arguments to support a ban on cloning and "empirical evidence" of "demonstrable harms." But how could there be wholly persuasive arguments in a domain new to human history and experience? Their invocation of reproductive rights as the premise for such arguments does, as an earlier critic noted, beg the issue of whether or not that is the appropriate, much less the only starting point for argumentation.

Nor is it reasonable to insist on "empirical evidence" of benefit or harm when the scientific outcomes are still in the future and wholly speculative in nature. Such evidence could become available only when human cloning was a reality; and then it could take years or decades after that to determine whether it had been a wise move to allow the research to go forward in the first place.

Our common problem, in any case, is to know how to make a judgment now about whether the research should go forward when no such evidence is available. Brock and Macklin have not, to use their own standards, demonstrated in some universally compelling, rational way that their acceptance of human cloning under some circumstances makes good sense. They have only shown that they like their reasons better than those of cloning opponents. Their reasons turn on their embrace of reproductive rights—surely contested terrain. Even if there is widespread acceptance of reproductive rights as a general category of rights, there is surely no agreement whatever that these rights entail a parental right to choose cloning as a means of reproduction. An independent case must be made for that entailment. The possibility of a relief of infertility is hardly sufficient for that purpose.

In their seeming inability to understand why anyone could feel repugnance at the prospect of human cloning, Macklin and Brock overlook or minimize why there was that reaction. Such cloning is perceived as a threat to individuality, a trait accorded a high status in western societies. Threats to it, even remote threats, are taken seriously, as well they should be. If we have learned anything from 20th century history, it is that dangers to individuality usually come disguised at first as progress and liberation. While sometimes excessive, even as well-meant an idea as school uniforms for children usually sets off a fierce community debate. We prize difference in people and take to the ramparts when it is threatened.

The key issue here is not, as Brock implies, genetic determinism or genetic identity but the preservation of individuality—by no means the same as genetic identity. Even so-called "identical" twins are not wholly identical genetically; that is well known. More to the point here is the issue of parents trying to use children for parental ends, procreating them with traits chosen by the parents for the purposes of the parents, not the welfare of the children. We happily accept twins when they are born, but no parents I have heard of go out of their way to procreate twins, or turn to assisted reproduction specialists to procreate twins.

If the cloned child shares no other trait than simply looking like the parents (give or take minor variations), then that child's individuality will be compromised. Is it too hard to imagine that a child might not choose to look like a parent, even if most of his other traits are different?

Analogously, don't most of us already feel repugnance at parents who excessively try to shape children to live out parental wishes, whether to follow in a parent's professional footsteps, to be pushed into professional tennis or soccer camps at an early age, or pressured academically for years in school in order eventually to gain admission to an elite college? If most of us tend not to like or approve of such conduct, why should we be expected to embrace human cloning, which raises the stakes many orders of magnitude? Arguments based on reproductive rights, it should be noted, are parent-centered and not child-centered. There is considerable interest these days in the welfare of children. Is there any evidence that what future children need is a right to be cloned, or that a world lacking in cloned children would somehow be a less worthy world?

As it happens I do not support a ban on cloning. I don't think it could be enforced. I will be satisfied if the federal government does not provide grant money for that purpose, and if most scientists, together with Ian Wilmut [who cloned the sheep Dolly], continue to feel repugnance at the idea (however badly they may articulate their reasons). As for Macklin and Brock, fine and conscientious philosophers, I would hope that they might cast a broader imaginative net as they continue to think about this problem.

REPLY BY DAN W. BROCK, PHD, AND RUTH MACKLIN, PHD

Dan Callahan takes both bioethics and us to task for having "few if any good methods for dealing with new and novel technologies." In particular, we are chastised for wanting "clear and persuasive arguments" and "empirical evidence" of "demonstrable harms" to support a ban on cloning. He then argues that this is an impossible standard to impose on radically new technologies. He is correct, of course, that we cannot show "demonstrated" harms from an as yet undeveloped and unused technology. But this is not to say we cannot impose reasonable standards on the speculations many opponents of new technologies offer about disasters the technology will bring.

There are two aspects to reasonable standards for claims about prospective harms. One concerns a showing about the probability or likelihood that the harms will occur, the other a showing that the feared effects would indeed be serious harms. Even in the absence of experience with the new technology, we can assess the likelihood of causal relationships between the technology and the feared harm, in part by reviewing experience with similar kinds of technologies in the past. For example, in the area of new reproductive technologies we can look to experience with artificial insemination to judge the likelihood of posited harms from a related technology like oocyte, or egg, donation.

However, even if people can come to agree about the probability of such posited harms, they may still disagree about the magnitude of harm. In the case of a new technology like human cloning, it is reasonable to demand of opponents that they identify tangible and serious harms of the sort generally required to support a prohibition of research on or use of the new technology. The language of repugnance, used by Leon Kass [1] and apparently endorsed by Callahan, makes clear that they find human cloning deeply offensive, but it does nothing to identify the harms, much less to establish that those harms are of sufficient magnitude to support a public prohibition of human cloning. In a free society, the burden of proof should be on those who wish to prohibit behavior, and mere offense to some people typically is not, nor should it be, sufficient to meet that burden.

What does Callahan offer as good reasons why human cloning should not take place? He argues that cloning would be a threat to individuality, on which our society places very high value. He takes this rather vague notion of individuality to be different from genetic identity and to be threatened even if a child should look like its father. But this is problematic at best. Even with genetic identity, phenotypic expression would be different, as would the personal history, relationships, and choices of the two individuals, and all of these would be the basis for distinct individuality. In Callahan's own example of a child cloned from the adult cells of its parent, the child would at most look like the parent looked two or more decades ago; the two would not look the same contemporaneously. Why would this seriously threaten individuality when the individuality of contemporaneous identical twins is not threatened by their looking alike? Why would it threaten individuality any more than that of a child conceived in the normal way who closely resembles a parent? This is an example of the kind of argument we were criticizing—the harm is neither sufficiently probable nor substantial to ground a legal prohibition of cloning.

But Callahan adds a second reason why cloning is repugnant: It represents the use of the child by the parents for their own ends, excessively trying to shape their children to live out parental wishes. We share Callahan's disapproval of extreme forms of such parental behavior, but there are at least two reasons to be skeptical about the import of this disapproval for public policy about cloning.

First, if human cloning becomes possible, many uses of it would not involve these undesirable parental behaviors or attitudes. If a couple used cloning to avoid the risk of transmitting a genetic disease, or to have a biologically related child in the face of their own infertility, no such objectionable motivation would be involved.

Second, we believe that in general, public policy and the state should not be in the business of evaluating people's motivations in reproduction and child-rearing. To do so could invite widespread abuse and be deeply invasive of both reproductive choices and family privacy. Public policy and the law appropriately intervene only when such motivations and attitudes result in behavior seriously harmful to the child, and it is worth noting that we impose a relatively high threshold of parental autonomy before intervening in other behaviors of the sort Callahan cites.

Finally, we are surprised at Callahan's conclusion that despite what he takes to be very strong reasons against human cloning, he does not support a ban on it because he believes it could not be enforced. Surely, a federal ban on human cloning would substantially reduce its use if and when it became possible to do it. It would not eliminate it entirely, and it could certainly go on in countries that choose not to ban it, but why should this be a reason not to support prohibition if cloning is as wrong as Callahan apparently believes? We believe our difference with cloning opponents like Callahan comes not from having failed to cast our imaginative net broadly enough, as he suggests, but from being unpersuaded by what we find in the imaginative nets of cloning's opponents.

NOTES

1. Kass LR. *The wisdom of repugnance. The New Republic* 1997;216(22):17–26.

☰ |||| |||| ☰

SHARON STEINBERG, RN, MS, CS

Ethical Issues of Egg Donation

Scientific advances have dramatically expanded human reproductive potential; it is now not unusual for one woman to donate her eggs to help another woman become pregnant. Recipients of donated eggs include women who have premature ovarian failure or age-related reproductive problems, or have had their ovaries damaged or surgically removed. Egg donation can also be appropriate for women who carry serious genetic disorders.

FUNDAMENTAL OBJECTIONS

The most fundamental objection to egg donation concerns using technology to create human life. Roman Catholic doctrine rejects fertilization outside the body and the use of donated eggs or sperm because it bypasses the unity of body and spirit thought to be present in the normal procreative process.

Islamic law encourages infertility treatment for married couples because of the importance of marriage, family formation, and procreation. However, egg donation is prohibited by Islam because it involves intervention of a third party.

Some feminists argue that women are exploited and pressured into seeking egg donation and other reproductive technologies because some women feel they have no value unless they bear children.

THE RISK TO DONORS

Fertile women normally produce one egg each month. To obtain multiple eggs for donation, women are injected with ovarian-stimulating drugs for approximately two weeks. When the eggs are mature, vaginal ultrasound is used to locate multiple ovarian follicles and the eggs are retrieved. These eggs are fertilized in dishes with the sperm of the recipient woman's spouse or partner. Usually, two embryos are placed into the recipient's uterus.

About 50 percent of these women deliver babies and multiple births are not uncommon; about 28 percent of women deliver twins and four percent deliver triplets.

Egg donors may be relatives or close friends of women who are unable to produce eggs, or they are "anonymous" donors. Young fertile women have the best quality eggs and donor programs target college students or aim advertising at young married women with children. Advertising commonly appeals to altruistic sympathies. One heart-shaped ad from a Boston reproductive clinic reads: "Our donor egg program is looking for women with something special . . . a generous heart. You have the opportunity to give the gift of childbirth to an infertile couple." Anonymous donors are reimbursed, not for their eggs, but for their "time and effort."

Despite recent discussion about a safe upper age limit for recipient women, virtually nothing has been said about the risks to the women who donate their eggs. Potential egg donors are screened to determine if they are fertile and in good medical and psychological health. They undergo a rigorous medical regimen involving hormonal stimulation, blood tests, and the retrieval of eggs. Although complications are infrequent, egg retrieval can cause injury to structures adjacent to the ovary, pelvic infection, or other problems.

A syndrome called ovarian hyperstimulation occurs in approximately one percent of cycles and can result in metabolic disturbances requiring hospitalization. Because egg donation is a relatively new technology, it is not known whether medically stimulated young women are at greater risk for late complications, such as ovarian cancer.

Egg donation carries with it a risk of regret, especially if the donor becomes infertile—for reasons related to or unrelated to the egg donation—before she has children of her own. While the medical and psychological risks seem relatively small for an infertile woman seeking a child through in vitro fertilization, these risks, along with the legal and ethical implications, need to be carefully considered by donors who volunteer for the benefit of infertile women.

Most women who donate eggs to their sisters believe that the benefits far outweigh any risks. In known donor situations, donors and recipient couples are advised to clarify the responsibilities and obligations of all concerned. Thoughtful counseling is essential.

THE BEST INTERESTS OF THE CHILDREN

It is now possible for postmenopausal women to become pregnant with donor eggs. In 2006, a 67-year-old woman who lied to doctors about her age gave birth to twins. Older women face more health risks during pregnancy; nonetheless, some believe that it is both ageist and sexist to say a woman is too old to bear a child. Older men have become fathers with little criticism. Some say it is unfair to a child to be born to older parents; others note that many children are successfully reared by their grandparents.

There is also a debate about the appropriateness of secrecy. Many mental health professionals believe that children have a moral right and a need to know about their genetic origins. They think secrecy about a child's origins inhibits intergenerational intimacy and trust. In addition, it is possible that children in different families, conceived from the same donor's eggs, could unknowingly marry their genetic half-sister or half-brother.

Many fertility programs provide extensive, though non-identifying, information to recipients about their egg donors. Some donors and recipients would also like identifying information to be available to potential offspring. However, some recipient couples choose an anonymous donor because they want to keep their infertility or use of egg donation a secret from the child and their family and friends.

Egg donation may generate complicated and confusing expectations within family relationships. For example, a sister who donates an egg is both mother and aunt. A daughter who donates an egg to a remarried mother is both mother and half-sister. Our understanding of what this means for family life and child development is incomplete.

Donor eggs are scarce and many believe that they should be reserved for younger women. Most agree that for women over age 42—the precise age is controversial—egg donation is not a medical necessity and should not be covered by insurance, since infertility beyond that age is normal.

In Massachusetts, assisted-reproductive technologies, including donor egg, are a mandated insurance benefit; however, Vermont, New Hampshire, and most other states do not mandate health insurance coverage. The cost of in vitro fertilization using egg donation is between $10,000 and $15,000 per cycle.

Where insurance coverage is available, guidelines for the number of covered cycles, medical appropriateness, age limits, and access to the limited supply of eggs need to be developed. Specific criteria are usually not included in legislation that mandates coverage.

RECOMMENDATIONS

Egg donation is virtually unregulated except by the rules of a free market society. Many issues beg for more discussion. Some clinicians advocate for developing a national registry that records and identifies all donors, recipients, and their children. This database could be available in the future to donors, recipients, or children who needed or wanted to find one another. Comprehensive longitudinal research studies on the psychological and medical impact of egg donation on young fertile women and recipient families are necessary. Public debate regarding the need for guidelines, regulations, or legislation will help to inform and protect egg donors, recipients, families, and children.

REFERENCE

Cohen CB, ed. *New ways of making babies—the case of egg donation.* Indianapolis: Indiana University Press, 1996.

☰ ⫼ ⫼ ☰

JOHN A. ROBERTSON BA, JD

Consent and Uncertainty in Egg Donation

Although some persons have called for regulation of egg donation and other assisted reproductive techniques, comprehensive legislation is unlikely, thus leaving discretion over many key aspects of egg donation to the professionals involved. With this power, the 160 centers offering egg donation have a duty to make sure that all participants are fully informed of the uncertainties of an unregulated environment.

An important feature of egg donation is that it is occurring in the absence of explicit legislative authorization. New Hampshire is one of only seven states with legislation that explicitly recognizes the recipient as the legal mother for all purposes and cuts off any rights or duties of the donor. No other New England states have this law. There is good reason to think that courts in other states would give effect to the parties' preconception intentions, as they generally do in the case of sperm donation. But there is some residual uncertainty here of which parties need to be informed. It would be helpful if more states passed laws that clarified legal rights and duties in resulting children, so that the enacted law explicitly matches the intentions of the parties.

Another important issue is protection of the egg donor. Most donors are young women of college age, who are paid for each cycle of donation. Donation is not a benign procedure. It requires a cycle of ovarian stimulation with powerful hormones, followed by surgical retrieval of the eggs. It is important that donors be fully aware of the physical burdens and risk of the procedure, including the risk of ovarian cancer. If they are truly informed, they will also know that they are most likely waiving any legal rights they would have in resulting offspring. This could be a cause of later regret and disappointment as might occur if they were later infertile and wanted contact with the child. In a largely unregulated environment, reliance on informed consent is the best ethical and legal protection for participants in this novel, but rapidly growing, procedure.

Fair dealing with the egg donor requires that she be provided with health insurance to cover the medical costs of any injuries that she suffers as a result of a donation. Some programs meet this need by accepting as donors only women who have their own health insurance. In cases involving uninsured donors, the program should purchase a health insurance policy for the duration of the donation, thus protecting the couple from later claims for injuries and assuring that the medical costs of injured donors are covered.

An important issue is whether children should be informed that their gestational and rearing mother is different than their genetic mother. Mental health professionals and counselors involved with assisted reproduction, generally advise that disclosure should occur, with the details of how and when to do it left to the couple. Non-identifying information about donors should be made available to the child. Disclosing the identity of the genetic mother, however, will require the advance consent of both donor and recipient. Egg donor programs should devise a system to allow donors and offspring to meet if both are agreeable. Until such registries are created, however, most children will not be able to learn who their genetic mother is.

Finally, social concerns have been expressed about paying young women for their reproductive labor. Although more onerous than sperm donation, egg donation is clearly distinct from surrogacy. Thus no state has banned paid egg donation, though several ban paid surrogacy. Perhaps the line is only symbolic, but most programs are careful to make the payment serve as compensation for the time and inconvenience of the donor, and not for her eggs.

In sum, the growing practice of egg donation raises several issues that need careful attention if it is to occur in a way that is satisfying for all parties. Recognition of the legal, medical, and social uncertainties is key to respectful treatment of the participants in this novel way of forming a biologically related family.

☷ ☶ ☵ ☳

CYNTHIA B. COHEN, PHD, JD

A Lesbian Couple Who Both Want a Biologic Link to Their Offspring

QUESTION: Two professional women have been in a stable lesbian relationship for five years and want to have children. Neither woman has a fertility problem. Ordinarily, pregnancy would be achieved with donated sperm and insemination could be performed at home or with a simple office procedure—intrauterine insemination. In this case, however, both women want a biologic link to their offspring similar to that of heterosexual couples.

Their plan is for the oldest, who is 36, to have one of her eggs retrieved and fertilized with donor sperm by in vitro fertilization (IVF) to produce an embryo that would be implanted in her 35-year-old partner who would become the gestational mother. When ready for their second child, they would switch roles and the younger woman's egg would be fertilized and implanted in the other woman.

The fertility team is concerned about using the complex medical technology of donor egg and IVF with the attendant costs and risks of ovarian stimulation, anesthesia, and a slightly higher chance of premature birth when there are no medical reasons for IVF. How would you advise the fertility team?

RESPONSE: Assisted reproductive technologies (ARTs) were originally developed to assist infertile married couples to have children. As their use has spread, and social practices regarding marriage and sexuality have gradually changed, a new question has emerged: Should lesbian and gay couples also be able to use assisted reproductive technologies? If the answer is "Yes," a follow-up question surfaces: To which of the ARTs should lesbian couples have access?

Three main arguments can be given in answer to the first question concerning any use of ARTs by lesbian couples. One is that this would violate the basic goals of medicine—to heal the sick and disabled. Neither woman in this case has a physical malfunction that renders her sick or disabled; both are fertile. It could therefore be argued that to provide each with artificial insemination by donor (AID) and egg donation would be to misuse medicine.[1]

Second, some maintain that giving lesbian couples access to the ARTs would be harmful to the resulting children.[2] These children, they hold, will have difficulty developing gender identity and sex-role behaviors. Critics further contend that they will not only have more adjustment difficulties than children born to heterosexual parents, but will be rejected and stigmatized by their peers. Some courts have denied custody of children to lesbian couples on such grounds.

Third, some would argue that giving lesbian couples access to the ARTs would have detrimental social effects, for it would weaken and ultimately destroy the role of the family in protecting basic social values. To this, others would add that such practices would lead to the objectification of children as manufactured products, the impoverishment of the meaning of procreation, and the perpetuation of degrading views of women.[1]

Yet the opposite answer to the initial question can also be given. Medicine is appropriately used, some argue, not only to heal those who are ill or disabled, but also to promote their well-being. Thus, we provide plastic surgery to those who are disfigured, but not sick or disabled. Similarly, some would hold, medicine is appropriately used to support the well-being of lesbian couples who desire to have children.

Further, there is some evidence that the welfare of children is not jeopardized by being brought up in a lesbian household.[1,2] Studies suggest that the sexual orientation of parents does not determine that of their children and that the development of children of lesbians is comparable to that of children raised in non-lesbian households.

Finally, those who would provide lesbian couples with access to the ARTs maintain that individuals should be allowed to reproduce in ways of their own choice, whether or not they are married. While a constitutional right to reproduce noncoitally, if one exists, would apply only to married couples, lesbians can also have "valid interests" in having children.[3] Cases are beginning to appear in which lesbian couples have sued clinics for discrimination on the basis of marital status or sexual orientation because they have refused them AID.[2,4] It is not clear, however, whether any of these suits will prove successful.

As a society, we are moving toward a greater acceptance of lesbian couples and an increased willingness to use the ARTs to assist them to have children. Indeed, the American Medical Association has stated that "it is not unethical to provide artificial insemination as a reproductive option" for lesbians.[5] Yet some caregivers disagree and believe they should be exempt as a matter of conscience from treating lesbian women with the ARTs.

Is it right for caregivers who are not opposed to providing the ARTs to lesbian couples to offer egg donation to these two women? Each is (presumably) unwilling to engage in sexual intercourse with men and can therefore be said to have what amounts to an inability to have children coitally. Egg donation, however, is not medically necessary to achieve pregnancy in their case. Indeed, there is good reason not to add this procedure to the repertoire of treatments for these women, for it bears greater medical risks than AID to them and to the resulting children. Moreover, it has a relatively low chance of success, especially in women of their age. Much as physicians are not required to provide computerized tomography (CT) scans or brain surgery to patients who suffer from simple headaches, physicians are not required to provide egg donation to women who can conceive in a simpler and safer way.

Should an infertility specialist decide to accede to this couple's desire for egg donation, he or she should consider developing procedures designed to give them a full picture of the risks and benefits and to protect the welfare of any resulting children. The National Advisory Board on Ethics in Reproduction recommends that physicians who provide egg donation to lesbian women (whom it presumes are infertile in such instances) should carry out their usual screening procedures for donors and for recipients beforehand, and should also have qualified counselors discuss with them special considerations that may arise.[2] These could include what support system they have, what they will tell the children about their origins, and who would have custody of the resulting children should the couple separate.

OUTCOME: The fertility team decided the risks were significant and did not honor the women's request for the use of IVF. The women then chose artificial insemination.

NOTES

1. Cohen, CB. Reproductive technologies: ethical issues. In Reich W T (ed): *The Encyclopedia of Bioethics*. New York: Macmillan, 1997;4:2233–40.

2. National Advisory Board on Ethics in Reproduction (NABER). Report and recommendations on oocyte donation. In Cohen CB (ed): *New Ways of Making Babies*. Bloomington, IN: Indiana University Press, 1996:67–9.

3. Robertson JA. *Children of Choice: Freedom and the New Reproductive Technologies.* Princeton, NJ: Princeton University Press, 1994:36.

4. New York State Task Force on Life and the Law. *Assisted Reproductive Technologies: Analysis and Recommendations for Public Policy.* New York, NY: New York State Task Force on Life and the Law, 1998:183–7.

5. American Medical Association, Council on Ethical and Judicial Affairs. Artificial insemination by an anonymous donor. *Current Opinions,* 2.05.

☰ ☷ ☷ ☰

DIANE BEESON, PHD

Social and Ethical Challenges of Prenatal Diagnosis

In the past three decades, the process by which new members are admitted to the human race has been undergoing a profound transformation. Prenatal diagnosis has made it possible to abort fetuses selectively on the basis of an increasingly wide range of characteristics. In the United States this process has decreased sharply the number of infants born with Tay-Sachs disease, Down syndrome, and neural tube defects. More significantly, throughout the world it has reduced by millions the numbers of females born and thus has significantly altered sex ratios in several countries. For many prospective parents, prenatal diagnosis is a miraculous solution that removes risks they perceive as totally unacceptable. Other young parents-to-be find that prenatal testing thrusts them into an emotional and moral quagmire, without providing adequate support or guidance. The proliferation of prenatal testing and our ability to detect an ever-wider range of conditions, including susceptibility to late onset disorders, calls us to reflect on the wisdom, consequences, and direction of these developments.

Amniocentesis, the first prenatal testing procedure to become widely used, can reveal conditions such as chromosomal disorders (including Down syndrome and trisomy 18), single gene disorders (including sickle cell disease and cystic fibrosis), and biochemical abnormalities (including those associated with neural tube defects). More recently, chorionic villus sampling offers earlier diagnosis but has a somewhat higher risk of procedural failure and fetal loss.

With the advent of maternal serum screening, a simple blood test of pregnant women has permitted the detection of neural tube defects and an increasing number of other conditions in the developing fetus. In pregnancies resulting from in vitro fertilization, genetic testing can be done prior to implantation, but this is not a procedure that can be used in natural pregnancies.

Despite promising developments, for the vast majority of fetal anomalies the only significant medical intervention is abortion. This close association between prenatal diagnosis, selective abortion, and the tension involved in the uncertainty is transforming the meaning and experience of pregnancy and making it increasingly difficult to avoid the social and ethical questions that are implicit in this process.

Support for prenatal screening, testing, and the accompanying use of selective abortion has broad acceptance among the general public, particularly among those who are young, white, and highly educated. They may view testing as an expression of reproductive liberty and choice, and some maintain that prospective parents have a responsibility not to bring a disabled child into the world—both for the sake of the child and for the sake of society.

Prenatal testing is based on the assumption that the vast majority of cases in which serious anomalies are identified will result in abortion. However, advocates like to point out that such tests also prevent abortion in some unplanned high-risk pregnancies by reassuring prospective parents that certain anomalies are absent. Few advocates of prenatal testing encourage or condone selective abortion for fetal sex selection or minor genetic problems, but they disagree about the extent to which abortion should be restricted for these factors. Some prefer legal restrictions or protections and others only moral suasion.

Powerful as arguments for the use of prenatal diagnosis of fetal disorders may be, there is deep concern among many in the United States about the social and ethical implications of these practices. The most widely recognized objections to selective abortion are based on the belief that all human fetuses are persons with attendant rights. Such objections typically reflect blanket opposition to abortion. But others, who are in principle strongly pro-choice, are increasingly uneasy about these practices as well. They see selective abortion becoming less an expression of personal choice and increasingly a socially determined response to a situation in which alternatives, such as assurance of good medical care and community support for children with special needs, are lacking. They point out that while we expand prenatal diagnostic services, social policies limit resources for children and for parents of children with disabilities. Then we use the rhetoric of individual autonomy to justify placing pregnant couples in the position of having to make difficult decisions.

The central assumption behind the deployment of prenatal diagnosis is that life with a disability is not worthwhile and is primarily a source of suffering. Yet, evidence suggests that those with congenital anomalies and disabilities view these as the normal condition of their lives, perceiving themselves as healthy. In fact, those with disabilities often achieve the same high levels of life satisfaction as non-disabled persons. Much of the suffering they do experience comes from the isolation imposed by inadequate social accommodations—which render their disability more salient—and the prejudice that treats the disability as the person's only relevant characteristic.[1]

It is dangerous to make assumptions that devalue the lives of those with disabilities when more than 50 million people in the United States have disabilities, and many of us will become disabled for a significant portion of our lives. Critics of selective abortion argue that negative attitudes toward those with disabilities are based largely on fear, prejudice, and an unwillingness to challenge—or even examine—discriminatory social arrangements. The tendency to reduce individuals to their disability is one that seems particularly prevalent among many healthcare providers whose work necessarily focuses them on that issue. In addition, mental retardation holds special stigma for the most highly educated, particularly in the United States.

These attitudes diverge sharply, not only from those of disabled individuals, but from the response of their family members as well. Parents of children with even severe life-threatening disabilities have been found to be much more likely to reject the idea of prenatal testing and selective abortion than parents without such experience.

In addition to the fact that our fears and biases limit our understanding of the intimate experience of disability, those biases have a major impact on our ability to counsel others or to decide ethically whether some people are better off never being born. Genetic counseling is usually offered as "unbiased" and "non-directive." However, Lippman and Wilfond have shown that "before-birth" information presented in obstetrical settings presents a different perspective on Down syndrome than "after-birth" information presented by pediatricians. The first is largely negative, while the latter tends to be more positive.[2]

From a disability-rights perspective, prenatal testing for fetal anomalies gives a powerful message that we seek to eliminate future persons with disabilities, fails to recognize the social value of future persons with disabilities, and conveys a devaluation of those now living with disability. Disability rights activist Marsha Saxton argues that the most serious problem the procedure poses may be the loss of the deeper experience of our humanity that comes from confronting, rather than attempting to avoid, our human vulnerability.[3]

Many women still would prefer not to expose their pregnancies to extensive testing even for small risks, and would not consider selective abortion. Recent research, however, indicates that many of these procedures have become so routinized that women often feel the choice to undergo testing is not completely voluntary. These women find it difficult to turn down testing when it is offered because acceptance seems to be the only option sanctioned by medical science.[4] Not surprisingly, research suggests that women who decline testing are more likely to be blamed by health professionals and lay groups for their child's disability.[5]

Women who "choose" prenatal diagnosis and selective abortion are inevitably responding to a social context in which medical care and social support for all children are recognized to be problematic at best, and one in which those with disabilities are not highly valued. For these women to have meaningful options, we first need to acknowledge that their decision to consider selective abortion reflects not only inherent qualities of the fetus, but social conditions as well.

Avoiding human imperfection by eliminating potential persons based on their phenotypes or genotypes is a strategy that leads us into ever more difficult quandaries, particularly as we expand the range of genetic conditions we can identify. Shall we eliminate fetuses with susceptibility to breast cancer or heart disease? What about Alzheimer's disease? How many years of good health does it take to justify one's existence?

At what point will we address the fact that it is not genes, but poverty, poor nutrition, and lack of prenatal care that cause the vast majority of illnesses and disabilities? By focusing so many resources on the elimination of potential persons with disability, we are drifting toward a eugenic resurgence that differs only superficially from earlier patterns. In the process, we are seriously distorting the historical purpose of medicine as healing. We are creating a society in which disability is becoming increasingly stigmatized, with the result that human imperfection of all kinds is becoming less tolerated and less likely to be accepted as normal human variation. We must question where the rapid proliferation of prenatal testing for an increasing variety of traits is taking us; and medical professionals, in particular, need to question the social policies that increasingly cast them, and the prospective parents they serve, as gatekeepers at the doors of life.

NOTES

1. Asch A. Prenatal diagnosis and selective abortion: a challenge to practice and policy. *Am J Public Health* 1999;89(11):1649–57.

2. Lippman A, Wilfond BS. Twice-told tales: stories about genetic disorders. *Am J Hum Genet* 1992;51(4):936–7.

3. Saxton M. *Prenatal Screening and Discriminatory Attitudes About Disability in Embryos, Ethics and Women's Rights: Exploring the New Reproductive Technologies.* Baruch EH, et al (eds). Haworth Press, New York 1988:217–224.

4. Browner CH, et al. Ethnicity, bioethics, and prenatal diagnosis: the amniocentesis decisions of Mexican-origin women and their partners. *Am J Public Health* 1999;89(11):1665.

5. Marteau TM, Drake H. Attributions for disability: the influence of genetic screening. *Soc Sci Med* 1995 Apr;40(8):1127–32.

☷ ☶ ☵ ☳

PETER SINGER, MA, BPHIL

Prenatal Diagnosis

Diane Beeson is right to draw our attention to the "Social and ethical challenges of prenatal diagnosis." These challenges will increase in complexity as our increasing knowledge of genetics enables couples to learn more about their unborn children. But there are some fundamental issues that I see very differently from Beeson. She goes astray when she asserts that the "central assumption" of prenatal diagnosis is "that life with a disability is not worthwhile and is primarily a source of suffering."

Before considering this claim, think for a moment about two related questions. First, how important is it to most parents to give their child the best possible start in life? Second, how serious a reason does a woman need in order to be justified in ending her pregnancy?

The answer to the first question is that, for most parents, giving their child the best possible start in life is extremely important. The desire to do so leads pregnant women who have smoked or drunk heavily for years to struggle to kick the addiction; it sells millions of books telling parents how to help their child achieve her or his potential; it causes couples to move out to suburbs where the schools are better, even though they then have to spend time in daily commuting; and it stimulates saving so that later the child will be able to go to a good college.

The answer to the second question must begin with the fact that, in accordance with the decision in *Roe v. Wade*, a woman in the United States can, in the first and second trimesters, or at least until the fetus is viable, terminate her pregnancy for any reason whatsoever. This does not, of course, mean that she is ethically justified in doing so. Some say that she is *never* ethically justified in terminating her pregnancy, and others that she is justified in doing so only to save her own life, or in cases of rape and incest. But Beeson is not arguing from this standpoint. She writes so as to appeal to those who are "in principle strongly pro-choice." So let me put my own cards on the table, and acknowledge that, as I have argued elsewhere, I do not think that a fetus is the kind of being that has a right to life.[1,2] Hence it is not hard to justify terminating a pregnancy. For example, suppose that a couple plan to have children, but an unplanned pregnancy has occurred before they feel ready to do so—let's say that at present they are sharing a studio apartment and cannot afford anything larger, but in five years they will be able to move to a larger home. In my view, they would not be acting unethically if they decide to obtain an abortion.

Now think about the case that Beeson discusses: a couple who are told that the child the woman is carrying will have a disability. Let's say, since this is the disability to which Beeson gives more attention than any other, that the child will have Down syndrome. Like most parents, the couple think it important to give their child the best possible start in life, and they do not believe that having Down syndrome is the best possible start in life. Is it true that this couple must be making the assumption that "life with a disability is not worthwhile and is primarily a source of suffering"? There is no more reason to believe that these parents make that assumption, than there is to believe that parents who terminate a pregnancy because they can't afford a larger apartment believe that "life living as a child in one room with one's parents is not worthwhile and is primarily a source of suffering." In both cases, all that the parents need assume is that it would be *better* to have a child without Down syndrome, or to have a child who can have a room of her own. After all, in neither case are the parents choosing whether or not to have a child at all. They are choosing whether to have *this* child or another child that they can, with reasonable confidence, expect to have later, under more auspicious circumstances.

Thus it is possible to justify abortion in these circumstances while accepting Beeson's claims that people with congenital disabilities "often achieve the same high levels of life satisfaction as non-disabled persons." A couple may reasonably think that "often" is not good enough. They may also accept—as I do—that people with Down syndrome often are loving, warm people who live happy lives. But they may still think that this is not the best they can do for their child. It is unfair to suggest, as Beeson does, that it is "stigma" that leads more highly educated people to wish to avoid having a mentally retarded child. Perhaps they just want to have a child who will, eventually, come to be their intellectual equal, someone with whom they can have good conversations, someone whom they can expect to give them grandchildren, and to help them in their old age. Those are not unreasonable desires for parents to have.

What of the "powerful message that we seek to eliminate future persons with disabilities" that Beeson tells us is sent by prenatal diagnosis and abortion to people with disabilities? Her concern seems highly selective. Every bottle of beer or wine sold in the United States bears the words:

GOVERNMENT WARNING: ACCORDING TO THE SURGEON GENERAL, WOMEN SHOULD NOT DRINK ALCOHOLIC BEVERAGES DURING PREGNANCY BECAUSE OF THE RISK OF BIRTH DEFECTS.

Does not that warning—much more visible to ordinary Americans than prenatal diagnosis—send out a "powerful message" that we should prevent the birth of children with defects? What about the message sent by programs that immunize girls against rubella? And if a person is injured in a motor accident, and would not be able to walk without extensive surgery, does the fact that she goes ahead with the surgery somehow "convey a devaluation of those now living with disability"? Have disability advocates ever called for government to stop supporting research into ways of overcoming spinal cord injuries? No, disability rights advocates focus on only one of the many ways in which people seek to prevent the existence of people with disabilities—and that happens to be the one where the disability movement can count on active support from the much larger and more powerful antiabortion movement. Perhaps that is just a coincidence.

We can and should have equal consideration and respect for people living with disabilities. It does not follow from this that we must deny the obvious truth that most people, disabled or not, would prefer to be without disabilities.

Does this mean that we are "drifting toward a eugenic resurgence that differs only superficially from earlier patterns"? If this is a veiled reference to Nazi policies that led to the murder of millions of people, it is indefensible. No state is ordering anyone's death; no one who wants to go on living is being murdered; no children whose parents want them to survive are being killed. These are not superficial differences.

NOTES

1. Singer P. *Practical Ethics*. Cambridge: Cambridge University Press, 2nd ed. 1993; ch. 6.
2. Singer P. *Rethinking Life and Death*. New York: St Martin's Press, 1994; ch. 5.

REPLY BY DIANE BEESON, PHD

Peter Singer and I agree that it is important to most parents to give their child the best possible start in life, and we both affirm the right of a pregnant woman to decide for herself whether it is best for her to continue a pregnancy or choose abortion.

The main source of disagreement appears to be that Singer is focusing on individual cases while I am concerned with newly developing norms that may themselves become coercive. This focus on individual cases fails to recognize the social realities of decision making. Very often, prospective parents faced with the decision of whether or not to abort, do so only after learning that few resources (services, educational programs, treatments) are available that might help a child with the condition in question—as well as the parents—to have a rewarding life. What Singer does not acknowledge is that individual choices are very sensitive to social context, including norms and values, as is illustrated by the fact that the vast majority of prenatal diagnoses and selective abortions worldwide are carried out, not to prevent serious disorders, but to prevent the birth of females.

Few of those who have gone through prenatal diagnosis followed by a second trimester abortion, or even those whose test results have been favorable, would compare this process, as Singer does, to more genuinely preventive measures for protecting the fetus, such as avoiding ingestion of toxic substances. Preventing a problem is not the same as preventing a person. Prenatal diagnosis is not a benign procedure. It disrupts the normal psychological process of pregnancy (as Rothman has shown),[1] requires vast medical resources, and even causes the loss of some normal fetuses.

Singer has ignored my major point, which is that those of us who participate in medical or policy arenas must question where this strategy of avoiding human imperfection is leading us. We must step back and look at the expanding range of qualities that can be predicted before birth. When we encourage placing many more prospective parents in the position of deciding which characteristics in a fetus are acceptable and which render it unworthy of being born, where are we really going? Wouldn't we be better off in the long run directing some of these vast resources into broader strategies for preventing disease and disability that are consistent with an ethic of caring, rather than following the chimera of human perfectibility?

NOTE

1. Rothman BK. *The Tentative Pregnancy: Prenatal Diagnosis and the Future of Motherhood.* New York: Viking, 1986.

☷ ䷀ ䷀ ☷

ERIK PARENS, PHD AND THOMAS H. MURRAY, PHD

Preimplantation Genetic Diagnosis: Beginning a Long Conversation

Preimplantation genetic diagnosis (PGD) was first described in 1989 as a means to help couples who carry disease-related mutations avoid creating babies with those diseases. The first step in performing PGD is to create embryos by in vitro fertilization. After two or three days, the embryos have cleaved into six to eight cells. One or two of those cells are removed and their DNA is amplified by the method known as polymerase chain reaction, or PCR. The DNA is then analyzed to ascertain which embryos carry, and which are free from, the disease-related mutations. Only those without the mutation are considered for implantation.[1]

This "embryo biopsy" has thus far appeared to be without short-term adverse physical effects—though, as an editorialist in *The Lancet* observed, "it is too early to exclude the possibility of later effects."[2] Cystic fibrosis, Tay-Sachs disease, sickle cell anemia, the thalassemias, phenylketonuria, spinal muscular atrophy, and myotonic dystrophy are among the disorders that have been analyzed with PGD thus far.[3]

The answer to the first ethical question in PGD turns on what one thinks about the moral status of a human embryo. If you regard embryos as having the same moral status as all other persons, then no form of PGD will be ethically acceptable for the simple fact that it entails destroying embryos—albeit embryos with mutations that cause severe, typically life-threatening, diseases. If instead you think that embryos, while they deserve respect, do not have identical moral status to, for example, children or adults, then the moral status of embryos will not be an insurmountable barrier to using PGD (or to using in vitro fertilization in general).

While the embryo's moral status may be the first ethical question, it is by no means the only one. People who do not object to in vitro fertilization may nonetheless have deep concerns about some possible uses of PGD. Although the line between acceptable and unacceptable purposes may never be bright or universally recognized, it is our responsibility, as citizens and as stewards of this technology, to try to articulate what divides ethically acceptable uses from those that are not.

Two kinds of reasons are usually offered to support the use of PGD to select against disease-related traits. The first kind has to do with avoiding the burdens associated with disease. That kind of reason can be expressed in terms of avoiding the harm to the person who would live with the trait, to the family of the person who would live with the trait, or to the society in which that person would live. That sort of reason will be well known to anyone familiar with the justification of prenatal genetic diagnosis and selective abortion,[4] which brings us to the second reason offered in support of PGD: it circumvents the psychological anguish and physical danger that accompanies selective abortion.

When many people imagine the ethically acceptable use of PGD, they have in mind a loving and healthy couple who wants to avoid having a child with a lethal disease. Tay-Sachs is often the example of choice. But PGD, of course, can be used for other, morally more complex, purposes. Two cases begin to make some of that complexity vivid.

The first case involves researchers helping a couple to have a child who would not be affected by early-onset Alzheimer's disease. In fact, it was the genetic profile of the mother—not the embryo—that put this case on the front page of major US papers. The prospective mother, who used PGD to create a child when she was 30, lost her own father to early-onset Alzheimer's when he was 42. It is likely that this child produced by PGD will, when she is still young, watch her own mother sink into dementia and die.[5]

It would be a better world if no young child ever had to live through the death of a parent; but, unfortunately, many children do. In this particular, real case, the couple thought exhaustively about the ramifications of their actions. Their genetic counselor told a *Time* magazine reporter that this couple was "10 times more thoughtful about what they chose to do than other people who have children."[6] Perhaps effective treatments will be found to keep dementia at bay; the child's father, presumably, is fully committed to loving and raising his daughter whatever happens to his wife. The child, in any event, will be spared the fate that struck down her ancestors.

Nonetheless, this case points to a larger question that we cannot continue to avoid. To what extent should medical professionals or the state become involved in attempting to protect the well-being of children produced by techniques like PGD? In this case, the parents were both thoughtful and loving. What if they hadn't been? Should professionals or the state have said no, as they do in adoption cases where the child's well-being is thought to be in jeopardy? On the one hand, we have reason to worry about professionals or the state becoming involved in such intimate and important decisions. On the other, leaving such decisions to the market alone has its own perils.

The second case involving PGD raises further questions, not only about the well-being of children, but about the nature of the society in which those children will grow up. Molly Nash was born with Fanconi anemia, a serious and eventually lethal blood disorder. When Molly's parents decided to have a second child with the help of PGD, they wanted that child to be free of anemia. They also decided to select an embryo that would be HLA (human leukocyte antigen) compatible with Molly—and thus a suitable cord blood donor. At first blush this case might appear to violate Immanuel Kant's famous dictum that a person should never be treated solely as a means, but always also as an end in himself or herself.[7] The "solely" is key here. All of the available evidence suggested that this child's parents—Adam is his name—would love and raise him with the same devotion they give Molly. So, yes, in one sense Adam is a means to help his sister Molly; but he is also valued—and loved—as an end in himself.

Although Adam Nash's parents had solid ethical reasons to use PGD as they did, nonetheless the Nash case is the first widely published use of PGD to select embryos based on a trait that was not pertinent to the health of the child that embryo would become. The clinician-researchers not only selected against Fanconi anemia, they also selected for a particular HLA haplotype.[8] That Adam had immune system markers similar to Molly was important for her health, but not to Adam's. It does not require Stephen King's baroque imagination to foresee a time when it will be possible to test for traits that have nothing to do with the health of either a tissue recipient or the person being created.

We must begin now to think about the prospect of using PGD to select for non-health-related traits, or, more colloquially, "enhancements." The relationship between genes and complex traits such as stature or intelligence is itself so complex that it may never be possible to predict precisely which set of genes will yield which traits. Nonetheless, given human nature, and the entrepreneurial spirit of some scientists and clinicians, we can soon expect to find professionals promoting PGD as a means to improve a couple's chances of having a child with some desired trait, as well as couples eager to purchase those services. One of the most important questions we face is what, if anything, is ethically problematic about selecting for such non-health-related traits or "enhancements"? After all, as individuals and a society we invest huge amounts of social resources to improve or "enhance" our offspring.[9] We believe that there are serious ethical concerns raised when PGD is used to attempt to genetically "enhance" children. We take each of these key concepts in turn.

The first concern regards using genetic means to try to enhance children. The worry here is that focusing on genetics would exacerbate a tendency in our culture to understand human beings in mechanistic terms. So even if we might welcome being treated "mechanistically" if our leg breaks or our heart stops, we might nonetheless want to resist vigorously the tendency to let the mechanistic understanding permeate all aspects of our lives.

The second concern regards using genetic technology to try to enhance children. If we assume for the moment that access to such enhancements will be unequal, perhaps left to the market, then we should worry about fairness: parents with access to resources could purchase the increased chances that their children will have traits that will enable them to be still stronger competitors for scarce resources, increasing further the gap between those who have much and those who have little.

If, instead, we assume equal access to "enhancements," we still will need to grapple with, among others, the problem of complicity with suspect norms.[10] For example, would it be acceptable to offer parents the option to select for the embryo with the greatest chance of becoming tall? In a society that favors tall people, parents might view PGD as a way to give their children the advantages that go with being tall. Using PGD for that purpose means bowing to—and thus becoming complicit with—the unjust norm of heightism. Do we want to live in a society that would sooner change the bodies of individuals than change the unjust and unjustifiable attitudes that give rise to the desire change those bodies? The third concern regards what it will mean to use genetic technology to try to enhance children. Would using PGD for the sake of enhancement exacerbate the tendency of parents to have unrealistic expectations of their children? Note: there is nothing new about this tendency. The question is, will PGD exacerbate it, and if it did, what would that mean for the well-being of children—and for parents?

The questions raised by PGD do not have easy answers. If anything, their difficulty reflects their complexity and significance. We are at the beginning of what will be a very long, important, and interesting conversation.

NOTES

1. Elias S. Preimplantation genetic diagnosis by comparative genomic hybridization. *N Engl J Med* 2001;345:1569–71.

2. [Editorial] Preimplantation donor selection. *Lancet* 2001;358:1195.

3. Elias S. Preimplantation genetic diagnosis by comparative genomic hybridization. *N Engl J Med* 2001;345:1569–71.

4. Parens E, Asch A (eds). *Prenatal Testing and Disability Rights.* Washington, DC: Georgetown University Press, 2000.

5. Towner D, Loewy, RS. Ethics of preimplantation diagnosis for a woman destined to develop early-onset Alzheimer's disease. *JAMA* 2002;287:1038–40.

6. Gibbs N. Dying to have a family. *Time* March 11, 2002:78.

7. Murray T. *The Worth of a Child.* Berkeley and Los Angeles: University of California Press, 1996.

8. Verlinsky Y, Rechitsky S, Verlinsky O, Masciangelo C, Lederer K, Kuliev A. Preimplantation diagnosis for Fanconi anemia combined with HLA matching. *JAMA* 2001;285:3130–3.

9. Buchanan A, Brock D, Daniels N, Wickler D. *From Chance to Choice: Genetics and Justice.* Cambridge: Cambridge University Press, 2000.

10. Little M. Cosmetic surgery, suspect norms, and the ethics of complicity. In Parens E (ed): *Enhancing Human Traits.* Washington, DC: Georgetown University Press, 1998.

☰ ☷ ☷ ☰

PAUL LAURITZEN, PHD

Heating Up the Conversation?

In his new book, *Our Posthuman Future: Consequences of the Biotechnology Revolution,* Francis Fukuyama suggests that there were two great dystopias of the 20th century, Orwell's *1984* and Huxley's *Brave New World.* Of the two, says Fukuyama, only Huxley's vision continues to haunt us. One reason is clear: the effects of the computer revolution and the emergence of the Internet have not had the sinister effect that Orwell might have predicted. On the contrary, if anything, these developments have undermined rather than strengthened totalitarian regimes. But how do we explain the enduring quality of Huxley's vision? According to Fukuyama, one reason that Huxley's vision always was, and continues to be, more worrisome than Orwell's, is precisely that, in Huxley's world, no one is obviously harmed.

I thought of Fukuyama's observations when reading the reflections on preimplantation genetic diagnosis (PGD) by Erik Parens and Thomas H. Murray. The authors wish to start a conversation on embryo screening by raising an important series of cautionary questions about PGD. Should decisions about PGD be left exclusively to the marketplace? Do medical professionals have a responsibility to consider the impact of PGD on the lives of the children who will be created using these techniques?

Is using PGD to select for so-called enhancement traits ethically acceptable? What kind of society will we create if we allow PGD to become widespread? These are all important questions, but one can almost hear the procreative entrepreneurs of reproductive medicine complaining to Parens and Murray: "But where's the harm?" The children wouldn't exist without in vitro fertilization; how is anyone harmed by selecting one embryo rather than another in the lab?

We are indebted to Parens and Murray, not to mention Aldous Huxley, for reminding us that sometimes we are harmed when we least suspect it. That is the real threat of PGD. It is hard to argue that screening an eight-cell organism to avoid the pain and suffering associated with, for example, Tay-Sachs disease is morally wrong. Yet, it is a short step from the paradigm cases that support using PGD to other more problematic cases, so short that we may fail to notice that we have crossed an important moral threshold. Consider, for example, the case cited by Parens and Murray, of the couple who used PGD to screen embryos to create a child who would not carry the gene for early-onset Alzheimer's, a disease from which the mother is likely to die before her made-to-order child is 10 years old.

In one sense, using PGD to screen against the gene for early-onset Alzheimer's is like using PGD to screen against Tay-Sachs disease. Both diseases are devastating and in both cases the motive for screening may well be one of beneficence. Still, as Parens and Murray properly ask: What about the child? Unfortunately, many fail to ask that question—or see it as secondary—when evaluating PGD. For example, writing in *The Wall Street Journal,* Jerome Groopman had little patience with the reservations raised by physicians and ethicists about screening in the case of early-onset Alzheimer's.[1] The fact that we are knowingly creating a child using PGD who will almost certainly have to watch her mother succumb to dementia and die seemed of little concern. To be sure, the couple in this case could have conceived a child without using PGD, so we cannot blame the PGD for the creation of a child whom we know will suffer. Still, the issue here is not merely what responsibility parents have in considering whether to procreate, but what responsibility physicians have in helping prospective parents pursue their desires. According to Groopman, however, only the parents' choice really matters. Those who would oppose the use of PGD in a case like this, Groopman wrote derisively, "do so primarily because of religious beliefs . . ."

Nowhere in their essay do Parens and Murray appeal to religious beliefs to oppose the use of PGD, but they do raise serious moral reservations about the growing and unqualified acceptance of PGD. Indeed, they seek to draw a line between acceptable and unacceptable uses of this technology. Specifically, they appear to endorse a distinction between using PGD to screen for health-related traits and screening for non-health-related traits.

I agree with Parens and Murray that we need to draw a distinction between treatment and enhancement, but a full moral discussion of PGD needs to be much more expansive than a focus on this distinction will permit. Notice, for example, that screening for the gene for early onset Alzheimer's is in fact screening for a health-related trait. Yet classifying this use of PGD as treatment related rather than enhancement related is hardly the end of the matter morally.

I am not, of course, suggesting that Parens and Murray would disagree with me about the need for expanding the framework in which we discuss PGD. Indeed, Thomas Murray has recently argued persuasively that almost all of the current debates about the ethics of reproductive technology are too narrowly focused on the theme of procreative liberty.[2] I certainly agree with Murray that, like so many other debates in bioethics these days, the terms of the argument about reproductive technology are too cramped. While autonomy is an important value, it is not the only or even the most important value.

Of course, the specific provenance of the framework of procreative liberty is a commitment to autonomy read through constitutional law. Essentially the reasoning behind the appeal to procreative liberty is as follows. Given that the Supreme Court has recognized a right not to procreate in its decisions upholding a liberty interest in contraception and abortion, it would likely recognize a right to procreate. If there is a right to procreate, the only reason to interfere with the exercise of that right would be to prevent direct harm to another. Because it is nearly impossible to harm someone by bringing him into existence, almost every restriction on reproductive choice, including the choice to use PGD for almost any purpose, is prohibited.

Just how impoverished the framework of procreative liberty is can be seen by considering how it would handle a variation of the second case discussed by Parens and Murray, that of the Nashes. As Parens and Murray explain, Molly Nash inherited Fanconi anemia from her parents. Hoping to avoid the same fate for their second child and seeking a good donor match for Molly, the parents conceived a second child using PGD to screen for embryos that would be HLA compatible with Molly and thus a good cord blood donor.

By all accounts, the Nashes were always committed to their second child and there was every reason to believe that they would love and cherish him. Yet, what if that were not the case? What if the parents decided to have a child merely to serve as a stem cell donor, with no intention to raise and care for the child? How would the framework of procreative liberty approach such a case?

For anyone who has read the work of John Robertson, the most well-known advocate of the procreative liberty approach, the answer is not reassuring. Indeed, recently Robertson and two colleagues, Jeffrey Kahn and John Wagner, have written about precisely this issue.[3] "As objectionable as such an action seems," they write, ". . . it is not clear that the parents have actually harmed the child, nor that they should legally be stopped from doing so." Although some people may apparently react badly to the prospect of creating children without any thought to their care, there are no moral grounds for opposing this practice and no legal grounds for prohibiting it. After all, nobody has been harmed.

Because I find the analysis of PGD offered by the framework of procreative liberty both wholly inadequate and disturbing, I very much welcome the thoughtful reflection on PGD offered by Parens and Murray. In the final analysis, however, I find their reservations too tepid and too restrained. I suppose that what I would like to hear from them is the kind of alarm Tom Wolfe sounds in his book *Hooking Up*, after exploring contemporary research on brain imaging technology and neuroscience. Noting the uncompromising determinism of the neuroscientific view of life, Wolfe wonders whether the notion of a self can survive in a world in which neuroradiologists can read a random list of words to a patient hooked up to a PET scan and see specific areas of the cerebral cortex light up when the radiologist hits a topic of interest to the patient. Wolfe's essay, entitled, "Sorry, but Your Soul Just Died," conveys the sense of urgency that he believes this technology ought to evoke.

I would not go so far as to say that we are about to lose our souls by embracing PGD. There are clearly uses of PGD that are morally acceptable, and it is certainly the case that most uses of the technology have so far been health related and designed to prevent pain and suffering. Nevertheless, it is perhaps worth noting that even in the highly secularized world of reproductive medicine, the road to hell is still paved with good intentions.

NOTES

1. Groopman J. Designing babies. *The Wall Street Journal* March 4, 2002.

2. Murray TH. What are families for? Getting to an ethics of reproductive technology. *Hastings Cent Rep* 2002;32(3):41–5.

3. Robertson JA, Kahn JP, Wagner E. Conception to obtain hematopoietic stem cells. *Hastings Cent Rep* 2002; 32(3):34–40.

MORAL RULES AND TECHNOLOGY

THE EDITORS

Paul Lauritzen implies criticism when he speaks of "creating a child who will almost certainly have to watch her mother succumb to dementia and die." He doesn't tell us whether this concern is relevant only when technology is used to make babies or whether he believes that women destined with high probability to have early-onset dementia should also not have children even when that is possible by natural means. If the use of technology produces an undesirable end, should producing the same end by natural means also be considered undesirable? Should the moral rules for having babies be different when technology is used?

REPLY BY PAUL LAURITZEN, PHD

The editors ask whether my implied criticism of creating a child whom we know will watch her mother die applies only when technology is needed to conceive or whether it also applies to conceiving naturally in such circumstances.

They have properly called me to task on this point because I intentionally attempted to sidestep this question in my response to Parens and Murray by focusing on the responsibility of physicians who assist couples to procreate rather than on the couples themselves. However, having now had my hand forced, my answer is that, of course, couples who conceive naturally must be every bit as concerned about the welfare of the child they conceive as couples who use assisted reproduction. Unfettered autonomy is no more to be encouraged among those who do not use assisted reproduction than it is among those who do. Whether in any individual case a couple should refrain from procreation will, of course, be highly contested, but if procreation is a bad idea when technology such as PGD is used, it is likely to be a bad idea without the technology as well.

A MEANINGLESS IMPLICATION?

PAUL J. REITEMEIER, PHD

Paul Lauritzen notes that some commentators make claims to the effect that "... it is nearly impossible to harm someone by bringing him into existence." Such claims do not need the qualifier "nearly" because the subject of the act of "bringing someone into existence" cannot already exist.

It is impossible to harm an entity that doesn't exist. Moreover, courts consistently dismiss wrongful life suits on the grounds that, while a damaged life has some value, nonexistence can have no value for there is no subject, or value holder.

☰ ☷ ☶ ☰

ERIC T. JUENGST, PHD

Genetic Enhancement: A Conceptual and Ethical Challenge for Gene Therapy Regulation

One of the fruits of the "genetic revolution" in biomedicine has been the ability to splice functional genes into the DNA of human cells to produce stable changes in the bodies of patients. The use of these "human gene transfer" techniques to treat genetic disease has been widely endorsed, as long as two lines are not crossed: no changes are made that would be passed on to the patient's children; and no attempts are made to exceed restoration of the normal, that is, to "genetically enhance" human traits like stamina, strength, beauty, memory, or intelligence. This second boundary is particularly interesting, because it captures an important moral intuition and, at the same time, is at constant risk of collapsing under the weight of basic conceptual arguments. If the boundary between gene therapy and genetic enhancement is to serve as a useful line for policy, we should be clear about what it is demarcating.

TREATMENT-ENHANCEMENT DISTINCTIONS

The treatment-enhancement distinction is often employed to argue that therapeutic uses of genetic engineering fall within the boundaries of medicine's traditional domain, while enhancement uses do not, and therefore are more problematic.[1]

There are several interesting rejoinders to this argument. Some argue that medicine has no essential domain of practice, so that a coherent distinction between medical and non-medical services never can be drawn in the first place. Others accept the distinction between treating and enhancing, but challenge the traditional values of medicine by arguing that privileging treatment over enhancement is itself wrong. Others argue that, in any case, for psychological and economic reasons, the line between treatment and enhancement will be impossible to hold in practice.[2]

There is another response to the distinction between treatment and enhancement, however, that is particularly relevant to gene transfer research. This response criticizes the distinction by showing how it dissolves in the use of human gene transfer techniques to *prevent* disease when such interventions involve the enhancement of the body's health maintenance capacities. For example, many new cancer protocols involve transferring genes that improve the ability of the human immune system to detect cancer cells, while other gene therapies already give their recipients better than normal abilities to lower cholesterol levels. To the extent that disease prevention is a proper goal of medicine, and the use of gene transfer techniques to enhance human health maintenance capacities will help achieve that goal, critics ask, how can we claim that we should be "drawing the line" at enhancement?

There have been a number of attempts to explain how the concept of "enhancement" can function as a boundary for medical practice and still include legitimate forms of preventive medicine. Some argue that any intervention designed to restore or preserve a "species typical" level of functioning should count as treatment, leaving only interventions that would create capabilities beyond the range of normal human variation to count as "enhancement." Others attempt to draw the line between interventions for diagnosable pathologies and those aimed at improvements unrelated to the individual's health.[3] All of these efforts, however, face a fundamental practical challenge: no matter how the line is drawn, most of the gene transfer interventions that could become problematic as enhancement interventions would not have to cross that line in order to be developed and approved for clinical use. Most gene transfer protocols with potential for enhancement uses first will emerge as therapeutic agents. Memory, intelligence, and other cognitive enhancement interventions, for example, are likely to be approved for use only in patients with neurological diseases. However, to the extent that they are in high demand by individuals who are merely suffering the effects of normal aging or want to increase their IQ, the risk of unapproved or "off-label" uses of these products will be high.

These realities press us to articulate the moral dangers of genetic enhancement more clearly. After all, personal improvement is praised in many spheres of human endeavor, and interventions such as cosmetic surgery are well accepted in our society as means of achieving personal improvement goals. Why should "genetic enhancement" mark a boundary for medicine?

ENHANCEMENT AS A FORM OF CHEATING

The idea has emerged that genetic enhancements are a form of social cheating. This is the view that taking a biomedical shortcut erodes the social practices that make the human achievement valuable in the first place. Thus, some argue that it defeats the purpose of the contest if the marathon runner gains endurance chemically rather than through training, and it misses the point of meditation to gain Nirvana through psychosurgery. In both cases, the achievements—successful training or disciplined meditation—add value to the improvements because they are understood to be admirable social practices in themselves. To the extent that biomedical shortcuts increasingly allow specific accomplishments to be divorced from admirable practices, the social value of those accomplishments— the runner's physical endurance or the mystic's visions—will be undermined. Not only will the intrinsic value be diminished for everyone who takes the shortcut, but the resulting disparity between the enhanced and unenhanced will call into question the fairness of the game. A runner genetically enhanced for endurance will hardly be a fair match for his genetically unenhanced competitor. For institutions interested in continuing to foster the social values for which they have been the guardians, this point has two ethically equivalent implications. Either they must redesign the game to evaluate excellence in admirable practices that are not affected by biomedical enhancements, or they must prohibit the use of the enhancing shortcuts.

ENHANCEMENT AS AN ABUSE OF MEDICINE

Unfortunately, some social practices, such as stigmatization and discrimination, are based on traits over which individuals have little control: skin color, stature, or physical ability. It is becoming increasingly possible to seek biomedical help in changing these traits with skin lighteners, growth hormone, and other enhancements to improve the recipient's social standing. Unfortunately, this only perpetuates the social bias under which they originally labored. When "enhancement" is understood in this way, as an attempt to use medicine to conform to unjust social norms, it warns of still another set of moral concerns.

What makes providing human growth hormone to a normally short child morally suspicious is not the absence of a diagnosable disease or the "species-atypical" hormone level that would result: rather it is the intent to improve the child's social status by changing the child rather than by changing the social environment. This is a moral mistake akin to "blaming the victim": it misdirects medical attention in an ultimately self-defeating way. For those faced with decisions about whether to attempt to enhance themselves or their children through gene transfer, this concept points to the real challenge: whether or not to collude in the injustice they are seeking to avoid.

CONCLUSION

The "enhancements" we envision in these discussions may never become technically possible: most of the interesting ones—intelligence, memory, beauty, stamina, strength—are complex traits influenced only remotely by many of our genes in collaboration. In practice, we may never have to worry about crossing the enhancement line towards those improvements. On the other hand, if we do, the issues raised by the "enhancement" concept will have to be addressed in policy. In doing so, three features of the genetic enhancement's regulatory environment will pose special challenges: the problem of "off-label" uses of interventions approved for therapeutic use, the entrepreneurial ethos of contemporary medicine, and the prospect of international access to enhancement where regulatory limits in the United States could be ineffectual. Each of these are social policy problems that have received negligible attention, but which will become increasingly crucial to address as genomic medicine matures.

NOTES

1. Anderson WF. Human gene therapy: Why draw a line? *J Med Philos* 1989;14:681–93.

2. Parens E. Is better always good? *Hastings Cent Rep* 1998;28(1):S1-S17.

3. Juengst E. Can enhancement be distinguished from prevention in genetic medicine? *J Med Philos* 1997;22:125–42.

☰ ☷ ☷ ☰

GLENN MCGEE, PHD

Genetic Enhancement

In his article on the problem of genetic enhancement, Eric Juengst points out that any attempt to describe and maintain a formal distinction between medical treatment and enhancement of human capacity will be riddled with philosophical and practical problems. So many of medicine's most important techniques blur the line between prevention and intervention, or between what is necessary and merely desirable, that any distinction between treatment and enhancement will necessarily rely on the values and judgment of medical institutions and the marketplace. For this and other reasons I agree with Juengst that the attempt to define a "species-typical" account of human flourishing may be doomed to the drawing board. There is too, an emerging consensus in bioethics that genetic enhancement is particularly problematic, both because genetic modifications seem so fundamental, and because germ line genetic enhancements might effect changes that could be passed to future generations.[1,2]

Juengst correctly intuits that medical and government institutions will be urged by state financial exigency and, in some cases, social pressure to identify some distinction between appropriate and inappropriate uses of genetic technology to improve human capacity. He suggests two possible problems: enhancements that defeat the purpose of the affected activities, such as an enhancement that increases a runner's endurance, or enhancements that treat the victim of some social problem rather than treating the social problem. I do not take issue with Juengst's description of these potential problems.

My purpose here is to ask a broader question: is specific policy on enhancement an important goal? It is frequently the case in the discussion of genetic technology by bioethicists that the debate begins and ends with what is to be permitted by the government. It is plain, though, that where genetic and reproductive services are concerned, legislation to prohibit or encourage behaviors is not only lacking, but is also the least important feature in the utilization of these technologies. A distinction between treatment and enhancement, or any cousin distinction aimed at a similar purpose, is likely to fail in large part because the public does not suffer such strong governmental intrusions, and because the U.S. Constitution is all but designed to prevent them.

The broad public fear is not that people might become exceptionally gifted, or cheat, or destroy their institutions through genetic enhancement. Instead, the fear of genetic enhancement reflects a broad sense that society is developing technologies that appeal to our more base desires, without simultaneously developing a dialogue about how to use those technologies responsibly. It seems to me that the focus in enhancement technologies has to be on developing institutional wisdom about how enhancements fit in to broader, pre-existing questions about how human beings can best flourish.

The agenda for a public debate of genetic enhancement is not really a genetics agenda at all. I have argued that the dangers of parental genetic enhancement are not related to how enhancements differ from "non-enhancement," but rather are related to broader social dangers faced by human beings any time they attempt to better their offspring. In particular, I focused on the dangers of calculativeness (emphasizing narrow, artificially defined traits), overbearingness (stylizing children along the lines of rigid parental expectation), shortsightedness (locking in the wrong traits in a changing world), hasty judgment (creating unexpected and disastrous ills), and pessimism (feeling the need to search for an exotic ethics of enhancement).

My purpose here is to highlight the fact that any exploration of enhancement must begin, not with the technology involved, but rather with the matrix in which people use that enhancement to solve problems or improve their lives. Parenthood is laced with the desire to enhance the experience and capacity of child and parent alike; any new technology must be situated in that context. Enhancements of adults in various situations play similarly complex roles: young people seeking cosmetic enhancement, aging people seeking enhanced sexual capacity, and generals seeking stronger soldiers each bring relevantly different contexts to the table. In only some of these situations will the moral issue be "cheating." Many times the moral issue in enhancement is really about other and more broad questions: Would tennis be a better game if everyone who plays could hit harder? Would life really be better for a society that could uniformly increase memory and intelligence?

The next step in the enhancement debate is to turn our creative attention toward the philosophical problem of refining our ideas about what it means to flourish in the various arenas where enhancement may become possible. No government policy can help with that.

NOTES

1. Parens E. Is better always good? *Hastings Cent Rep* 1998;28(1):S-1-S-17.
2. McGee G. Parenting in an era of genetics. *Hastings Cent Rep* 1997;27(2): 16–22.

REPLY BY ERIC T. JUENGST, PHD

Glenn McGee does the discussion a service by reminding us that, in the final analysis, the problem of "genetic enhancement" is not so much a challenge to public policy as it is to public attitudes. It is the ethics of parenting and self-improvement, not the moral boundaries of professional medicine, that drives the issue and deserves the attention of more "sermons and self-help books"—or even more ethical analysis! And since the "enhancement" flag does seem to warn of so many different moral shoals, from parental short-sightedness to social prejudice, it would be silly to enshrine one of its uses in public policy and too draconian to try to cover them all. Nevertheless, there is an analogy here to the practice of gene transfer research itself. Most would agree that best strategies for combating heart disease, cancer, and AIDS are preventive: "sermons and self-help" designed to forestall the problems before they fulminate. But there is still room for research attempting to develop treatments for those already sick, such as gene therapies.

By analogy, public policy-makers will be faced with the need to develop policies addressing the availability and use of fulminating "enhancement" technologies, even while the broader public discussion of human flourishing proceeds. My purpose was to illustrate the challenges policy makers will face in that task, regardless of whether the resulting policies are permissive (e.g., provide any enhancements on demand as part of a fair, client-centered, health plan) or restrictive (e.g., limit certain enhancements to those who can pay for them out of pocket at private offshore clinics).

☰ ☷ ☷ ☰

DAVID MAGNUS, PHD

Genetically Modified Organisms

Debate among policy makers and experts about genetically modified organisms has tended to frame the issue in terms of risks and benefits; this circumscribes the role of values in the debate and transforms the issue into a largely scientific one that should be restricted to experts. Scientists tell us what the benefits and risks are and whether the new technology is worthwhile. Critics often respond by noting that values can play at least some role even within this framework. The questions of how much risk is too much, what sorts of benefits are worthwhile and to what extent are they valued, and, above all, how much uncertainty is acceptable are all issues that allow values to be introduced. Even so, the role of values is fairly limited in this way of framing debates.

There is little doubt that the creation of genetically modified organisms can offer many advantages. Current genetically modified organisms have included crops that are largely of benefit to farmers and are not clearly of broad public value. That situation will soon change as future genetically modified organisms will include: foods that have far greater nutritional benefit, crops that can grow in regions with poor soil that currently cannot support subsistence agriculture, cattle whose milk offers pharmaceutical benefit, foods that are more desirable in terms of traits that the public wants (e.g., Brussels sprouts that taste like chocolate). The market forces that largely determine which of these products are developed are complicated. For example, the traits that may be needed to feed a starving world are different than the traits that farmers in the US want, and both may differ from the characteristics that the paying public supports.

Most criticisms have focused on two issues. First, there is concern about food safety. What impact will genetically modified organisms have on the health of those who eat them? The new technology makes it possible to cross species barriers with impunity. Will a shellfish gene placed in a tomato cause allergic reactions? The recent scare over StarLink corn is instructive. "Bt corn," a common genetically modified organism, includes a gene from Bacillus thuringiensis, which produces a pesticide that kills the European corn borer. One of the problems with Bt corn is that it is likely that insects will soon develop resistance. StarLink is a new variation of Bt that includes a protein, Cry9C, that does not break down as easily in the body. It may therefore postpone resistance. However, it also has some characteristics of food allergens.

The fact that it will remain in the body longer increases the risk of allergic reactions (though there are no verified cases). StarLink corn was approved for animal feed, but not for human consumption. It is difficult, if not impossible, to keep the food supply for animals and humans separate. The feed is often in the same silos and at least some of the corn from one field can send seed to another.

The result has been the discovery of small amounts of StarLink corn throughout the food supply. In addition to allergic reactions, some critics worry that each new generation of pesticide-producing genetically modified organisms could lead to a buildup of harmful poisons in the body that might, for example, cause mutations or cancer.

A second set of concerns focuses on the environmental impact. First, there are worries about gene flow—the movement of genes from one population to another. The same genes that may one day make it possible for plants to grow in poor, salty soil or in relatively arid regions could create an ecological nightmare if they should be introduced to other plants. This can happen through interbreeding between genetically modified plants and plants from different but closely related species (out-crossing). For example, genetically modified wheat could cross with native grasses in South America to alter the makeup of the ecosystem and potentially create "super weeds." Even in the absence of gene flow, the genetically modified organisms themselves could become super weeds as a result of the traits that make them better suited to new habitats.

Another environmental trade-off for technology that makes it possible to produce sustainable agriculture in regions where it cannot "naturally" flourish is a significant risk of loss of biodiversity (a desirable seed is likely to be planted over millions of acres leading to monoagriculture) and the unchecked spread of plants into unintended regions. In addition to these concerns over the ecosystem and the creations of super weeds, there is a worry over the potential impact of some genetically modified organisms on non-target organisms. Cornell University researchers found that pollen from Bt corn could kill the larvae of monarch butterflies who ingested it. This raised the fear that these engineered crops could kill butterflies and other non-target organisms. The result of subsequent field research to determine whether Bt corn really represents such a threat outside the laboratory have been mixed.

Similarly, creating genetically modified animals and fish could lead to problems. Genetically engineered salmon could lead to the widespread introduction of new genes into wild fish runs. If the genes spread sufficiently (the very large number of fish normally introduced to rivers from "fish farms" tend to swamp the relatively smaller number of "wild" fish), they could introduce new vulnerabilities to disease and create unanticipated problems. The problem of "killer bees" was a result of laboratory organisms that escaped into the wild. Genetically modified mice and other mammals could create pests that will be much more difficult to eliminate.

Genetically engineered microorganisms present even greater environmental and health concerns. It will soon be possible to engineer bacteria and viruses to produce deadly pathogens. This could well open a new era in biological weapons in addition to the environmental problems that could result from the release of organisms into the environment. It has been a number of years since the Supreme Court allowed the patenting of genetically modified bacterium that could eat oil. The environmental assessment of the widespread introduction of engineered microorganisms has only barely begun to receive attention.[1]

There are inadequacies in the regulatory framework that exists for genetically modified organisms. The present system is quite complex—organisms that have been modified to give off a pesticide fall under the jurisdiction of the Environmental Protection Agency (EPA), while an organism produced to express a gene to provide a nutritional benefit falls under the Food and Drug Administration (FDA). There is a growing sense that the FDA, Department of Agriculture, and EPA are not sufficiently rigorous or consistent in how they regulate genetically modified organisms and that there should be a single set of standards that more closely resembles the way the FDA handles drug development. The single most important factor for the differences between European and American attitudes in this matter (there is much more widespread opposition in Europe) is the amount of confidence in the regulatory institutions that protect the food supply. After "mad cow disease," Europeans do not trust their governments to provide safe food. A similar loss in confidence among US consumers could have a similar effect.

There is much that can be said about the arguments in favor and against each potential risk and benefit. However, this way of framing the issue is not the way people seem to think about genetically modified organisms (or biotechnology generally). There seems to be a moral and even religious aspect to this debate that may be more important than a simple risk and benefit analysis can capture. When a sheep named Dolly was cloned from an adult cell, the widespread hysteria over cloning had very little to do with any analysis of the risks and benefits of the technology. Rather, there was a clear sense of "moral repugnance" that was expressed in a variety of ways. Similarly there is evidence that the fundamental framing of the genetically modified organism issue is in similar terms (and in fact is a related response). The term "Frankenfoods" suggests the modern Promethean myth—human hubris in the pursuit of knowledge can lead to our own unwitting destruction. Talk of "playing God" permeates and underlies the genetically modified organism debate just as it does the cloning controversy.[2] Indeed there is at least some empirical evidence to back up the claim that people are primarily motivated by moral concerns when they oppose genetically modified organisms Those who think in terms of risks and benefits tend to be at least cautious supporters of the technology.[3]

Leon Kass and others have argued that, in the context of cloning, we should give great weight to the moral repugnance of the public.[4] On this view, the visceral response is either significant for its own sake or, at a minimum, a way of capturing a whole set of objections that are difficult to articulate but clearly perceived. On the other hand, there are those who object to this type of concern as irrational. This type of visceral response tends to be ephemeral—as people become used to the technology, the concern dissipates. On this view, concern over "playing God" is nothing more than prejudice against the new and unfamiliar.[5]

I would argue that the truth lies in between these two views. Clearly, it is a mistake to think that a sense of moral repugnance or anxiety is sufficient to end debate. However, it is not irrelevant to the debate either. Analysis of these moral concerns and using them as a way to frame issues may be useful in a way that a simple risk-benefit analysis will miss. For example, an important source of concern is not merely risk, but such questions as, who is exposed to the risk? Who has the power to make decisions about that risk? Is the scientific community accountable to the public? These and other questions must be addressed as central to debates over genetically modified organisms. The sources of moral concern must be explored and addressed if we are to move forward with a technology that offers both promise and pitfall.

NOTES

1. Cho MK, Magnus D, Caplan AL, McGee D. Policy forum: genetics. Ethical considerations in synthesizing a minimal genome. *Science* 1999;286:2087–90.

2. Pollan M. Playing God. *The NY Times Magazine,* Oct. 25, 1998.

3. Gaskell G, Bauer MW, Durant J, Allum NC. Worlds apart? The reception of genetically modified foods in Europe and the U.S. *Science* 1999;285:384–7.

4. Kass LR, Wilson JQ. *The Ethics of Human Cloning.* Washington, DC:AEI Press, 1998.

5. Pence GE. *Who's Afraid of Human Cloning?* Lanham, MD: Rowman and Littlefield, 1998.

☰ ☷ ☷ ☰

DANIEL CALLAHAN, PHD

Reason and Repugnance

David Magnus is correct and sensitive in concluding that while "it is a mistake to think that a sense of moral repugnance or anxiety is sufficient to end debate" … "it is not irrelevant to the debate either." We are, after all, creatures of feeling and reason. The problem is to know how to use reason to evaluate emotion and no less to know how to pay attention to our emotions when they challenge our reasoning. John Rawls has argued convincingly for what he has called "reflective equilibrium," whereby we go back and forth between our reasoning and our intuitions, playing each off against the other to achieve an equilibrium—but one is always subject to further adjustment. Leon R. Kass does invoke repugnance—against human cloning, for instance—but immediately follows up with reasons against cloning; his critics usually ignore that.[1]

The common mistake in rejecting our emotional reactions in favor of reason is to misunderstand our emotions. Psychology has long showed that most of our emotional responses—fear, anxiety, and repugnance among them—embody cognitive judgments, and that our cognitive judgments no less embody emotional components. It makes no sense, then, to draw a sharp distinction between reason and emotion. They form a continuum rather than discrete categories. The challenge is to let each of them tutor our thinking and decisions in an appropriate way.

The failure of much risk-benefit analysis is not simply that it tries to set aside value judgments (as Magnus appropriately notes), but that it ignores the hidden emotional content of the analysis. Such an omission helps explain why those who use that kind of analysis more often come out on the side of technology than on the side of caution: their excitement or enthusiasm (both emotions, but unacknowledged) favors going forward. Their anxiety, by contrast, is slight or non-existent. This phenomenon can be seen again and again in many current biotechnology controversies. The prospective benefits of human cloning are touted enthusiastically—but those who worry about the long-term consequences are dismissed as irrational and anxious (Gregory Pence's tactic).[2]

Taking account of emotion becomes all the more important at those junctures of history when change, scientific or social, is in the air and where there is little rational precedent to work with. The early opponents of slavery, in the 16th and early 17th centuries, felt great repugnance toward it. They were disgusted by what they saw and they felt it was wrong. Yet they had no "rational" support for that feeling at a time when science held blacks to be inferior, the church approved of slavery, and many of the economic institutions of the day made it seem a necessary institution.

Nonetheless, they trusted their repugnance, gradually finding a rational basis for their opposition.

Those prescient Jews in the early years of Naziism who fled Germany could not rationally prove that the early instances of anti-Semitism would lead to the holocaust—and they had many practical reasons to stay—but they had a sense that disaster was a possibility. In his splendid book *Lest Innocent Blood Be Shed*, the late philosopher Philip Hallie wrote about a small French Protestant community in France that, at direct risk to their own lives, hid Jews in their homes. Most remarkably, Hallie found, was that they could offer no "rational" reason for their action, and for their courage. They simply knew—"in their hearts" as the old saying had it—that it was the right thing to do.[3]

After many years of thinking about it, I have concluded that my initial untutored repugnance (at the age of 15) at the development of nuclear weapons and my corresponding judgment that they should never have been deployed was right. But I was beaten down for a long time by the risk-benefit argument that it shortened World War II, saved hundreds of thousands of American soldiers from death, and that, in any event, "if we didn't do it, the Germans or Japanese would have." Better, now I think, that those lives would have been lost than to burden future human life with such weapons of destruction.

I mention these instances because they are almost always overlooked when it is argued that our emotions tell us little of value, or when examples of repugnance dissipated or overcome are advanced to show their flawed qualities. Of course that happens from time to time, and we look back wondering how we could have felt such resistance to something that now seems utterly benign. But for every example of that kind, I suspect one could find another that showed how spontaneous repugnance had been numbed and then excised for altogether bad reasons. I think here of the atrocities committed in war by soldiers who could never have imagined themselves doing such horrible things in peacetime. Or those who knew slavery was wrong but allowed themselves to be persuaded by the reasons of the era that they were wrong. Those contemporary Germans, fearful of genetic developments and suspicious of smooth assurances that it will not go sour, show more wisdom than they are given credit for. Maybe it is better to be kicked and dragged into the "new genetics" (as it is called) than to be persuaded by confident "reason" to forget how it all went wrong earlier.

Magnus made a shrewd choice in picking the debate over genetically modified food as his example of the clash between reason and emotion. It is an almost perfect case study, full of cost-benefit analysis of the rationalist kind and emotional outbursts of the visceral kind. As it happens, I am part of a European–North American project at The Hastings Center examining why Europeans have been so hostile to genetically modified food and North Americans so receptive. The fact that—as, analogously, with the German eugenic history—Europeans have had a recent history of food problems and government cover-ups is a partial explanation: once burnt, and so on. Yet it also needs noting that Europeans have been much quicker to regulate, and ban, various forms of human genetic research than Americans.

I bring to the project a kind of idiosyncratic response. I have felt anxiety, and sometimes repugnance, at many of the genetic developments with humans—but am almost totally devoid of an emotional response to genetically modified food. When I go to the supermarket, I always pass over the "organic" vegetables in favor of the pesticide-loaded, genetically manipulated variety if the latter are cheaper. I do not lose sleep over the possibility of wild "super-weeds." Meanwhile, I have testified before our Congress on a bill in favor of a ban on human cloning research and I look with suspicion upon germ-line therapy (a kind of genetic therapy that would pass all changes down through the generations).

Am I simply (a) irrational, (b) uninformed, (c) inconsistent, or (d) right on? I can't answer that question but it is clear (at least to me) that I exclusively apply risk-benefit analysis to genetically modified food and some broader standard to human genetics (including but not limited to risk-benefit analysis). There is, in short, no good equilibrium in my overall thinking about genetic interventions, human and agricultural. Is there a better way? Well, my theory about such matters, if not my consistent practice, is that four elements need to be blended in trying to think about novel technologies with no clear historical precedents.

The first is to consult my emotions, looking for what lies below the surface; if I have no emotional reaction (as with genetically modified food), then I need to ask myself why. The second element is to use my imagination, attempting to visualize the long-term implications and possibilities of new technologies, medical, social, and cultural, taking care to watch out for blatant bias of a Luddite or progress-enthusiast kind.

The third is ordinary risk-benefit analysis, but making certain that risks and benefits are understood more broadly than matters of safety and physical health. The fourth element is to consider the history of technological and scientific developments, and what became of them. The Europeans have a good reason to be more wary of genetically modified food than we are and, by virtue of the Nazi misuse of genetics, to be wary of optimistic talk about using genetics to improve human traits. We Americans would be wise to draw upon their experience, perhaps profitably coming to feel some of the repugnance we might not naturally feel because of our more sheltered history.

NOTES

1. Kass LR. Preventing a brave new world. *New Republic* 224:21 (May 21, 2001), 30–9.

2. Pence GE. *Who's Afraid of Cloning?* Lanham, MD: Rowman & Littlefield, 1998.

3. Hallie PP. *Lest Innocent Blood be Shed.* New York: HarperPerennial, 1994.

Daniel Callahan's thoughtful commentary presents a very complex and subtle approach to the issues involved in cognitive and emotional responses to new technologies. He points out the falsity of the dichotomy between emotion and reason and highlights the fact that there are usually good reasons for our emotional responses.

Things become complicated by the fact that different groups can and do respond differently to developments in technology (and other institutions). How do we determine which responses should be respected and which rejected as mere prejudices? As Callahan notes, institutions like slavery elicited both acceptance and repugnance in different individuals. Similarly, in the past (and unfortunately possibly even today) racial integration of schools also produced a sense of moral repugnance in many individuals and groups.

From this, two things follow. First, as Callahan points out, even if we do not share a sense of repugnance, we should respect the fact that others do—though I do not personally share the emotional opposition to either cloning or genetically modified organisms, the fact that others do, is significant.

Second (and here I may diverge from Callahan) the mere fact of moral repugnance, while significant, is not sufficient to reject a technology. In the end, there must be reasons to offer and values that are at stake and these must be articulated to explore whether a response is justified or a mere prejudice. These values may well be compelling even when they do not fit within the framework of a cost-benefit analysis. In the debate over genetically modified organisms, considerations of justice (who has control, who is exposed to risk, who benefits), of concern with human hubris, and the appropriate balance of perspective in our relationship with nature are as important as the harms and benefits the technology can produce.

☷ ☶ ☶ ☷

GARRATH WILLIAMS, PHD

Human Gene Banks

The past five years have seen a new wave of interest in the storage of human genetic materials. This interest partly reflects increased knowledge of genetics and partly the hope of further understanding and new applications.

On the one hand, states—and especially their police forces—have seen that quite basic existing genetic knowledge is of great use to them. The ability to identify individuals in terms of a near unique "genetic finger-print" has already proven forensically very valuable. As the number of samples held in police databases increases, so too does the usefulness of these databases for linking samples found at crime scenes with individual identities. On the other hand, medical and scientific interest in genetics begins with the fact that we have barely begun to decipher the meaning of this identifying data. We can identify some mutations of single genes that result in rare and extreme diseases—a good example is Huntington's disease. But in most cases the connections between human genetic variability and health remain hidden, and we have hardly any knowledge concerning the interaction of large numbers of genetic variations. Given our poor understanding of gene expression, the best weapon to study these is sheer statistical force—to compare health outcomes across large numbers of people with their genetic variations. To do this, new human gene banks orders of magnitude larger than the many well-established gene banks dedicated to the study of particular diseases are needed.

Not only is banking "genes" important—we also need information about the health or phenotype of the sample donor. In the large-scale research gene banks that have attracted much recent attention, this personal information is meant to be continually updated. This has the significant implication that samples cannot be made fully anonymous; otherwise, we could never link new data back to the original sample. Our ability to identify individuals on the basis of genetic samples means that gene banks pose significant privacy issues that will only increase as we become better able to decipher genetic information.

Bioethics has given the most attention to human gene banks for medical research. This is natural, in that bioethics is especially concerned with research and human health. Also much more publicity has surrounded these projects. But something is odd about this emphasis, because the biggest, best funded and most effective human gene banks are forensic ones. The UK National Police Database, for instance, includes samples from 2.75 million people (September 2004)—twice as many as it did two years ago—and is still growing.[1]

By contrast, the gene banks that have attracted recent attention remain more promise than reality. The two best known examples are the Icelandic Health Sector Database[2] and UK Biobank,[3] neither of which has yet gathered any genetic samples. In the US, an interesting third example is First Genetic Trust,[4] a private company that essentially mediates between researchers and individual donors.

The Icelandic database has been controversial for several reasons. Meant to include the entire population of Iceland—270,000 people—it features medical data on an "opt-out" basis: that is, individuals are not asked for their consent, but may register their dissent and withdraw from the database. So far, only a small minority of the Icelandic population has opted out. Moreover, the database has been licensed, by act of Parliament, for a twelve-year period to the company deCode Genetics,[5] closely linked with Hoffman La Roche. As many see it, the genetic heritage and health data of the Icelandic people have been sold to a private company at a low price and with scant regard for the principle of informed consent. However, although the license was granted in 1998, deCode has yet to gather any genetic samples.

By contrast UK Biobank is intended to include more samples— 500,000—from only a subset of the British population, 45- to 69-year-olds (the age range when many common diseases of Western societies set in). Research subjects, who must specifically consent, will complete lifestyle and health questionnaires as well as grant access to their healthcare records. Funded by the UK government and its Medical Research Council as well as the Wellcome trust (the world's largest medical research charity), UK Biobank will be open to both public and private researchers on terms yet to be announced.[6]

Two obvious issues for human genetic banking are posed by these cases: commercial exploitation and the consent of individual research subjects. Samples and information have often been spoken of as gifts by the donor (the reference is to Titmuss's work on blood donation in the context of a publicly funded healthcare system).[7] "Gift" is ambiguous, though. Donation is a free and consensual act; the sample is donated supposedly with no thought of return or recompense. Yet while people may be happy to give to public health research, this may be because they receive ongoing benefits from that system—so that gifts are not quite so one-sided as may be thought. It is less clear that people are, or should be, so willing to "give" to profit-making entities.

Consent is problematic because these proposed gene banks promise a new form of health research, one that is essentially collective and peculiarly open-ended—aiming to learn more about the relations between genetic variation and health. This seems to render informed consent impossible: researchers cannot tell donors in advance what their sample and data will be used to research. The sheer scale of the projects also makes asking donors about each individual study quite impractical—something one might anyhow think burdensome to individuals and problematic from a privacy point of view. Commentators and policy documents, therefore, tend to speak of "blanket" or "broad" consent.

Beyond this, it is not clear that these massive new biobanks represent a sensible priority for research. Gathering high-quality data for such a large number of people seems impractical. Perhaps the best that the large gene banks can do is to facilitate the identification of a much smaller pool suitable for intensive investigation of a particular drug or condition. In this case, how important the gene bank was in the first place is open to question;

the many much smaller disease-specific banks would serve just as well. Likewise, the promise of technologies for population genetic screening is unlikely to be realized or to represent a sound public health investment. We already know that most chronic ill-health and premature death in Western societies owes to factors such as diet and exercise patterns, not to mention wealth inequalities. Testing individual genetic predispositions can only be the most minor supplement to addressing those factors.

Doubts of this sort may have slowed private investment in large-scale, open-ended biobanks over the past couple of years—resulting in the failure of deCode to begin collecting genetic samples. Markets and private companies are unlikely to sink large sums into projects whose payoffs are so uncertain. This leaves biobanking in the hands of public and charitable concerns—where one may think ensuring that investments are directed to public health benefits is much more important. But because a project like UK Biobank is so enormous—a £60 million budget ($120 million), which many suspect is only the beginning—it has escaped the usual processes of scientific peer review. Yet if we are going to place less weight on informed consent than we do for standard medical research—as it seems we must if such projects are to be practicable—then clearly we must place much more weight on scientific and public scrutiny. That is, we must be sure that the projects are both scientifically well conceived and reflect proper public priorities for research. My own view, in line with the doubts sketched in the preceding paragraphs, is that such a case has simply not been made.

Interesting parallels and illuminating differences exist between forensic and medical biobanks. Costly as forensic biobanks are, they are certainly much cheaper overall, because they do not require the same sort of detailed data collation as research biobanks. Their benefits, in terms of crime detection if not crime prevention, are much clearer and more immediate. Consent has not been thought an important principle in the case of forensic banks—it would be plainly absurd for police forces to have to require consent from someone they have good basis to suspect of a serious crime. At the same time, it is disturbing that forensic databases have attracted even less debate than research biobanks—despite the fact that they pose serious privacy issues and represent a huge potential growth in state power.

While few bioethicists are willing to endorse the Icelandic example and bypass consent entirely, it now seems clear that individual consent is not the most important issue posed by this new form of collective and prospective medical research. Much more central is whether research biobanks represent a well-conceived priority.[8] This question may be even more difficult to debate than in the case of the forensic databases; yet it surely deserves to be debated more vigorously and more widely than it has so far.

NOTES

1. Williams R, Johnson P, Martin P. *Genetic Information & Crime Investigation.* London: Wellcome Trust; 2004. Available at http://www.dur.ac.uk/p.j.johnson/

2. http://www.wellcome.ac.uk/doc_WTD003280.html

3. http://www.ukbiobank.ac.uk/

4. http://www.firstgenetic.net/

5. http://www.decode.com/

6. See the excellent briefing papers on UK Biobank by Genewatch: http://www.gene watch.org/

7. Titmuss, RM The Gift Relationship. Oakley A, Ashton J, eds. Rev ed. New York: The New Press; 1997.

8. See also Ruth Chadwick "The Icelandic Database—Do Modern Times Need Modern Sagas?" Br Med J 1999;319:441–444.

☰ ☷ ☷ ☰

JON F. MERZ, MBA, JD, MD

Are Human Gene Banks Worth It?

In "Human Gene Banks," Dr. Garrath Williams raises a fundamental question about recent efforts to build general population human DNA banks for research: Is the money needed to develop these resources worth it? Looking at a broad sample of efforts around the world suggests that the answer is a resounding "no."

There have been numerous efforts to develop population-based DNA and data banks. In addition to those discussed by Dr. Williams in Iceland and the UK, projects were announced in Tonga, Sweden, Latvia, Singapore, Estonia, and Sardinia, and several have been started in the United States.[1] Most of these efforts combine public or quasipublic (e.g., nonprofit hospital) resources with commercial interests. In the US, numerous firms are in the business of procuring and storing human biosamples for research including, but by no means limited to Ardais, GeneLink, First Genetic Trust, GenomicsCollaborative, DNA Sciences, Integrated Laboratory Services, Zoion Diagnostics, Novagen, the National Disease Research Interchange and Phylogeny. With the exceptions of the MRC/ Wellcome project in the UK and the Marshfield Clinic's Personalized Medicine Research Project (PMRP), the population efforts have been driven by commercial firms.

In most cases, these efforts have failed relatively early due to financial and political problems. A look at some examples of what has worked and not worked so far supports Dr. Williams's contention that the best route to take for genetics research is smaller, narrowly focused repositories. Two successful efforts at building and operating a repository include that in Umeå, Sweden, and Marshfield's PMRP. Uman Genomics is a company established to commercialize an existing tissue bank and related medical records held by the Medical Biobank of Umeå. The bank was created as part of a large population study of cardiovascular disease and diabetes, and is owned and operated by Umeå University and Västerbotten County Council.[2] The company has exclusive commercial rights to the bank, which includes blood and plasma from more than 100,000 individuals and counting.

The second success is the Marshfield Clinic's PMRP. This effort is focused on the prospective collection of DNA, with broad consent, from people in the Clinic's mid-Wisconsin catchment area. The PMRP was funded by state and federal grants.[3] Since its start in 2002, more than 20,000 individuals have agreed to participate.

In contrast, two efforts to build or operate a repository that failed may be compared and contrasted to the above. First is that of Framingham Genomics, a company started to commercialize the extremely rich research data (including blood samples) on people in the 57-year-old Framingham Heart Study. This large epidemiological study has collected information over time on two generations of residents of Framingham, Massachusetts, encompassing over 10,000 individuals.[4] The study, funded by the NIH's National Heart, Lung, and Blood Institute (NHLBI), has a DNA repository including over 5,000 of the subjects. Framingham Genomics banked on securing exclusive commercial access to the project's resources and data; the project was abandoned when the NHLBI refused to grant such broad rights, suggesting such exclusivity conflicted with their public mission.

Second is the population effort by Iceland's deCODE Genetics. deCODE proposed legislation allowing the compilation of the population's medical record data (going back some 15 years, plus comprehensive prospective collection) into a centralized Health Sector Database (HSD). An exclusive license was granted to deCODE allowing the company to build and operate the HSD, and, critically, to link the HSD with an extremely complete genealogy on the Icelandic population and with a proprietary dataset of genetic markers (this last developed with consent from subjects). This combined database, called the Genealogy Genotype Phenotype Resource (GGPR) could be used for research. The HSD has not been built, and it is not clear that it will be. Independent of its efforts to conceptualize the GGPR, deCODE has performed smaller studies targeted on a range of specific diseases. They have developed rich databases and networks of clinicians that enable them to do gene discovery as well as other types of research, now even including clinical trials. For example, deCODE's genetic studies identified a gene, defects in which put patients at high risk of heart attacks. Knowing the mechanism of disease, they identified and licensed a drug candidate from Bayer, and are now running a clinical trial in Iceland on the drug.[5] Given the success of their smaller, disease-focused research, the estimated $100 million it would have cost them to develop a computerized medical record system, install it in clinics and hospitals across the country, and pay for the past abstraction of medical records is not likely worth it.[6]

These four projects, perhaps exemplary of the kinds of human DNA banking activities that have been pursued, suggest several things. First, consent is generally seen as an ethical imperative for the compilation of human DNA and medical data banks. deCODE, which proceeded with a waiver of consent but an opportunity to opt out (totally or by individual doctor visit), is the lone exception to this. Even for some retrospective efforts (using tissues collected in years past), researchers have ensured that the scope of past consent would encompass the types of things proposed in the future, and, if not, required a new consent from subjects for new uses that exceed those disclosed in the original informed consents.

Of course, consent can be problematic, because it adds to the cost of research, it can impute biases if some people are more or less likely to participate (for example, in Iceland, it was reported that psychiatric patients were more likely to opt out; in other cases, women are more likely to opt out of having their medical records included in research), and it can result in low participation rates. Nonetheless, consent is the best way to show respect for persons and their rights to privacy and to choose whether and in what ways they will participate in research.

Second, privacy is universally acknowledged as requiring protection, particularly for research involving human genetics. Methods of protecting privacy range from anonymization (stripping all links and identifying information), use of firewalls to prevent subject identification, data smoothing to help mask identities, and data (or linking code) encryption. In Europe, researchers are required to use Data Protection authorities, which are governmental boards that ensure adequate protections are in place for use of many different types of private information. Third, commercial pressures and intellectual property ownership issues can determine whether a project succeeds or not. Firms that have been highly involved in official gene banking efforts often demand exclusive commercial rights to the resources (the DNA banks and related databases) developed at their expense. Exclusivity is exclusionary, and it cuts against the grain for public institutions and for academic or clinical researchers to agree to such conditions. The exclusivity demanded by Framingham Genomics was a deal breaker, and the exclusivity granted to deCODE was a sore point for many critics.

As suggested by the numerous efforts described here, many believe there is money in human genes, but few efforts have succeeded thus far in developing generalized population based research human gene banks. Patents on human genes, while arguably necessary to foster downstream research on therapies, are far removed in technology and time from a profitable product. Thus, the investments have largely proved thus far to be commercially too risky and may only proceed if development costs are supported by public or foundation grants, as seen with both Uman Genomics and the Marshfield Clinic. This does not imply that no commercial entities are or will be successful, but it is too soon to predict whether firms—such as Ardais[7]—will be around for the long haul.

NOTES

1. Merz JF. On the intersection of privacy, consent, commerce and genetics research. In Knoppers BM, ed., *Populations and Genetics: Legal Socio-Ethical Perspectives*. New York: KluwerLegal Int'l, 2003.

2. http://www.umangenomics.com/.

3. http://www.mfldclin.edu/pmrp/.

4. http://www.framingham.com/heart/.

5. http://www.decode.com/.

6. Merz JF, McGee GE, Sankar P. "Iceland Inc."? on the ethics of commercial population genomics. *Soc. Sci. Med.* 2004;58:1201–1209.

7. http://www.ardais.com/.

≣ ⫼ ⫼ ≣

ELLEN M. MCGEE, PHD AND
GERALD Q. MAGUIRE, JR, PHD

Implantable Brain Chips: Ethical and Policy Issues

The future may include the reality of science fiction's "cyborgs," persons who have developed some intimate and occasionally necessary relationships with a machine. It is likely that computer chips implanted in our brains and acting as sensors or actuators may soon not only assist the blind and those with failing memory, but even bestow fluency in a new language, enable "recognition" of previously unmet individuals, and provide instantaneous access to encyclopedic databases.

Developments in nanotechnology, bioengineering, computers, and neuroscience are converging to facilitate these amazing possibilities. Research on cochlear hearing and retinal vision has furthered the development of interfaces between neural tissues and microcomputers. The cochlear implant, which directly stimulates the auditory nerve, enables totally deaf people to hear sound. An artificial vision system, the "Dobelle Eye," uses a tiny television camera and ultrasonic distance sensors mounted on eyeglasses and connected to a miniature computer worn on a belt. This invention enables the blind to navigate independently, "read" letters, "watch" television, use a computer, and access the Internet.[1] These "visual" activities are achieved by triggering pulses from the microcomputer to an array of platinum electrodes implanted on the surface of the brain's visual cortex. In March 1998, a "locked in" victim of a brainstem stroke became the first recipient of a brain-to-computer interface, enabling him to communicate on a computer by thinking about moving the cursor.[2]

Used for therapy such as remediating retardation, replacing lost memory faculties, or substituting for defective sensory abilities, implantable brain chips are noncontroversial and desirable interventions. The issues that arise with such therapeutic uses of implantable brain chips primarily involve questions of equity and the costs of implementing this technology.

Questions that are far more difficult are raised by the potential for enhancement. The linkage of smaller, lighter, and more powerful computer systems with radio technologies that involve low-frequency electromagnetic waves widely used for wireless communication will enable future users to access information and communicate anywhere or anytime.

Through miniaturization of components, systems have already been developed that are wearable and nearly invisible, so that individuals supported by a personal information structure[3] can move about and interact freely, as well as share experiences with others through networking.[4] The wearable computer project envisions users accessing a large communally based data source.[5] The next step in this development is use of the implantable brain chip and direct neural interfacing.[6]

As intelligence or sensory "amplifiers," the implantable chips will generate at least four benefits: (1) increasing the range of senses, enabling, for example, seeing infrared light, ultraviolet light, and chemical spectra; (2) enhancing memory; (3) enabling "cyberthink"—invisible communication with others when making decisions; and (4) facilitating access to information where and when it is needed. These enhancements will produce major improvements in quality of life or in job performance. The first prototypes for these improvements in human functioning should be available in five years, military devices within 10 years, adoption by information workers within 15 years, and general use in 20 to 30 years.

A myriad of technical, ethical, and social concerns should be considered before proceeding with implantable chips. The most obvious and basic problems involve safety. Evaluation of the costs and benefits of these implants requires a consideration of the surgical and long-term risks. The question of whether or not the difficulties with development of non-toxic materials will allow long-term usage should be answered in studies on therapeutic options and thus not be a concern for enhancement usage. However, the issue of whether there should be a higher standard for safety when technologies are used for enhancement rather than therapy needs public debate. Because of the enormous potential for societal impact, it is debatable whether the informed consent of recipients should be sufficient for permitting implementation.

Consideration needs to be given to the sociological and psychological effects of enhancing human nature. Will the use of computer-brain interfaces change our conception of man and our sense of identity? If people are actually connected via their brains, the boundaries between self and community will be considerably diminished. Not only may the boundaries of the real and the virtual worlds blur, but the pressures to act as a part of the whole, as a "collective consciousness," rather than as an isolated individual would be increased. The sense of self as a unique and isolated individual might be changed. Modifying the brain and its powers could change our psychic states and our understanding of what it means to be human. The borders between me "the physical self" and me "the perceptory intellectual self" could change as the ability to perceive and interact expands. Whether this would lead to bestowing greater weight to collective responsibilities and whether this would be beneficial are unknown.

Since usage may also engender a human being with augmented sensory capacities, the implications need consideration. Supersensory sight will see radar, infrared, and ultraviolet images; augmented hearing will detect softer and higher and lower pitched sounds; enhanced smell will intensify our ability to discern scents; and an amplified sense of touch will enable discernment of environmental stimuli like changes in barometric pressure. These capacities would change the "norm" for humans. As the numbers of enhanced humans increase, today's normal might be seen as subnormal, leading to the medicalization of another area of life. Thus, substantial questions revolve around whether there should be limits placed upon modifications of essential aspects of the human species.

Changes in human nature would become more pervasive if the altered consciousness were that of children. Will parents in our intensely competitive society be able to secure implants for their children, and if so, how will that change the already unequal lottery of life? Will the inequalities produced create a demand for universal coverage of these devices in healthcare plans, further increasing costs to society? Or will implanted brain chips be available only to those who can afford a substantial investment, thus further widening the gap between the haves and the have-nots? Of major concern should be the social impact of implementing a technology that widens the divisions not only between individuals, but also between rich and poor nations.

Beyond these more imminent prospects, British scientists have concluded that in about 30 years, "it will be possible to capture data presenting all of a human being's sensory experiences on a single tiny chip implanted in the brain."[7] These data would be collected by biological probes receiving electrical impulses and would enable a user to recreate experiences, or even to transplant memory chips from one brain to another. Combined with cloning technologies and given the possibility of continually recording and editing our lives, novel meanings of the self would be generated.

The most frightening implication of this technology is the grave possibility that it would facilitate totalitarian control of humans. Using such technology, commercial interests or governments could control and monitor citizens. In a free society this possibility may seem remote, although it is plausible to project initial compulsory usage for children, for the military, or for criminals. Policy decisions will arise about this usage, and also about mandating implants to affect specific behaviors. A paramount worry involves who will control the technology and what will be programmed; this issue overlaps the uneasiness about privacy concerns and the need for secure communication links. The prospects for sinister invasions of liberty and privacy are alarming.

In view of the potentially revolutionary implications of the implantable brain chip, should its development and implementation be prohibited or, at the very least, regulated? This is the question that open dialogue needs to address. Certainly, it appears that moving towards implantable brain chips can be a positive step in the evolution of humans. Nevertheless, the issues as described in this paper are weighty and need international consideration. Disagreement exists even between the authors of this paper: Gerald Maguire thinks there should be no limits placed on how people can choose to modify themselves; Ellen McGee thinks that, at least initially, when used for enhancement, the technology should be regulated, treated as research on human subjects, and closely monitored for its effects. Both authors are worried about uses in the military and for children or other individuals whose choices might be compelled. McGee is particularly troubled by the inequities, especially on an international level, that will arise if this technology is left to a market economy. Our discussions have convinced us that public debate and multidisciplinary evaluation from thinkers in the fields of computer science, biophysics, medicine, law, religion, philosophy, public policy and international economy are urgently needed.

NOTES

1. Artificial vision system for the blind announced by the Dobelle Institute. Press Release. *Science Daily* http://www.sciencedaily.com/releases\2000\01\000118065202.htm.

2. Headlam B. The mind that moves objects. *The New York Times Magazine* June 11, 2000:63–4.

3. Mann S. Wearable computing: A first step toward personal imaging. *Computer* Vol. 30, No. 2, February 1997. http://www.computer.org/co1997/r2025abs.htm.

4. Mann S. Wearable, tetherless, computer-mediated reality (with possible future applications to the disabled). http://wearcam.org/tetherless/.

5. *Augmented Memory* http://www.media.mit.edu/projects/wearables/augmented-memory .html. June 1997.

6. Thomas P. Thought control. *New Scientist* March 9, 1996.

7. Dawley H. Remembrance of things past—on a chip. *Business Week* August 5, 1996.

☷ ☶ ☶ ☷

DANIEL C. DENNETT, PHD

Implantable Brain Chips—Will They Change Who We Are?

What are your boundaries? Where do you stop and where does the world begin? If you are a violinist, your bow is already an eloquent, feeling part of you. If you drive racecars, you feel the grip of the tires on the road as if you were running barefoot. If somebody steals your eyeglasses, you are temporarily disabled as surely as if they punch you in the eye. Take away my computers and I might as well have brain damage.

The skin is an important membrane, for most purposes the natural boundary between a person and the rest of the world, but it lost its role as the edge of agency when our ancestors first began to make and use tools. Is there really that much difference between a tool you put inside your body and a tool you enclose in the palm of your hand or wear on the bridge of your nose? Most, if not all, of the conceptual issues—the ethical dilemmas and the other deep revisions in our way of life—have already been confronted time and again, in simpler versions. Implantable brain chips—if they really do become widespread (which I doubt)—will intensify problems and opportunities we are already trying to cope with. Will this intensification move us into altogether new territory? Let's consider the prospects.

Predictions about the spread of new technology have a dismal track record, so we will probably both overestimate some problems and underestimate others by a wide margin. But we should try. McGee and Maguire say "these enhancements will produce major improvements in quality of life or in job performance," and although they probably didn't mean "or" to be exclusive, it may well turn out that we will indeed have to choose. Which do we want, improved quality of life or improved job performance?

Why would anybody suppose we couldn't have both? Because we have already seen many instances in which improving job performance does diminish quality of life. Consider first a relatively trivial case, and then an ominous one. Thanks to global positioning systems (GPS), it is no longer possible to have the thrill of navigating your little boat across the ocean, relying on sextant and chronometer. You would be foolish to the point of criminal negligence to leave port on such a voyage without availing yourself of the best practical technology, and that technology takes the task of navigation out of your hands, routinizes it to the point where "job performance" is well nigh perfect, but job satisfaction is well nigh invisible. It's too easy a task to care about, so there is one less adventure opportunity in the modern world. You can "rough it," locking your GPS in a box to be opened only in case of emergency, but that's an exercise in make-believe, like camping out in a theme park. The risks are all packaged.

Much the same future looms for the practice of medicine: as diagnostic technologies get better and better, the satisfactions will correspondingly evaporate. "You" caught your patient's cancer early enough to treat it successfully, but hey, all you did was order a few obligatory tests, and one came back positive. Anybody could have done it. More to the point, anybody would have been obliged to do it. A miracle of modern medicine has happened, but the "art" has been distributed throughout a huge network of technology, leaving only relatively routine activities for the human participants. Where there are few opportunities for heroism, for genuine, risky adventure, the quality of life is diminished. But from the patient's point of view, this is just as it should be: may all my medical care be as routine and risk-free—and, yes, boring—as possible!

This trend towards improved job performance with decreased grounds for satisfaction shows every sign of growing indefinitely with or without implantable brain chips. Imagine a brain chip specialized for anesthesiologists; all the outputs from all the monitoring equipment that now confront the doctor in the operating room are collected in a radio device that transmits them to the chip, for handy distribution to various appropriate cortical areas. Bad idea. Instead, just slap some earphones on the anesthesiologist and code the information about vital signs into an appropriately modulated ensemble of sounds that form a natural system that can be readily understood and internalized, and you've accomplished a superb impedance match; your anesthesiologist is optimally "wired" without any wires in the brain. (This is not a fantasy; just such a device has been patented and will soon be in production.)

Implantation is an extreme measure that probably will never be warranted except in very special cases, where people have lost the function of some part of their nervous system. But even here, it is still not clear that implanted interfaces will be more effective than external, wearable interfaces that avail themselves of some underutilized part of the extraordinary bandwidth of the total human sensory surface. But this may change, so let's consider the range of outcomes that might confront us if implantation becomes a highly desirable course of action.

Whenever a new technology is created, it has the potential to create a new disadvantaged group: those who for whatever reason cannot avail themselves of it. When the highly visual desktop and mouse interface revolutionized human-computer interactions, a large corps of blind programmers lost their livelihoods. They could keep up with sighted programmers as long as everybody was using old-fashioned line editors which moved text around by multiple-keystroke commands, but highlight-and-drag was beyond the capacity of Braille displays to convey to their fingertips. Some activists went so far as to urge outlawing the desktop and mouse, on the grounds that it was a violation of the Americans with Disabilities Act. It is certainly possible (however unlikely) that some equally enhancing brain chip will be developed that can only be implanted in brains that have some currently negligible feature—a deeper-than-average central sulcus, for instance. Then we'll have created a new ethical problem: what to do about the 50 percent of the population that are ineligible for the new boon.

There is no way to avoid such problems. Any technology worth developing enhances some valued ability, and hence is almost certain to magnify some differences in ability. In some arenas of human competitive action we particularly prize equalization of ability, and in some we don't. If some violinist wants to take drugs to enhance her performance, or insists on wearing some hearing-enhancing device to improve her pitch, ensuring herself a position in the orchestra, that's her business; she may ruin her health in the quest for artistic glory (and the increasing use of beta-blockers by musicians raises some troubling issues), but we currently have no ethic that insists that she give less radically dedicated musicians a "sporting chance" to compete with her.

The use of technology in enhancing the abilities of athletes, in contrast, is a fascinating battleground for our intuitions of fairness. High-altitude training camps are okay, but achieving some of the same physiological effects by stockpiling the athlete's own blood and retransfusing it is beyond the pale—according to some people. The coach may call instructions from the sidelines (and a hearing-impaired athlete can wear a hearing aid to take advantage of this advice) but a radio receiver tuned to the coach's transmitter is out—in some sports, but not in others.

What resources may a competitor bring to an examination or quiz? A calculator? A laptop? A cellular phone? Once again, the issue of implantation doesn't seem to me to raise new problems. If you can "phone a friend" to get the answer, it doesn't much matter whether your cell phone autodials from its home in your cingulate gyrus.

Very few people today know how to calculate square roots by hand, and why should they? Why memorize the list of state capitals or Tudor kings or amino acids when these can be retrieved in a few seconds from a Web site (or an old-fashioned multi-volume encyclopedia)? We tend to prize the skills we had to learn in school, even as they become utterly obsolete, and we tend to import the sports ethic into other arenas even when it is of dubious relevance. These heartfelt convictions may be wise or foolish, but we can't just jettison them all. We do need to agree to live by some relatively stable and mutually acknowledged set of rules, and as technology changes the background conditions, we have to revise these understandings. Equality of opportunity is an elusive goal worth striving for, however the sands may shift beneath our feet as we do so.

What, finally, of the "sinister invasions of liberty and privacy" that McGee and Maguire warn about? They are already upon us, without the need for implants. A bracelet locked on a child's or convict's ankle will do as well as an implanted chip. For that matter, a credit card or a cell phone with GPS will do as well. The prospect of implantable brain chips may dramatize the issues for us, but we shouldn't make the mistake of thinking that the unlikely prospects of developing such chips shows we may safely postpone decisions about them.

REPLY BY ELLEN M. MCGEE, PHD AND GERALD Q. MAGUIRE, JR., PHD

Professor Dennett's intriguing response to our paper claims that brain chips add nothing new to the ethical concerns raised by technology in general, and that "there is no way to avoid such problems." Essentially, he seems to assume that the endeavor of reflecting upon and controlling technologies is futile. Our paper did not claim that brain chips will raise uniquely new ethical issues; rather our point is that there are ethical problems inherent in the proper human uses of technologies, that brain chips are a likely future technology, and that it is both possible and necessary to formulate policies and regulations which will mitigate their effects.

There are differences between harnessing the power of fire and harnessing that of nuclear energy, between the use of carrier pigeons and the direct transmission of thoughts via wireless brain waves. That these differences are ones of degree rather than of kind, does not imply that they are insignificant. A "tool" such as implantable brain chips collapses the traditional separation between the tool and the subject using the tool, and necessitates mechanisms to ensure that it is a tool that one can choose not to use. Concerns about autonomy, privacy, and the just allocation of benefits are not ethical issues that will suddenly become real with the advent of brain chips; rather the technology will put new forms of stress on privacy, autonomy, and justice, and the task of applied ethics is to look for practical ethical responses to such posited problems. It is more than probable that brain chips will be used since they will very significantly reduce the power required and provide for a highly efficient system. To adopt a fatalistic attitude towards this development is irresponsible, and will leave the decision making in the hands of technocrats, corporations, and governments.

☰ ☷ ☶ ☶

ROBERT M. VEATCH, PHD

The Fight over How to Allocate Livers

If people need a liver for transplantation, it makes a huge difference where they live. For example, in New York City the mean waiting time is 511 days, but across the river in northern New Jersey it is only 56. The reason has to do with the allocation system put in place by the United Network for Organ Sharing (UNOS), the private organization that holds the federal government contract for the organ procurement and transplantation network in the United States.

UNOS classifies patients by the severity of their illness, Status 1 being the most serious. Status 1 patients have acute fulminant liver disease with a life expectancy of fewer than seven days. Status 2 patients are also seriously ill, usually hospitalized. (Patients with serious, chronic liver disease, including alcoholic cirrhosis, have recently been moved from Status 1 to a new sub-category called Status 2A, while those previously in group 2 are now categorized as 2B). Status 3 involves less serious illness, usually homebound patients. UNOS allocates organs in order from the most to the least serious status. Within the same status, waiting time is also considered.

In addition, the allocation system takes geography into account. There are 61 local organ procurement organizations (OPOs) in the United States. Before a recent modification, an organ acquired by an OPO was used locally, if possible, even if it went to a Status 3 patient. Only if it could not be used locally did it get transported outside the area. It then went to others in the same region, one of 11 geographical areas, again allocated in order of severity. Finally, if no one in the region could use it, it was allocated nationally. This meant that less ill local people had priority over the most urgent cases at the regional or national level. Within each status locally, persons in the same blood group as the liver donor get priority. This combination of preference for the sickest patients, local priority and blood group preference explains why it is plausible that Mickey Mantle, who was in Dallas, Texas, got a liver so quickly even though several thousand people had been on the national waiting list longer.

In April 1998, while this locals-first system was in place, the federal Department of Health and Human Services (HHS) issued a mandate that organs be allocated based on uniform medical criteria and over a large enough area so that organs would go to people who need them most. In effect, HHS was responding to the widely publicized disparities insisting that there be greater equity in the allocation system, giving organs on the basis of need rather than geography.

THE UNOS UTILITARIAN RESPONSE

The leadership of UNOS has resisted going to a more national list. Their arguments have been utilitarian. They believe more good can be done in the organ transplantation system if much of the local priority in allocation is retained. They make several claims. First, they have claimed that using organs locally encourages more donations. They think people will be more willing to donate organs if they believe their neighbors will get them. Several states, including Louisiana, South Carolina, Wisconsin, and Oklahoma, have, in fact, passed laws requiring organs to be kept within state boundaries if they can be used there. Second, they point to the potential deterioration in organs with the longer ischemia time (time that tissue is without blood flow) that would be required for transport to more distant patients. Third, they claim that placing organs in the sickest patients will be less efficient because patient survival will be less. All of these are meant to be arguments that local priority results in more favorable consequences even if it means allocating organs inequitably, because patients who are equally ill have radically differing prospects for getting an organ.

THE HHS RESPONSE

The HHS and other defenders of the mandate disagree with some of these empirical claims. They point out, for example, that it is not clear that family members will be less willing to donate if organs will go to more needy persons in a more distant city. They point out that some transport of organs to a different region may not involve significant increases in ischemia time compared with allocations within an OPO catchment area. Some hospitals where organs are procured may be hours away from the site where transplantation will take place. The data about greater graft and patient survival times if transplants go to less sick patients are also controversial. HHS has claimed that one computer model led to the conclusion that 300 lives a year could be saved with broader allocation areas.

These efforts to refute the UNOS utilitarian arguments on utilitarian terms challenge the claims about which type of allocation will do the most good. The real ethical dispute, however, is over whether the national organ system should necessarily strive for the absolute maximum number of years of life from the organs procured. If maximizing years of life-added comes at the expense of significantly greater inequities, the defenders of the non-utilitarian principle of justice are willing to forego some efficiency, particularly if the added benefits from an inequitable system are controversial or modest, and the unfairness is profound; justice-based approaches intentionally sacrifice utility to make the system more fair. In this case, that would mean moving away from an exclusive priority for local allocation in the direction of a more national list in which the sickest category of patients gets organs before those whose need is less urgent regardless of geography. In fact, as HHS Secretary Donna Shalala has pointed out, this probably would not actually require a single national list, but rather exchanges within a region or perhaps across certain regional lines. The HHS requirement is that the geographical areas be reconfigured so that waiting times are made more fair.

THE ECONOMICS OF THE CONTROVERSY

Not all local transplantation centers support the locals-first priority. The University of Pittsburgh has, in fact, been the most visible promoter of the reallocation. It has even been suggested that Pittsburgh had a hand in the HHS action. At the December 1996 HHS hearings that opened the discussion of reassessment of liver allocation, at least 20 of the 110 people who testified had an association with Pittsburgh, either as surgeons, researchers, or other personnel, or as transplant patients or family members. The University of Pittsburgh would have its interest served by a reallocation. Because of the fame of its program and its willingness to take difficult cases, it has many very ill patients waiting for organs. The local Pittsburgh procurement organization cannot possibly meet its need for organs, while other OPOs have enough organs so that patients in lower status groups can get them. Organ transplantation is big business for hospitals. More organs mean more work for surgeons and more income.

The smaller programs that dominate the UNOS decision-making process also have a significant financial and clinical interest in maintaining the current local priority. If other OPOs lose organs to Pittsburgh and other large programs, the number of transplants they can do will decline, income will decrease, and, in some cases, programs may actually cease to be economically viable. Some programs may not even be able to continue to meet the numerical requirements necessary to continue their training programs. Thus both the large and the small programs have substantial economic and clinical interests in how this ethical and policy debate turns out.

The ethical stances are not only related to the economic interests of the various institutions; they are also related to the professional identities of the participants in the debate. It is clear that UNOS, which is influenced by the large number of relatively small programs, is also dominated in many of its policy processes by transplant surgeons, while HHS is more heavily influenced by nonphysicians. It is clear that physicians, especially surgeons, have strong tendencies toward ethical reasoning based on consequences. Their Hippocratic tradition focuses on benefits and harms for patients. When they shift to more policy-oriented questions, they continue to tend to be consequence maximizers. The most relevant evidence is the vote of the UNOS ethics committee in which all the physicians voted for the consequentialist positions. Conversely, the nonphysicians voted as nonconsequentialist proponents of a more liberal political philosophy. They were more concerned about matters of respect for autonomy and fair distribution of scarce social resources.

Therefore, the debate between HHS and UNOS tends to mirror the controversy between the commitment to maximizing good consequences that prevails in the UNOS structure and the more robust commitment to equity even at the expense of efficiency that is more central to the current Democratic administration.

At this writing, a preliminary adjustment has been made by UNOS to attempt to respond to the HHS mandate. In June 1999, it rearranged its priority list for liver allocation so that regional Status 1 patients come before local patients of lower degrees of urgency. This will mean that OPOs with few Status 1 patients will have to ship their organs to other centers within their region if those centers have qualifying Status 1 patients awaiting organs. UNOS has recently announced that it proposes to replace the current Status 2A, Status 2B, and Status 3 levels of urgency with a continuous numerical scale based on the patient's risk of mortality calculated from a model developed by the Mayo Clinic that utilizes the prognostic factors of creatinine, bilirubin, prothrombin time and disease etiology.[1]

It remains to be seen whether inequities will remain among waiting times from one region to another, and whether inequities in waiting times will continue to exist from one local OPO to another for lower status patients. One suspects that HHS may not be satisfied with the relatively modest change UNOS has made thus far. One thing is clear, however: the debate is not only pitting one transplant patient against another and one OPO against another, it is also pitting consequence-maximizers against those willing to sacrifice good outcomes to make a national organ system more equitable. I have spent my career arguing that consequentialist ethics must be subordinated to certain deontological ethical duties, including the duty to allocate scarce resources to the worst off. Hence, as an egalitarian, I would favor the minimizing of the influence of local priority and endorse the HHS position. If I were a consequentialist, I would be ambivalent because the data seem to pull both ways.

NOTES

1. Heiney DA. Memo to UNOS members and interested persons Re: UNOS policy proposal for public comment and announcement of a UNOS public forum on liver allocations. August 24, 2000.

FURTHER READING

United States Department of Health and Human Services. Organ Procurement and Transplantation Network: final rule, 42 CFR Part 121. *Federal Register* 1998; 63:16296–16338.

UNOS News Release, February 27, 1998; UNOS. *Response to HHS Concerns about UNOS Statements Regarding the Regulations.* September 17, 1998. www.unos.org.

UNOS Policies 3.6.4.1 www.unos.org.

Veatch RM. Urgency vs. geography: the controversy between UNOS and Donna Shalala. In Veatch RM. Transplantation Ethics. Washington, DC: Georgetown University Press, 2000:363–387.

☷ ☶ ☵ ☳

DAN W. BROCK, PHD

Equity in Liver Allocation

In his article, "The fight over how to allocate livers," Robert Veatch describes the conflict between the U.S. Department of Health and Human Services (HHS) and the United Network for Organ Sharing (UNOS). HHS wants to move towards a national list for allocating scarce livers in order to reduce regional differences in waiting list times. UNOS has employed a system giving local organ procurement organizations significant priority for scarce organs. This is sometimes seen as a conflict between large programs treating the sickest patients—who would be benefited by a national list—and the smaller programs who benefit from local priority. Veatch correctly understands it also to be an ethical conflict between those who use consequentialist reasoning to support allocating livers to produce maximal benefits from a scarce resource and those who seek a more equitable distribution even at some cost in overall benefits. Whatever one's view of equity, it does not seem equitable or fair that where one happens to live should greatly affect how long one waits for an organ, particularly since a long wait can sometimes mean not getting it at all; many persons die each year while on waiting lists for a liver transplant. So the current system that HHS is seeking to change is difficult to defend on grounds of equity.

Even on consequentialist grounds, as Veatch notes, the data are ambiguous about whether local priority increases overall benefits through higher levels of donation and reduced organ deterioration from shorter ischemia times (length of time blood supply is deficient), but, for the sake of argument, I will assume that some local priority does increase overall benefits. Veatch is then correct that the conflict is one between equity and maximizing overall benefits. However, I want to broaden the debate some by questioning the account of equity that Veatch and HHS appear to share.

Both Veatch and HHS criticize the current system of local priority because it can result in patients with less severe illness receiving priority over sicker patients. For example, organs may go to Status 2 patients, who are seriously ill and usually hospitalized, instead of to sicker Status 1 patients with acute fulminant liver disease and a life expectancy fewer than seven days. Veatch favors giving priority to the sickest patients as an expression of the priority to the worst off that equity or justice requires. If we assume that Status 2 patients also have liver disease that will ultimately prove fatal without a transplant, then the difference between Status 1 and 2 patients is a matter of urgency—how quickly must the patient get a transplant to avoid dying? Veatch and HHS appear to assume that urgency is the proper criterion for equity. But is it?

To assess the moral importance of urgency in organ allocation, we need to distinguish between temporary and persistent scarcity. In temporary scarcity, there may be a period in which available resources are insufficient to meet the need, but that period is temporary and over time resources will be sufficient to meet the full need. When a lifesaving resource is temporarily scarce, it is reasonable to treat the most urgent cases first to avoid their dying before the scarcity is relieved; it will be possible to treat the less urgent cases later. This is simply a way to increase the number who can be treated.

Persistent scarcity, on the other hand, limits how many can be treated, and so giving preference to the most urgent cases determines who will be saved and who will die, but does not change the number who can be saved. It is hard to see why the fact that one's case has reached Status 1 urgency when a liver happens to become available would make it equitable that one gets it. In persistent scarcity, urgency should have little weight in selection of patients all of whose lives are threatened by their disease.

What other factors does equity require that we give weight to in allocating scarce livers? There is not space here to try to provide a full answer, but let me suggest one other important consideration. Imagine two Status 1 patients of equal urgency who each need the one organ we have available for transplant and who are otherwise similar except that one is age 25 and the other is age 65. Does equity or fairness require that we give each an equal chance to receive the scarce organ? Suppose the 25-year-old patient is Status 2 because he is expected to live for more than seven days, but less than one month, without a transplant. Does equity or fairness now require that the 65-year-old Status 1 patient receive the scarce organ? Many would say that in both of these cases the younger patient should receive priority. Why? Consequentialists might argue that we get a greater benefit in expected life-years by treating the younger patient, but that will not always be so and, in any case, I agree with Veatch that consequentialist reasoning should not be decisive here. Equity or fairness also favors the younger patient who will have had so much less life than the older patient if not treated.

I have argued elsewhere that equal opportunity to live a full life requires favoring the younger patient who will have been denied so much more of a full life without treatment than the older patient.[1] Alan Williams has characterized this as the fair innings argument—the older patient has had many more years of life and it would be unfair to give additional years to him while denying more years to the younger patient who has had so many fewer.[2] Frances Kamm supports a notion of need according to which the patient who will have had less life if not treated has the greatest need for the treatment.[3]

However the argument is formulated, the point is that equity or fairness is in significant part a backward-looking consideration—it looks back at how much the candidates for a resource have already had of what the resource can provide. Urgency, on the other hand, is a forward-looking consideration—how soon will a person suffer the loss that a scarce resource can prevent. In organ transplantation, persistent scarcity differences in the backward-looking consideration of how much life a patient has had will often be much greater, and more important morally, than differences in how quickly a patient will die without treatment. Equity or fairness requires that greater weight be given to age than to urgency.

So I am on Veatch's side in the consequentialism/equity conflict, though I do not believe that concern for equity should always outweigh aggregate benefit, but I have tried to suggest one important respect in which equity is more complex than the appeal to urgency.

NOTES

1. Brock DW. Justice, health care, and the elderly. *Philosophy and Public Affairs* 989 Summer;18(3):297–312.

2. Williams A. Intergenerational equity: An exploration of the 'fair innings' argument. *Health Economics* 1997:117–32.

3. Kamm F M. *Morality, Mortality. Vol. 1: Death and Whom To Save From It.* New York: Oxford University Press, 1993.

REPLY BY ROBERT M. VEATCH, PHD

Dan Brock adds clarity to complex issues. We agree that the fight over allocating livers involves disagreement between those who would allocate based on consequences and those who would include justice. From the justice perspective, if the most urgent patients beyond a local area are worst off, they have claims on organs even if that allocation would not maximize outcomes.

Brock challenges us to think more carefully about whether those with most urgent needs (Status 1) are necessarily the worst off. If less urgent patients are just as likely to die and die just as miserably, then Status 1 patients are not worse off, but merely further along their life trajectories. If less urgent patients eventually face equally awful lives, then their justice claims are equal.

When I suggested Status 1 patients were worst off, I did not spell out why. Consider three reasons. Since less urgent patients have longer times before their cases become critical, they are more likely not to die for lack of transplants. Their disease could fail to progress. Other technologies (xenografts, artificial organs, and new therapies) may negate the need for homografts. They may receive organs when no Status 1 patients are available.

It is reasonable to calculate how poorly off someone's life is by calculating the life's expected total quality-adjusted life years. This suggests Brock is right about age being a legitimate consideration. I have argued that younger persons have greater justice-based claims for organs for this reason.[1,2] But it also means that less urgent cases are more likely to avoid miserable outcomes and can reasonably be considered better off.

Two other reasons exist why Status 1 patients *might* have stronger justice claims. Some people believe that presently identified suffering persons have greater justice claims than unidentified persons who will eventually suffer just as much (the "identifiable lives problem"). That claim is controversial, but may be justified. If Status 1 patients are more certain to be among the worst off, they may also have justice-based claims for this reason.

Finally, justice is sometimes used to support a policy of "first come first served" when other criteria cannot be identified for just allocations. If a first-come policy is a valid criterion for resolving ties among people who are worst off, then giving Status 1 patients priority may be a crude marker for who has reached this status first. That claim will not always be true, but it is a good approximation. It may be more defensible than attempting to determine when less urgent patients have become among the worst off. Other justice-based considerations (such as age or waiting-list time) could also be factors in fair allocation. What is critical is that the discussion between Brock and me focuses on the complexities of determining who is worst off. If less urgent patients have justice-based claims, it is not because they will benefit more, but because somehow we can argue that they are as poorly off as Status 1 patients. I am convinced that, in general, they are not.

NOTES

1. Veatch RM. Winslow GR, Walters JW (eds). How age should matter: Justice as the basis for limiting care to the elderly. In *Facing Limits: Ethics and Health Care for the Elderly*. Boulder, CO: Westview Press, 1993:211–229.

2. Veatch RM. The role of age in allocation. In *The Ethics of Organ Transplantation* Washington, DC: Georgetown University Press, October, 2000:336–51. (Author note: This reference shows how my view differs from that of Frances Kamm.)

PART FOUR

In the Clinical Arena

DAVID STEINBERG, MD

Introduction: In the Clinical Arena

There are two types of decisions in clinical practice, medical decisions and non-medical decisions. Medical decisions pertain to diagnosis, the specifics of treatment, and prognostication and should be made by healthcare professionals. Non-medical decisions can be relatively mundane and may involve, for example, selection among qualified surgeons to perform a procedure, or selection of an approved nursing home for convalescence. They also can be value laden and vital; for example, determining whether the quality of a person's life justifies continued medical treatment.

This section is concerned with decisions in the clinical arena that are not entirely medical because important non-medical values are at stake. Who should make these "ethical decisions" and how should they be made? Many of these decisions involve moral values beyond the realm of medical expertise and therefore are not the exclusive prerogative of healthcare professionals. As Fischer and Arnold note, "healthcare providers have no claim to special expertise regarding what makes life worth living."

RESPECT FOR PATIENT AUTONOMY

In the US it is generally accepted that patients have the right to make medical treatment decisions that concern their own body; this ethical principle is formally known as respect for personal autonomy. To act autonomously a patient must be adequately informed, must understand the relevant information, must act without manipulation or coercion and should have the mental capacity to adequately process the relevant facts. One limitation of respecting a patient's autonomy is that patients do not always want autonomy. Some patients don't bother to read consent forms before agreeing to treatment, ask few or no questions, and simply decide to trust their doctor's judgment.

In some cultures patient autonomy may be withheld. Ethicists from Beijing, China, note "the key element of clinical decision making is not the will of the patient;" a traditional belief within Chinese society is that the patient deserves care and love and should be free of the responsibilities of decision making. To spare the patient from this burden, making medical decisions is delegated to the patient's family. The previous emperor of Japan, Hirohito, died without being told that he had stomach cancer. Some cultural preferences are worthy of respect, while others are not. When I was a medical intern in 1964 it was not unusual for a family to debate whether to tell their relative of a cancer diagnosis. Autonomy has subsequently been elevated to a primary moral principle in the US and patients are now generally told the truth about their condition—notwithstanding there are many ways to tell the truth—and given the right to make decisions that affect their own body.

In clinical medicine ethical conundrums arise when ethical principles conflict. For example, the principle of beneficence, which calls for healthcare professionals to do good, may conflict with the principle of respect for patient confidentiality. Should a doctor allow a patient to keep secret genetic information that is of life-saving importance to her sister? Should a doctor ever inform a spouse that a patient is HIV positive over the patient's express refusal to consent to that disclosure?

There are limits to patient autonomy. A patient cannot demand a brain biopsy when a brain biopsy is not medically indicated. Doctors must not simply acquiesce when patients make decisions against their medical best interest. Though it may require difficult conversations, doctors should strive to convince their patients to do what best serves their health and well-being. The conscientious physician may risk an accusation of paternalism, but in this context medical paternalism suffers undeserved disrepute. Genuine autonomy includes the right to make dumb decisions and, as I've learned from experience, medicine is an uncertain enterprise in which a doctor's advice is not always correct. With few exceptions, the patient should be allowed the last word.

ADVANCE DIRECTIVES

For patients who lack decision making capacity, there may be conflict or uncertainty over who is the appropriate surrogate decision maker. In most states selection of a surrogate decision maker (the proxy) can be made in advance of illness. Two standards have been set for surrogate decision makers. Whenever possible, surrogates should make the choices the patient would have made; this process is called substituted judgment. Unfortunately, studies have demonstrated that surrogate decision makers often misjudge the patient's preferences;[1] therefore, it's important for people to discuss their healthcare preferences with their designated proxy before they get sick. When the patient's wishes cannot reliably be discerned, the second standard calls for the proxy to act in the patient's best interest; the best interest standard suffers because what decisions are in a patient's best interest is not always obvious.

A living will is an alternative means of expressing one's wishes concerning medical treatment choices when one cannot actively engage in making decisions. A living will is a set of written healthcare treatment instructions intended to assist surrogate decision makers. Living wills suffer from two major faults. Not all future medical circumstances can be anticipated and living wills often express preferences in vague language using terms such as *heroic, extraordinary,* or *futile,* which can be difficult to interpret accurately.

Living wills can also be conflicting or confusing and may reflect clinically important misunderstandings. One of my patients, an older man who was responding nicely to treatment of a low-grade malignant lymphoma with chemotherapy, sent me a living will that said he would not want to be treated if he had an incurable disease. When I reminded him that he already had an incurable disease and was responding nicely to therapy he tore up the living will.

UNCERTAINTY

End-of-life scenarios are prone to ethical conflict because it may be uncertain whether the end of life is inevitably at hand and the time has come to allow a patient to die peacefully, free of needle sticks, tubes, and intravenous lines. It may also be uncertain whether the patient, now unresponsive, would have wanted continued treatment because his or her living will employs language that is difficult to interpret.

The much discussed concept of medical futility did not live up to expectations. It was hoped that if a treatment could reliably be deemed futile it could be stopped regardless of the patient's or surrogate's wishes to the contrary; however, the concept of medical futility proved to be more nuanced than was first appreciated. For example, the goal of a mechanical ventilator is to oxygenate circulating blood in a patient; if it performs that function its use is not, in terms of physiological value, futile because it achieved the desired outcome of improved oxygenation. If the mechanical ventilator sustains the life of an inevitably doomed patient, it may be considered futile in relation to a different set of values. Both withholding and withdrawing medical treatment in ethically appropriate circumstances are deemed acceptable; but crossing certain boundaries such as allowing physician-assisted suicide or euthanasia remains controversial.

If it could be known that a patient's death was both inevitable and imminent, continued treatment would make no sense. Similarly, if good quality survival was nearly certain, then stopping treatment would be a mistake. There is no consensus on the point between a zero and a 100 percent probability of recovery that should serve as the boundary separating reasonable from unreasonable treatment. Should we treat someone with a 40 percent chance of recovery? What if the probability of recovery is only 10 percent or 2 percent? The uncertainty of clinical medicine often makes prognostication difficult and further complicates these decisions. An ethics consult was requested by a critical care physician who was troubled because a patient's family insisted their relative be given cardiopulmonary resuscitation even though that seemed a futile effort. While we were discussing the case the patient suffered a cardiac arrest and was successfully resuscitated by the doctor who only moments earlier had predicted such an effort would be futile. Although the patient died later the same day this case illustrates how medical uncertainty can lead to conflicts.

Most hospitals have either ethics consultants or ethics committees to help patients, their loved ones, and healthcare professionals who believe they have an ethical problem. Ozar and Orr describe the value of ethics consultation. I have two strong feelings about ethics consultation: Ethics consultants should help clinicians define the nature of an ethical problem, identify the relevant values at stake, help with a well-reasoned analysis, and provide suggestions that hopefully will lead to the best available solution, however, the ethics consultant should not relieve clinicians of their professional responsibility for ethical decision making. Managing ethical conflict is a basic responsibility of the clinician and should not be outsourced to experts.

As Gert notes "there is no special expertise in ethics; everyone knows everything there is to know about their own moral principles." Clinical ethicists can be very helpful but at decision time they are no more skilled at telling the difference between right and wrong than anyone else.

The articles in this section that begin with a question are our "Ask the Ethicist" columns. In each issue of the *Lahey Clinic Journal of Medical Ethics* a case is presented to an ethicist. Although minor details have been changed to protect patient confidentiality, these are actual cases and outcomes. Before reading the ethicist's answer to a question think about your own response; if you disagree with the ethicist, remember, they're not authoritative and you're not necessarily wrong.

NOTE

1. Shalowitz David I; Garrett-Meyer, Wendler David. The Accuracy of Surrogate Decision makers *Arch Intern Med* 2006; 166: 493–497

☷ ☶ ☶ ☷

DAVID OZAR, PHD

The Value of an Ethics Consultation

Most hospitals and health systems now have either an ethics committee or trained ethicists on staff to provide ethics consulting assistance. In most institutions, such assistance is available to caregivers, patients, families, and anyone else involved in an ethically complex decision. Most ethics consultation programs are less than 10 or 15 years old, but healthcare ethics scholars and professional societies like the American Society for Bioethics and Humanities have begun to study ethics consultation carefully. This essay is the fruit of such study.

What is the value of an ethics consultation? Why would someone ask for this kind of assistance and what do those who offer ethics consultations aim to provide?

James Rest,[1] a psychologist of ethical development, has identified four components of ethical decision making and implementation and to these I will add two more. The six factors are: ethical sensitivity; ethical reasoning and judgment; ethical motivation; practical implementation; shared rather than isolated ethical wisdom; and fitting ethical decisions into our lives.

The first component of every ethical decision is being aware of what is ethically at stake. Rest calls this ethical "sensitivity." It is the ability to understand all that is ethically significant about a situation so it can be assessed from the perspective of various values, ethical principles, rights, virtues, and duties. It also entails appreciating the perspectives of the stakeholders.

Sometimes we overlook something that is ethically significant because we have a pattern of blindness to that kind of thing. For example, we might discount certain kinds of reactions or feelings as not important, or we might discount all of the experiences or feelings of a certain kind of person. But whether such deficits are situational or a more stable part of our makeup, if we want to make a good ethical decision, we need to rectify them. An ethics consultation can help with this, revealing a gap in our awareness of what is ethically at stake—either some ethical data that we are overlooking or the perspective of someone whose point of view we are not adequately attending to. Correcting a deficit of ethical sensitivity is one possible value of an ethics consultation.

Suppose, for example, a patient or a family requests life-extending treatments with serious side effects and little likelihood of benefit because they fear a lonely and painful death and see it as the only alternative. If they cannot hear caregivers' offers of good palliative care and assurances that they will not abandon them, an ethics consultation might get this message across.

A second thing that goes into good ethical decision making is good judgment about ethical matters. A person whose sensitivity is well attuned to a situation will often have a lot of ethical data to process; good ethical decision making depends on having the necessary skills for processing that data and using them to reach a sound judgment.

Most adults have some skill at processing ethical data, but very few have thought much about how ethical judgments are reached, much less about the thought patterns by which different kinds of ethical judgments are formed (e.g., the differences between judgments based on character and virtue, those based on maximizing values and minimizing harms, those based on principles or duties or rights, and so on). Few are truly skillful in determining when an ethical judgment is defective because it doesn't process the ethical data coherently. An ethics consultation can assist a decision maker in drawing a sound conclusion from the ethical data. Ethics consultants are also often able to offer helpful concepts and distinctions, such as those developed in the scholarly literature of healthcare ethics that can clarify the elements of a puzzling situation and render a difficult situation easier to comprehend. In addition, they are often able to clarify ethical judgments by being knowledgeable about the standards of professional ethics that are relevant to the situation.

Suppose a physician caring for a neurologically damaged patient feels confident that life-extending care is best for the patient, but has not asked what intervention the patient would choose if he or she could do so. An ethics consultation could help the physician attend to this important ethical principle for patients incapable of decision making.

A third element of good ethical decisions is motivation to do what one ought to do. Even when a person is sensitive to what is ethically at stake in a situation and judges well about what ought to be done, the person may not be motivated to act accordingly. The elements of motivation—a person's habits and patterns of living according to certain values, principles, and ideals—typically develop and grow only over time. So it would be inappropriate to expect an ethics consultation to magically rectify a deficit of motivation if that is the problem. But straightforward description of appropriate motivation and straightforward discussion of people's actual motivations can be very helpful. Occasionally it prompts significant change in decision makers' motivations and, in any case, it can at least assist the others involved in "calling a (motivational) spade a spade."

The fourth component of a good ethical decision is knowing how to implement it in a practical way and being emotionally able to do so rather than being hindered by feelings of fear or hopelessness. On the practical side—especially in complex institutional and professional settings like contemporary health care—people sometimes discover they do not know how to do what they ought to do. They may lack the needed expertise and do not know how to get assistance, or perhaps they do not know how to work the institution's systems. On the emotional side, they may have to confront powerful fears or a sense of hopelessness in order to carry out the action they have judged appropriate. Ethics consultations often contribute by educating the person on how to make it happen or helping the person handle his or her fears or sense of hopelessness. In many situations, for example, patients, family members, or caregivers are quite thoughtful in determining what they ought to do, but are overwhelmed that their choice is a choice between tragedies. An ethics consultation can help them deal with the hopelessness of such terrible choices and the fear that often attends being responsible for choosing the least bad outcome for someone else.

Throughout this essay, the decision maker has been spoken of as if the decision maker is always an individual. However, very frequently, the "decision maker" is a group of people acting as a unit. For example, if a patient is incapable of decision making, several family members may need to come to a consensus about treatment, even if one of them is formally and legally the official spokesperson. The nursing staff or the residents caring for a particular patient, or the entire interdisciplinary team may, in a given situation, function as a unit in deciding the ethically right intervention for the situation.

It is sometimes assumed that ethics consultations are there to serve ethics, to make sure people act ethically, as a sort of ethics police force. This view of ethics consultations is deeply mistaken. Ethics consultations are done for the sake of decision makers, to help them in their desire to make the best ethical decisions they can, not for some more abstract purpose.

This means that when deciding whether to seek an ethics consultation, those wanting assistance should stop to figure out who the decision maker is in the situation. Is this my personal decision? Is it my ethical questions with which I need help? Or is this a collective decision? Obviously, making this clear to those providing the ethics consultation will also help them in serving the decision maker or group effectively.

This takes us to a fifth component of good ethics consultations. Judging difficult ethical matters can be a very lonely business (whether the decision maker is an individual or a group) because we humans make our ethical decisions, in an important sense, before all the world. While no one else can be responsible for our actions, it is consoling to know that other thoughtful people are sharing in what may be a particularly difficult process or ethical judgment. This means that an ethics consultant—whether a committee or an individual—cannot walk out of a consultation thinking that everything that happened rested solely on the shoulders of the decision maker. Unless the decision maker chooses to ignore what has been shared in the consultation, the judgment about what ought to be done must be viewed as a shared judgment between decision maker and consultant. This sharing of responsibility, this gift of *consolation,* is often a very great gift for a decision maker.

Sixth, good ethical choices should make sense to the one making the decision. Furthermore, the decision maker should be able to explain it so it makes sense to others. When the story is told of what was ethically at stake in the situation, of the judgments this led to, of the motivation to carry out the decisions, the efforts taken to implement the decision and overcome hindrances, and of the actor's recognition of being the responsible party for what was done—that story needs to make logical, cognitive sense and affective, emotional sense.

WHY WOULD SOMEONE ASK FOR AN ETHICS CONSULTATION?

Since we know that these six characteristics of good ethical decision making are sometimes very hard to achieve, if there are people who can help us achieve them even a little better than we could on our own, that is a good thing. Many of us have friends or family members to whom we can turn to for assistance with ethical decisions in personal matters. What healthcare ethics committees and individual ethics consultants can do is provide similar assistance for difficult ethics decisions that need to be made within the institutional setting. That is the value of ethics consultation.

NOTE

1. Rest JR. The major components of morality. In Kurtines W, Gewirtz J (eds). *Morality, Moral Behavior, and Moral Development.* New York: Wiley, 1984.

SUGGESTED READING

Aulisio MP, Arnold RM, Youngner SJ. Health care ethics consultation: nature, goals, and competencies. A position paper from the Society for Health and Human Values-Society for Bioethics Consultation Task Force on Standards for Bioethics Consultation. *Ann Intern Med* 2000;133:59–69.

Freedman B., Francoicse B (ed). *The Roles and Responsibilities of the Ethics Consultant: A Retrospective Analysis of Cases.* Hagerstown, MD: University Publishing Group, 2000.

Ozar DT. Professions and professional ethics. In Reich W (ed). *Encyclopedia of Bioethics, revised edition.* New York: Macmillan, 1995.

Rest JR. Background: theory and research. In Rest JR, Narvaez D (eds). *Moral Development in the Professions.* Hillsdale, NJ: Lawrence Erlbaum, 1994:1–26.

☷ ☲ ☵ ☳

ROBERT D. ORR, MD. CM

Dialogue: Who Does the Ethics Consultation Serve?

An ethics consultation service is supposed to do just that—to provide a service. When I receive a request for an ethics consultation, whether from a member of the healthcare team (most commonly), or from a family member, or directly from a patient, my first question to the requestor is, "How can I be of help?" The conversation that ensues is intended to help me articulate "the ethics question" that will appear prominently at the beginning of the typed ethics consultation report, part of the patient's permanent record. This is often the most difficult part of the entire consultation process because the person making the request commonly perceives some distress, or discomfort, or conflict, but may not be able to articulate a classically understood ethical dilemma.

Notice that I did not open the consultation by asking, "How can I help you?" but "How can I be of help?" There is a subtle difference. The former would imply that the ethics consultation is expected to, or even intended to, serve the requestor. While that is often the case, sometimes the service the ethics consultant provides is for another of the three entities mentioned (team, family, patient), or even for "ethics" per se.

David Ozar has clearly articulated six potential values of an ethics consultation. This expansion on James Rest's components of morality[1] is useful in understanding the process of consultation and is also affirming for the ethics consultant. In his essay, however, Ozar says something that some professionals and some patients or families may find quite surprising: "Ethics consultations are done for the sake of decision makers, to help them in their desire to make the best ethical decisions they can, not for some more abstract purpose." The ethics consultant must occasionally point out that the course of action proposed or chosen by the decision makers is outside the bounds of accepted ethical standards. They may not be thrilled that "the best ethical decision" is not the decision they would make, and thus they might construe that the consultation was not done for their sake, but for the sake of some abstract purpose.

While I agree with Ozar that the ethics consultant must not be perceived to be either the ethics police or the ethics judge, proclaiming "Thou shalt . . ." or "Thou shalt not . . ." there are occasions when the ethics consultant must articulate standards and must try to ensure that these standards are met. For example, if the parents of a newborn girl with duodenal atresia refuse consent for standard lifesaving surgery because the infant also has Down Syndrome, and they request an ethics consultation to support their claim of parental discretion, the consultant is obligated to support the professionals and serve the infant by protecting her from this unethical request.

Some ethicists believe the ethics consultant should always maintain a neutral stance, acting only as a mediator in resolving conflict. In contrast, and more correctly in my estimation, Marsha Fowler has said the ethicist should ". . . analyze the case, explore acceptable alternatives and exclude wrong options."[2] The ethicist is sometimes obligated to establish some boundaries, such as that options A and B are ethically permissible, but option C is outside the bounds of accepted practice.

Dennis deLeon and I have argued elsewhere that the role of the ethics consultant varies in conflict resolution, serving in the three different roles understood in alternative dispute resolution, or sometimes serving a role not clearly representing any of these.[3] Sometimes the consultant does act as a mediator—facilitating the discussion, reframing the question, helping the parties develop creative alternatives. At other times he or she acts as a negotiator, actually "taking sides" after thoroughly evaluating a dispute and determining that one perspective is morally obligatory, then trying to persuade the other party to understand and relent. In other situations, the consultant is called in as an arbitrator to give guidance about the substance of the dilemma. Sometimes the ethics consultant changes roles as new information comes to light. And sometimes the ethics consultant "serves" without clearly fitting into any of these three roles.

The roles—mediator, negotiator, arbitrator—vary in at least two different ways. They vary first in the issue of partiality. The mediator enters the discussion as an impartial third party and remains neutral as he or she guides the process. The negotiator enters the discussion at the behest of one party to act as his or her advocate, and is thus partial from the outset. The arbitrator, on the other hand, is invited in by both parties to be an impartial analyst of the situation, ultimately giving an opinion as to the merits of both parties, and often "taking sides" at the conclusion.

The roles vary also in terms of standards. The mediator applies standards of process, insisting that both parties have a fair hearing, encouraging each to present his or her argument as clearly as possible, searching for common ground, or helping create a new solution, etc. The negotiator applies personal or professional standards in deciding whether to accept the request to advocate for one side, but once he or she accepts that role, pursues that goal with dedication. The arbitrator is expected to apply external standards of substance—standards that may come from medicine, ethics or law.

While I believe Ozar's statement that ethics consultations are done for the sake of the decision makers is most often correct, there are situations where the consultant (or committee) may be called upon to advocate for the patient who no longer has capacity to participate in the decision at hand. At other times, the consultation may articulate standards of ethics that may run counter to the wishes of one or more of the decision makers.

MEASURING THE VALUE OF ETHICS CONSULTATION

When researchers are trying to measure the value of a particular intervention, they must choose an objective end point, most often mortality, morbidity, quality of life, or cost. Assessing the value of ethics consultations is not so easy or precise. The end point most often chosen in such research is satisfaction—satisfaction of the professionals or satisfaction of the patient or surrogate. It is an interesting curiosity that healthcare professionals have generally found ethics consultations more helpful (71–90% of the time) than have patients or surrogates (57%).[4] In our earlier study, one family member queried about the usefulness of an ethics consultation done a few weeks earlier said, "The doctors and nurses may have found it helpful, but we didn't see the need for it."

Recently a multicenter study expanded the research to include cost and resource utilization. In a randomized comparison, Schneiderman et al. found that ethics consultations were associated with reductions in hospital days, and in the use of life-sustaining treatment without affecting mortality.[5] Their study again found that 90% of professionals and 80% of families found the consultations helpful.

THE DISVALUE OF ETHICS CONSULTATION

After providing bedside ethics consultations for about 15 years, I have a nagging concern about a potential problem with this whole endeavor. Mark Siegler, director of the fellowship program where I learned how to do ethics consultation, said at the end of our training, "You should work yourselves out of a job. Teach clinicians how to properly struggle with these ethical dilemmas so they will not need to request future consultations." I think that does actually happen in some settings and with some clinicians.

My fear, however, is that just the opposite happens in other situations. Some clinicians encounter a difficult situation and immediately request an ethics consult without taking the time or effort to dive into the dilemma themselves. The complexity of modern medicine, compounded by the pressure from payers to be efficient in providing health care, encourages some clinicians to "let the ethicist worry about it." Such a knee-jerk response to these profoundly important issues in medicine can further erode the vitally important patient-professional relationship.

Clinicians should continue to strive to provide whole person care. Rather than becoming merely medical technicians, they should seek to identify and resolve the physical, psychological, social, spiritual, and ethical needs of their patients. This sounds overwhelming in our current healthcare delivery system. Consultations are available in each of these domains and are clearly "of value." However, the availability of consultants does not relieve the clinician from the responsibility of addressing ethical dilemmas.

NOTES

1. Rest JR. The major components of morality. In Kurtines W, Gewirtz J (eds). *Morality, Moral Behavior, and Moral Development*. New York: Wiley, 1984.

2. Fowler MD. The role of the clinical ethicist. *Heart Lung* 1986;15(3):318–9.

3. Orr RD, deLeon DM. The role of the clinical ethicist in conflict resolution. *J Clin Ethics* 2000;11(1):21–30.

4. Orr RD, Morton KR, deLeon DM, Fals J. Evaluation of an ethics consultation service: Patient and family perspective. *Am J Med* 1996;101:135–41.

5. Schneiderman LJ, Gilmer T, Teetzel HD, et al. Effect of ethics consultations on nonbeneficial life-sustaining treatments in the intensive care setting. *JAMA* 2003;290:1166–72.

☰ ☲ ☲ ☷

JAMES E. SABIN, MD

Should I Lie to the Insurance Company?

QUESTION: A forty-eight-year-old male is becoming progressively incapacitated from the type of multiple sclerosis known as *chronic progressive MS*. He has fallen on a number of occasions, and his disease is interfering with his ability to work at his job and to participate in activities he finds pleasurable.

Within the recent past, ß-interferon has been demonstrated to reduce the number of new attacks and the incidence of new lesions in another form of the disease called *exacerbating-remitting MS*. Although patients with the chronic progressive disease are currently being studied, there is no current proof as to whether ß-interferon would be effective or not.

There are many neurologists, including myself, who believe that the two forms of the disease differ only in the ages at which they present, and that the ß-interferon should work as well for the one as for the other. That being the case, I feel a moral obligation to provide it to my patient, and I have prescribed it for him.

The cost to deliver it is approximately $10,000 per year, however, and the patient's managed care plan has requested a letter from me documenting that he has the exacerbating-remitting form of the disease. If I am honest, they will certainly deny him coverage. I am torn between my desire to be honest and my desire to help my patient. What is an ethicist's reading of this dilemma?

REPLY: Thank you for raising such gripping questions—they take us right to the heart of several major ethical issues.

We should start by probing the premise that you have "a moral obligation" to provide ß-interferon to your patient. Suppose your patient is poor, has no insurance, and you happen to have $10,000 to spare in your checking account. Would you truly feel morally obliged to withdraw the funds to purchase the ß-interferon for him? Doing so would be an admirably generous act, but do you believe that you would be violating a moral obligation by not doing it? I don't. Given your belief that ß-interferon might be of great benefit to your patient, you are correct in your decision to inform him of that possibility, but I doubt that you really mean to endorse the view that you are yourself obliged to provide it.

Many physicians, however, would advise you that even though you are not personally required to provide the ß-interferon through your own funds, you would be justified in lying to the insurance company to get it for him. I disagree.

Health insurance is a social mechanism by which groups of people pool resources to pay for health care. Because the resources are limited, insurance administration requires rules and regulations to determine how the available money will be spent. The entire insurance system ultimately depends on trust between the involved parties—patients, doctors, insurers, and the corporate and government entities that purchase the insurance for employees or groups of citizens.

You might argue, however, that your patient's suffering is so severe and, in your view, the likelihood of benefit to him is so great that lying is justified. After all, honesty is not an absolute value. If the Gestapo asked us if we were hiding Jews, the correct answer would be "no" whether we were or weren't. And if your patient's insurance program covers a million people, a $10,000 treatment for your patient will cost each member only a penny, so the funds your lie would commandeer from each subscriber are trivial.

If we physicians lie to insurers when we believe that doing so will benefit our patients, the system—and ultimately the common good—will deteriorate in several ways. Insurers aren't dumb. They will implement new ways of checking up on us or will decide to limit coverage. Other doctors will lie for less defendable reasons than yours. And when our patients see us lying to the insurer, their overall trust in the integrity of our profession will go down.

Managed care plans don't print money—they manage the collective funds of those who purchase the insurance. They may do this well or poorly, but that is their job. They are not simply deep pockets for us to raid as Robin Hoods in white coats.

I recommend the following course of action to you:

(1) Tell the patient that although ß-interferon is not a validated treatment for his disease, you believe it might benefit him, and explain why.

(2) Explain the insurance restrictions, and what the cost of the treatment would be to him.

(3) Tell the truth to the insurance company, and explain why you think the policy is wrong and the treatment should be provided.

(4) Since the same question will come up for other patients and neurologists, work with colleagues and MS advocacy groups to promote your perspective on coverage policy.

In countries where collective budgets provide insurance coverage to all citizens (almost all first world economies except for the US), it is easy to see that trade-offs and hard choices must be made. If ß-interferon is not a validated treatment for chronic progressive MS, I doubt that other countries would cover it because doing so would mean not covering something else of more potential benefit. Your wish to see the policy changed is totally legitimate, but it would be unethical to pursue your objective by lying to the insurance company and commandeering the pooled resources in the insurance fund without the consent of the subscribers who create the fund.

☷ ☶ ☵ ☴

DAVID GOLDBLATT, MD

Conflicting Advance Directives

QUESTION: A 68-year-old woman was admitted for treatment of a large cardioembolic left hemispheric stroke in the setting of atrial fibrillation. Several years previously, she had named her husband her Durable Power of Attorney for Health Care (DPAHC). She had annotated this document to state that if she were ever permanently incapacitated and unable to communicate, she wished all treatments including artificial hydration and nutrition (AHN) to be discontinued. Basing their conclusion on MRI findings after two weeks, the neurologists informed the family that she would have permanent aphasia and right-sided paralysis. Her physicians offered placement of a feeding gastrostomy tube. When her husband learned that she would die without it, he consented to the surgery. Their two daughters were upset that their mother's expressed wishes were being ignored. The physicians then were uncertain whether they should respect the patient's previous written directive or the current directive of her DPAHC. How would you advise them?

REPLY: A DPAHC may make any treatment decision on behalf of an incapacitated patient that the patient could previously make. Neither a patient with capacity nor a legally appointed surrogate may demand a specific treatment, but both may refuse even life-sustaining treatment. The "living will" portion of a Health Care Proxy and annotations on a Durable Power of Attorney are written advance directives stating the patient's wishes. They are best regarded as the patient's advice to her legal surrogate and her professional caregivers. State proxy laws vary: a DPAHC who lacks knowledge of the patient's wishes may usually make a decision about AHN in the patient's "best interests." Institutional pressures may make it difficult to justify failure to place a feeding tube, but physicians must never act against what they consider to be the best interests of the patient. If the treating physician favors AHN and no proxy decision is available, a court must consent to surgery on the patient's behalf.

Two weeks after an embolic stroke, a prognosis of permanent loss of ability to communicate and permanent paralysis is difficult to make. Moreover, failure to regain the ability to take food by mouth is unusual after unilateral hemispheric insult. The physicians are obliged to indicate a reasonable range of possible outcomes, to be sure that the proxy's consent or refusal of treatment is "informed." They should explore the husband's understanding of the patient's advance directive in detail. Perhaps he believes she meant permanent, total inability to communicate or complete hemiplegia. Neither of those conditions is a likely outcome of an embolic stroke. He should also understand the handicap imposed by lesser degrees of dysphagia, dysphasia, and hemiparesis. Because good ethics begins with good medicine, the patient or DPAHC must receive accurate medical information and must understand it. Otherwise, consent or refusal cannot be truly informed.

The efforts of the patient's attending physician or an ethics consultant should be directed at helping her husband to understand and accept his role: he is to decide as the patient would decide, not as he thinks best or in response to his anticipatory grief at losing his wife. If he accepts the physicians' prediction, he must also be helped to understand that his wife has chosen not to prolong her life under such circumstances. If he continues to insist on the feeding tube, it may be helpful to assure him that there is no legal or moral difference between refusing and withdrawing a treatment. He will be able to decide at a later date to discontinue the treatment if his wife does not become self-sufficient or recover her ability to communicate.

The patient created a written advance directive that her husband was obliged to follow. If in the years following the creation of this directive she had told her husband that she had changed her mind and would accept AHN, he could conform to her oral instruction. In practice, the DPAHC often fails to decide in accordance with the patient's expressed wishes. In this case, one or both daughters could seek to remove their father from his role as legal surrogate through court action. A physician responsible for the patient's care may also seek to have a legal guardian appointed to replace a DPAHC who appears to be acting against the patient's instructions. A court, however, is not likely to replace as DPAHC a spouse who is able to demonstrate his understanding of the situation the patient faces and the predicted consequences of various treatment decisions.

Physicians are not obligated to respect the wishes of family members who have not been appointed to be the patient's proxy, but they are understandably mindful of the rifts among family members that often follow on the death or incapacitation of a loved one, and may try to preserve family unity, reasoning that their patient would wish for that outcome. Family dynamics are complex, however; even the principals in a conflict may not fully understand them. It seems most prudent, therefore, to offer information and mediation, but not attempt to manage the disagreement or impose unwanted treatment. In this instance, the physicians merely offered the tube feeding, as they should. They did not try to force-feed their patient. This was a wise decision.

OUTCOME: After several days, the daughters succeeded in persuading their father that a feeding tube should not be inserted. The patient died approximately a week later.

SUGGESTED READING

Bernat JL. *Ethical Issues in Neurology,* 2nd ed. Boston: Butterworth-Heinemann, 2002:79–104;157–81.

Goldblatt D. A messy necessary end. Health care proxies deserve our support. *Neurology* 2001;56:148–52.

Goldblatt D. Who's listening? Advance directives are not always directive. *The Neurologist* 2001;7:180–5.

☰ ╟╢ ╟╢ ☰

DAVID STEINBERG, MD

What Information Should Be Disclosed to Patients?

Most people agree that patients should be given adequate information about their health and any planned medical interventions. The difficulty is defining what constitutes adequate information. Three standards of information disclosure have traditionally been used. All of them are flawed.

The professional standard requires disclosure consistent with the standards of other professionals in the same community acting in the patient's best interest. Standards defined in this manner risk disproportionately reflecting the values of professionals, not patients. Also, the question of how professional standards were justified in the first place is left unanswered.

The reasonable person standard calls for the provision of information that a reasonable person would want. This standard suffers because of the difficulty gauging the needs of a hypothetical reasonable person; also, reasonable people may differ in their information needs.

The third standard—and my preference of the traditional models—is the subjective standard, which calls for information to be tailored to the needs of each patient. Physician and patient engage in dialogue; if more information is requested, it is given. The subjective standard is, however, fragile because it depends on the skill and willingness of the physician to engage in this sort of information exchange and on the ability of the patient to ask the right questions.

The existing disclosure standards are based on what professionals, reasonable people, and individual patients choose to know or disclose. Little attention is paid to the characteristics of information itself. Why should a physician decide to disclose certain information and not other information? Why should a patient want certain information and not other information? A challenging case illustrates the inadequacy of the currently used standards and will serve to demonstrate a different way of analyzing disclosure decisions that considers the characteristics of information.

The American Red Cross notified a hospital blood bank director that a unit of blood shipped to his hospital a year earlier and transfused to a patient came from an apparently healthy donor who subsequently developed Creutzfeldt-Jakob Disease (CJD). Because CJD has a long incubation period, the donor probably harbored the causative agent at the time of donation. The letter noted that the American Red Cross, the Centers for Disease Control, and the New York Blood Center "strongly discouraged" sharing this information with the recipient of the blood transfusion because there was no screening test and no treatment and because the information would cause the patient "tremendous stress." The letter also noted that representatives of the hemophilia community, a highly transfused group, disagreed with this position and at public meetings expressed their expectations that recipients of possibly tainted blood be notified.

CJD is a rare, rapidly progressive fatal brain disorder that has been transmitted to humans by hormones derived from cadaveric pituitary glands, corneal transplants, dura mater grafts, and reusable deep brain electrodes. A variant of CJD has been transmitted with the ingestion of beef and is popularly known as "mad cow disease."[1] The transmission of CJD by blood transfusion is theoretically possible but there have been no documented cases.[2] We might expect the increased use of blood products in recent decades to be associated with an increase in CJD if CJD were transmitted by blood; but that has not been the case. Confounding this reassuring data is CJD's long incubation period, which can be decades; heavily transfused people may not survive long enough for us to observe manifestations of the disease. The rarity of CJD limits our ability to obtain a reliable number of observations and there is no laboratory test to determine whether the causative agent has been transmitted.

There is reason for the blood bank director not to notify the recipient of the CJD blood. There is no proof that blood transmits the disease, there is no test similar to HIV testing that would indicate whether the agent has been transmitted, there is no treatment for CJD, and notification could be psychologically devastating to the recipient. However, CJD might be transmitted by blood, the illness is horrendous, the patient might want this information, and although there is no treatment for CJD, it would be prudent for the recipient to know he should avoid donating any of his tissues or organs.

How should the blood bank director analyze this case? The traditional disclosure standards are not helpful. Decisions concerning the notification of CJD blood recipients are so unusual—and there are no clearly analogous situations—that no community professional standard exists. In several informal surveys, about half of the presumably reasonable people I questioned would want to be informed if they had received blood from someone who developed CJD and half would prefer they not receive this information. In the wake of a CJD scare in Canada involving the transfusion of albumin from a donor who subsequently developed CJD, 68 percent of presumably reasonable Alberta residents favored notification of recipients and 32 percent did not.[3] Because some reasonable people favor notification and others do not, the reasonable person standard is not helpful.

The subjective standard would be difficult to implement because the blood bank director could not call the patient a year after the transfusion without explaining the reason for the call—which would lead to notification of the patient independent of the patient's wishes. If there were a physician who knew the patient, that might to some degree obviate this problem.

Another approach to information disclosure discussions examines eight characteristics.[4] Consideration of these factors may not make the blood bank director's decision easier, but they provide a useful framework for thinking about the problem.

Relevance is a threshold criterion. CJD is an infectious disease and its transmission by blood is theoretically possible; therefore information about the transfusion is relevant to the recipient. If the blood donor had glaucoma, that information would not be relevant because there is no reason to believe glaucoma can be transmitted by blood.

Probability is an important factor because an event that occurs with a probability of 1 in 10,000 does not have the same claim on disclosure as an event that occurs with a probability of 10 percent. It is a reasonable guess that the probability of CJD transmission by blood transfusion is very low.

The significance of information is important because omitting insignificant information is less ethically troublesome than materially significant information. For example, an evanescent rash does not demand disclosure as strongly as heart or kidney failure. The factor of significance is high in this case because CJD destroys the brain and is fatal.

The availability of interventions can in some instances trump all other factors. There is no diagnostic test for CJD and no treatment. The recipient of CJD blood would be well advised not to donate blood, a kidney, a lobe of liver or, when he dies, his corneas. Notification now might be advised so the patient can be alert to tests or treatments developed in the future. At this time the availability of CJD-related interventions should be considered relatively low.

Does the patient have a subjective need for this information? Faced with the prospect of a fatal illness, even if the probability is low, some people might alter their lifestyle, take a long anticipated trip, or resolve a festering family dispute. We do not know the recipient in this case, therefore his subjective needs must be considered unknown.

The disclosure of information can cause harms. The knowledge that you have received blood from someone who developed an awful and ultimately fatal brain disease can cause anxiety and depression. Some Canadian recipients of CJD albumin were "scared silly every time they forgot a number or a key." If you inform a recipient of CJD blood, you may cause considerable harm.

Patient autonomy should be respected. If a patient has made it clear that he doesn't want certain types of information, that wish should be respected. However, if a patient has indicated a desire for detailed information about his or her condition, even trivial details, to the extent possible those wishes should also be respected. Clinicians who routinely solicit information preferences from their patients are better equipped to gauge the factor of patient autonomy.

The decision maker's perspective cannot be ignored. A transfusion service director who, in the wake of the AIDS crisis, promised full disclosure in all cases would be under self-imposed pressure to inform the CJD recipient. A decision maker in a different professional culture that frowns on delivering bad news is likely to be more restrained. When the disclosure decision is difficult, as in this case, my perspective is to err on the side of disclosure. That's why I would inform the recipient of CJD blood.

When there is a substantial probability of a significant future event and beneficial interventions are available, a patient who would want the relevant information and use it to modify his life without suffering mental turmoil should receive it. Of course, difficult cases will not be this straightforward. Information about some of the eight characteristics may be unknown or controversial and it may be unclear how to weigh contradicting factors, which differ qualitatively, one against the other. Despite these limitations, disclosure decisions are best made by including an analysis of the characteristics of the information in question rather than resorting to the flawed traditional professional, reasonable person, and subjective standards. The identification of eight characteristics—relevance, probability, significance, availability of interventions, subjective needs, harms, autonomy, and the decision maker's perspective—will hopefully provide a framework for this analysis.

NOTES

1. Rhodes R. *Deadly Feasts: The Prion Controversy and the Public's Health.* New York Touchstone, 1998.

2. Dodd RY, Sullivan MT. Creutzfeldt-Jakob disease and transfusion safety: tilting at icebergs? *Transfusion* 1998;38(3):221–3.

3. Sibbard B. Features. *Can Med Assoc J* 1998;159:829–31.

4. Steinberg D. Informing a recipient of blood from a donor who developed Creutzfeldt-Jakob disease: the characteristics of information that warrant its disclosure. *J Clin Ethics* 2001;12(2):134–40.

☰ ☰ ☰ ☰

HEATHER J. GERT, PHD

The Characteristics of Information and Avoiding Surprises

In his article "What information should be disclosed to patients?"[1] David Steinberg notes that none of the traditional standards for determining what information patients should receive is wholly satisfactory. Instead of these standards, Steinberg suggests that physicians consider eight characteristics of the information they are thinking about disclosing.[2]

I agree with Steinberg that his list of characteristics can be a useful tool for thinking about when to disclose a certain bit of information, and that the traditional standards he discusses often don't work. I also applaud the fact that he would give patients more information than traditional standards require. Unfortunately, although consideration of his characteristics may be a useful guide, I doubt that it can serve as a standard for judging when withholding information is permissible. Before looking at Steinberg's suggestion, I will present my own principle. This is the principle of avoiding unsurprising surprises.[3]

According to the principle of avoiding surprises, what physicians should aim at is not merely that patients have sufficient information to give (or withhold) informed consent—as traditional standards require—but at protecting their patients from being surprised by anything having to do with their healthcare situation.[4] So, for instance, patients should be told about the discomforts they'll probably experience while recovering from surgery. And this is so even when no one in their right mind believes that the information will affect the patient's treatment decision. Most people simply like to know what to expect, and this is especially true when they are going into situations that are already scary.

But to demand that physicians tell patients about every possible outcome that might surprise them, no matter how unlikely, is to demand too much. It would also mean overloading patients with information, much of which physicians are certain will not actually protect them from any surprises. Therefore, if a possible outcome is so unlikely that the physician himself would be sincerely surprised if it occurred, then the physician isn't required to disclose that possibility. In short, this principle says that unless a physician would be willing to say that he was unprepared for a given outcome, he should ensure that his patient is prepared for it as well.

Now let us return to Steinberg's characteristics, and compare them with my principle. His characteristics are: (1) relevance, (2) probability, (3) significance, (4) availability of interventions, (5) subjective need, (6) harms of telling, (7) patient autonomy, and (8) the decision maker's perspective. We will consider them in turn:

We might first collapse Steinberg's first characteristic into his second. A fact is relevant insofar as it has a bearing on the probability that the patient will suffer a certain harm, or gain a certain benefit. If the director of a blood bank learns that the donor of a unit of blood has recently been arrested, he clearly has no obligation to provide the recipient of that blood with this information. This is because the information is irrelevant, and it is irrelevant in the sense that it has no bearing on the probability that the recipient will develop or avoid any medical problems.

Of course, the principle of avoiding unsurprising surprises takes relevance and probability into account as well. But it also gives a reason for this: Relevance and probability are important because, among other reasons, it is important to help patients avoid surprises. Whether or not a physician must pass along a given bit of information depends on how probable it is that doing so will ensure that the patient avoids being surprised. If the probability is high enough that the physician would not be seriously surprised by an outcome, then she should give the patient that information. To use Steinberg's example, if what the director of the blood bank has learned is that a donor has developed Creutzfeldt-Jakob Disease (CJD), and he would not be surprised that CJD can be contracted in this way, then he is obligated to inform the donor that she may have contracted CJD.

Significance is important as well, and this is Steinberg's third characteristic; developing a rash is less significant than developing CJD. But significance will also affect whether or not a patient is surprised, and how surprised he is. It is much more surprising to discover that you have CJD than that you have a rash. But patients are surprised by rashes, and should be warned of them. Thus, whereas talk of characteristics encourages us to think of significance as a continuum, I am inclined to see it as a threshold. If an outcome is significant enough to cause surprise, then the patient should be informed about it.

One of the main reasons patients want information is so that they can use it to make informed decisions. This fact is reflected in Steinberg's fourth and fifth characteristics, availability of interventions and subjective need. In talking of subjective need, Steinberg reminds us that information about one's prognosis, what to expect during recovery, etc., can affect many decisions beyond those about medical interventions; the decision to reconcile with a family member or friend, for instance, or when to schedule an important meeting. The need to make decisions such as these is what Steinberg calls subjective need.

One way of putting the gist of the principle of avoiding surprises is to say that patients often have a legitimate subjective need for information, even when that information will not affect any decisions in or out of the medical context. That is, they have a subjective need to avoid surprises. For instance, patients often feel tricked or betrayed when they experience unexpected pain while recovering from surgery, or even when they are surprised by less than pleasant aspects of hospital routine. Again, this is true even when they acknowledge that the information would not have affected their decision regarding treatment *or any other decisions.*

The sixth characteristic Steinberg discusses is the harm that being informed might cause the patient. As with most other moral principles, the fact that someone might die, or be permanently disabled—and has not voluntarily accepted this risk—is normally overriding. So I agree that this consideration can also override the principle of avoiding surprises.

Nonetheless, the fact that bad news will harm by causing anxiety does not weigh strongly against informing a patient. That Steinberg's seventh characteristic is autonomy hints at this, but I would stress it more strongly. He also notes that sometimes patients don't want information, and that in these cases autonomy requires not telling. This is also consistent with the principle. As with other obligations, the person to whom the obligation to inform is owed can waive it. So a patient can tell her physician that she waives protection from surprises, and prefers not to have certain information. But merely preferring not to be told is not the same as waiving the obligation to tell. Thus, the physician's sense that her patient does not want information is not enough to justify withholding it. She should get explicit permission.[5]

Finally, Steinberg's eighth characteristic concerns physician- rather than patient-centered considerations. He notes that medical professionals working in a setting that frowns on delivering bad news will find it diffi-cult to deliver such information. That is true, but the principle of avoiding surprises encourages us to criticize the culture of such a setting. This seems a good thing to me. As I hope it's easy to see, I agree with Steinberg that healthcare workers should take the characteristics he lists into ac-count. But I think his suggestion is vulnerable to one of the same worries he expressed about the subjective (conversation) standard: it depends on the good will of physicians. In the odd case where a patient or ethics com-mittee is dealing with a physician who does not believe that patients should be informed, a requirement to *take into account* characteristics is simply not enough. Such a physician can truly take characteristics into ac-count and still always decide to withhold information.

The principle of avoiding surprises, on the other hand, provides some recourse. This is because most of the time there is general agreement about which possible outcomes would be surprising. Moreover, if the pa-tient is surprised, that is some—albeit inconclusive—reason to believe that the physician should have provided the information. Also, a physi-cian who fails to warn a patient must be willing to say that he was unpre-pared for that outcome, and so may be open to the criticism that he should have been. Granted, there will be instances in which it is not clear that the physician should have been prepared for an outcome, or should have found it unsurprising. But these correspond with the instances in which it simply is not clear whether the physician had the obligation to provide that information. There are gray areas. Although Steinberg's characteristics will be helpful for physicians sincerely looking for guid-ance, my concern is that they cannot provide a standard, and would not allow criticism of those rare physicians who stubbornly refuse to inform their patients.

NOTES

1. www.Lahey.org/Ethics/Newsletter/ Fall2002.asp

2. In the interest of space, I will use the term *physician*. But I really have in mind health care professionals more generally.

3. Gert HJ. Avoiding surprises. A model for informing patients. *Hastings Cent Rep* 2002;32(5):23–32. For simplicity's sake, in what follows I will usually drop the "unsurprising" and refer to this as principle of avoiding surprises.

4. Steinberg does not explicitly represent these standards as specifically concerned with informed consent, but this is how they are usually discussed in the literature.

5. It might even be an explicit condition of treatment or testing that a patient waive that obligation. For instance, testing done to detect a specific genetic malady can result in information about paternity. Many believe that it is best to have an explicit policy noting that such information, collected inadvertently, will not be provided. If the patient freely releases the physician from this obligation, she is no longer obligated to provide the gath-ered information.

Although I listed the characteristics of information I thought warranted consideration, Gert is correct in noting that I did not provide a standard or formula to weigh and balance those characteristics to make a disclosure decision. To her credit she attempts this next step. Gert does this using the notion of surprise.

This is an intriguing but problematic solution. She is judging an action with moral content—disclosing medical information—by a psychological reaction. Some patients are inattentive, forgetful, or prone to denial; information can be appropriately disclosed yet the patient will nonetheless be surprised by a disclosed event. Other patients have an innately pessimistic view of life and may suffer an expected, untoward event that was not disclosed, yet they will not be surprised because they believe that bad things happen. In both cases the reaction of surprise would incorrectly judge how appropriately information was disclosed.

Physicians are also subject to the vagaries of human behavior; what surprises one physician might not surprise another. For the notion of surprise to be a useful concept it cannot be subject to the whims of human psychology. This forces us to ask the question, when should a physician be surprised? If a side effect randomly occurs once in every 25,000 patients who receive drug X, should the physician be surprised when it happens to his patient? He should not be surprised because the event is known to occur and, because it is a random event, there is no reason for him to believe it could not happen to one of his patients. However, the physician might be surprised in the way I would be surprised if I won the lottery. I know it is possible for me to win, but I'm surprised because I won despite long odds. If the physician should be surprised at an event that occurs once in every 25,000 patients, should he be surprised at an event that occurs once in 150 patients? What is the threshold for surprise?

To make the notion of surprise useful, we need a developed ethics of surprise that provides the rules for determining when a patient or physician should be surprised. Because Gert has not yet developed this, the notion of surprise, although useful in many instances, cannot serve as the final arbiter of disclosure decisions.

Some of the characteristics of information I've identified may in some cases clearly trump the others. However, disclosure decisions are often made within a hazy web of complex and conflicting factors. We often have to weigh one against the other and struggle to make the most defensible decision. I do not see a simple universal solution on the horizon.

☷ ☶ ☵ ☳

JOHN A. BALINT, MD, FRCP

The Man Who Wouldn't Be Shocked

QUESTION: In 2002, a 67-year-old man with a history of myocardial infarction was admitted to the hospital because of an episode of life-threatening ventricular tachycardia. To prevent sudden death from future episodes of cardiac arrhythmia, his physicians recommended—and the patient agreed to—placement of an implantable cardioverter-defibrillator (ICD). The device produces a shock in response to a dangerous arrhythmia.

In 2003, he had another life-threatening episode of ventricular tachycardia, successfully treated by a single discharge from the ICD. In 2005, however, the patient asked to have the ICD removed. He felt that it never had been necessary and said it was causing abdominal discomfort and insomnia. He refused deactivation of the device, insisting on removal.

He was told that removal would result in a two to three percent risk of serious infection, and that, without the device, there would be a 30 percent risk of recurrent arrhythmia and possible sudden death within the next few years. Despite repeated efforts by his physician to convince him of the importance of leaving the ICD in place, the patient continued to insist on removal, and eventually retained an attorney. A psychiatrist found the patient capable of decision making.

The patient's cardiologist thought it was medically inappropriate to remove the device; on the other hand, he recognized the patient's right to make decisions concerning his own body.

How would you advise the cardiologist?

REPLY: The issues in this case can best be examined in the contest of the "four boxes" described by Jonsen, Siegler and Winslade.[1]

1. Medical Indications,
2. Patient Preferences,
3. Quality of Life, and
4. Contextual Issues.

The medical issues clearly indicate that retention of the ICD would have benefits. Therefore, the medical indications are for retaining the ICD.

The patient's preference, however, is clearly for removal. We are not given any clear indications as to the patient's values that might explain his demand for removal of an apparently effective device. Is he truly so discomforted by the presence of the ICD that he would rather face the risk of sudden death? Is there some psychological factor which makes reliance on such a device an intolerable burden? This area would need exploration.

The issue of patient competence or capacity for decision making was resolved by psychiatric consultation and found to be in good order.

In trying to deal with refusal of beneficial care, it is worthwhile to address the issue of a therapeutic trial of defined duration. Perhaps a trial of medication for control of his discomfort and insomnia, or even of changing the placement of the device on the abdominal wall, might be an option.

The patient's preferences are closely tied to considerations of quality of life. Lack of sleep and chronic discomfort, as already noted, may make living with the ICD too burdensome. It may also be that concerns about how well the device will function are causing an unacceptable level of anxiety.

The contextual factors in this situation may relate to the family dynamics. Does he have a wife, children, or siblings who are there for support? Has there been a recent death in the family, perhaps from heart disease, that precipitated the patient's wish to have the ICD removed? If the family is close and supportive, they must be brought into the discussion if at all possible.

In the final analysis, patient autonomy, if based on competent consideration of the options, even if apparently irrational from the physicians' viewpoint, must take precedence over the physicians' beneficent advice. In this case, if the patient is indeed competent, has rational reasons for his decision and family support, I would advise removal of the ICD.

OUTCOME: Efforts to help the patient adjust to the ICD involved his family and psychiatrist and were unsuccessful. The device was removed. The patient remains alive and well 32 weeks after removal of the ICD.

NOTE

1. Jonsen AR, Siegler M, Winslade WJ. *Cllinical Ethics 3rd Ed.* McGraw-Hill, 1992.

☰ ⠇⠇⠇ ⠇⠇⠇ ☰

DAN W. BROCK, PHD

The Case of the Unresponsive Hermit

QUESTION: An 83-year-old woman did not answer the door for Meals on Wheels. She was found on the floor, unresponsive. She had no known relatives or friends and no one knew anything about her beliefs or values.

She was hospitalized with an elevated serum calcium and impaired function. A CT Scan showed a large pelvic mass and a chest X-ray revealed multiple nodules consistent with metastatic disease.

The clinical diagnosis was metastatic cancer. A gynecologic oncologist was consulted. It was his opinion that a meaningful response to treatment was unlikely. He advised comfort measures only.

Despite correction of her serum calcium, the patient remained unresponsive. The primary care physician agreed with the advice to keep the patient comfortable; however, the physician felt uneasy making an important decision for an incompetent patient in the absence of a surrogate decision maker. A psychiatrist confirmed that the patient was not competent and advised the primary physician to ask the court to appoint a legal guardian.

Other colleagues, however, advised the primary physician against seeking a legal guardian. They believed "comfort measures only" was the right treatment and that physicians have the training and responsibility to make decisions of this type and should be trusted to do so.

How would you advise the primary physician?

REPLY: Incompetent patients without natural surrogates can present special problems when decisions must be made about whether to employ or forgo possibly life-sustaining treatment. The first question, in this case and generally, is whether the patient is incompetent. I shall assume that the psychiatric evaluation established that there was no significant possibility that the patient could become able to make decisions about her care.

The central ethical issue is who should decide about the patient's care. Could the physician take responsibility as her colleagues urged, or should she apply to the courts for legal guardianship? Both alternatives have significant drawbacks.

There is a potential for abuse if physicians make decisions on their own to forgo life-sustaining treatment for incompetent patients. For example, the possibilities of treatment that would be of significant benefit may not be adequately explored because no one else is serving as an advocate. Or discrimination may take place against patients without funds or against members of minority groups.

On the other hand, going to court to have a legal guardian appointed can be a time-consuming and expensive process, and the result can be an attorney with little interest or ability to serve effectively as surrogate for the patient.

Better than either of these alternatives is for the healthcare institution to anticipate cases like this—they are hardly rare—and to have procedures in place to provide the attending physician with further review of the decision.

One possibility used by some hospitals is to require consultation with the chief of service, who is charged with the responsibility of deciding what further review or measures, if any, are necessary before any decision to forgo life-sustaining treatment is made.

Another possibility is to require consultation with the institution's ethics committee, which can provide an exploration of the ethical aspects of the decision from different perspectives. The general point is that the health-care institution should have some established practice in place to ensure that someone beyond the attending physician reviews the decision before it is carried out, and that the practice is flexible enough to permit different responses to different cases. Sometimes the decision may be sufficiently troubling, controversial, or legally problematic that the courts should become involved, but in my view, that is neither desirable nor required in all such cases, and probably would not be found to be necessary in this case.

OUTCOME: A guardian was appointed by the court. Communication between the guardian and the primary physician was difficult. The order for "comfort measures only" was given; the patient expired.

☷ ☶ ☵ ☳

STUART J. YOUNGNER, MD

Live Organ Donation: Determining the Mental Age of Consent

QUESTION: Robert L. contacted the renal transplant coordinator stating that he wished to donate a kidney to his older brother George who was on dialysis for end-stage renal failure. Robert is a 42-year-old mentally retarded man with an IQ between 70 and 80. He lives independently without a guardian and has a job.

Robert's psychologist, who has known him for 10 years, submitted a letter stating that he believed Robert was capable of giving informed consent for the donation. The renal transplant psychiatric social worker found that Robert came from a close-knit family, had a warm relationship with George, and concluded that he was capable of making an informed decision. There were several meetings with the transplant nephrologist. Robert met with him alone as well as with his family. The nephrologist's evaluation concluded that Robert understood that his donation was voluntary and that he was capable of giving informed consent.

On the day of surgery the anesthesiologist, who did not know Robert, was reluctant to provide anesthesia in this circumstance. When the prior evaluations were reviewed with the anesthesiologist, he agreed to proceed but the surgery was canceled because of an infected mosquito bite. To reassure everyone that the donation was appropriate, a psychiatrist who had not previously seen Robert was consulted. This psychiatrist disagreed with the previous evaluations and concluded Robert should not be allowed to donate a kidney to his brother.

How would you advise the kidney transplant team faced with one dissenting opinion?

REPLY: As the waiting list for organs grows, our society has turned more often to living donors, persons who give one of paired organs, the kidneys, or part of an unpaired organ such as the liver. The problem with living organ donation is that the donors expose themselves to risk of harm. For single kidney donation, the risk of death (0.04% as reported by the Organ Procurement and Transplantation Network[1]) or serious morbidity is small and the benefits for the donor can be considerable.[2] Still, an otherwise healthy person must undergo major surgery in order to donate and even if things go as well as possible, there is certainly temporary pain, discomfort, disability, lost work or social opportunity, and the risk of living with only one kidney. Nonetheless, living donation is increasingly common and in 2001, the number of living kidney donors exceeded the number of dead donors.[3]

If donors are going to be exposed to the unavoidable morbidity of surgery and the risk of even more serious harm, we want to be sure they give full, informed consent. This means receiving adequate information about the risks, having adequate mental capacity to process that information, and finally, not being coerced or unduly pressured. In evaluating the appropriateness of Robert L. as a donor for his brother George, there is reason for questions about two of these three issues (I will assume that the transplant team has given him enough information). While we are not told specifically why the psychiatrist dissented, the following issues should be considered.

First, was there undue pressure on Robert to donate? Some argue that being a family member, by its very nature, puts one in a coerced position. How can you say no to a family member without being made to feel disloyal or worse? Nonetheless, our society has generally accepted the notion of live donation within families. In fact, we have traditionally been more comfortable with family donation than we have with donation by friends, acquaintances, and certainly, outright strangers (although each of these categories is becoming more acceptable as well). I believe that the "coercive" aspects of being part of a family are considered by most of us to be part of the perceived obligations that come in many forms simply from being a family member. Of course, there can be coercion beyond that, and the most vulnerable to excessive coercion within families are children or adults who are emotionally, physically, or financially dependent.

Robert is not a child. While retarded, he has a degree of social and financial independence. The family is described as close-knit and loving. He seems to have a good relationship with them and his brother, the recipient. Robert himself came forward with the donation offer. Unless the dissenting psychiatrist has information to the contrary, undue coercion does not seem a reasonable justification for denying Robert's request to donate.

The second issue that must be considered is that Robert has some degree of mental retardation.[4] We must ask if he was capable of giving informed consent even though he is able to get along pretty well. He works, lives alone, and from what we know, makes important life judgments every day. We have no information that he has ever been judged incompetent to make important life decisions. He has, from all that we know, a loving and supportive family. To discount his ability to consent to donation, we would have to have specific information about how his intellectual deficits impair his ability to understand the nature of the surgery, its risks, etc. Because the most serious risks (death and disability) are extremely unlikely, the threshold for judging his ability need not be as exacting as it would be if he were facing a high likelihood of serious risk.

The evaluation was quite thorough prior to the second, dissenting opinion and the psychiatrist has not given us any specific information to make us doubt Robert's ability to make the decision to donate and to take responsibility for it. If important new information is brought forward by the psychiatrist (for example, that Robert had revealed that his family had threatened him with rejection, or that Robert thought they could take his kidney without surgery), the team should reconsider. Until the dissenting psychiatrist has provided such information, we can reject his or her opinion.

OUTCOME: The patient was subsequently seen by a psychiatrist at another institution who was experienced in the evaluation of potential organ donors. All parties agreed that the decision of this psychiatrist would be determinative. The psychiatrist concluded Robert was capable of making the decision to donate and the kidney transplant was successfully performed.

NOTES

1. In a three-year period from 1999 to 2001, of 15,782 kidney retrievals from healthy live donors seven deaths were reported for a rate of one death for every 2,255 donors (0.04%).

2. Johnson EM, Anderson JK, Jacobs C, et al. Long-term follow-up of living kidney donors: quality of life after donation. *Transplantation* 1999;67:717–21.

3. United Network for Organ Sharing (http://www.unos.org/).

4. Consensus Statement on the Live Organ Donor. *JAMA* 2000;284;2919–26.

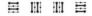

JOSEPH J. FINS, MD

A Time for Reflection

QUESTION: A 21-year-old college student, while inebriated after a party, dove headfirst into a shallow pond fracturing his neck and severing his spinal cord. He was pulled out of the water by companions and given artificial ventilation because he did not appear to be breathing. Upon arrival in the hospital approximately 30 minutes later, he was found to be totally quadriplegic and could not breathe. He was intubated and placed on a ventilator. Neurological assessment concluded with a high degree of certainty that both the quadriplegia and inability to breathe would be permanent. He was able to communicate, despite the artificial ventilation, by a device that temporarily interrupted the ventilator.

From the first moments of awareness of his plight, he demanded that the ventilator be stopped to permit him to die. Family members, friends, and treating physicians urged him to "hang in there" and permit a rehabilitation program to proceed before making such a draconian decision. Psychiatrists found him to be depressed, but no more so than would be expected after such an injury and loss of function. His treating physicians were uncertain whether to respect his right to refuse treatment and allow him to die by discontinuing the ventilator or to continue to treat him against his will. The ethics committee was asked to review the case.

REPLY: Viewing this case simply as the right of a patient to refuse unwanted care mistakes ethical theory for good clinical practice. This patient's desire to be removed from the ventilator requires more than a nod to his self-determination: it demands careful assessment, time, and prudence.

As a quadriplegic survivor of an alcohol-related accident, we can only imagine this young man's state of mind. Does he feel guilty about his drinking and view his injury as just punishment? Or, does he believe that his quadriplegia destines him to a life of incontinence, impotence, and institutionalization? Until we explore his beliefs and outline his future prospects, it would be premature to accede to a request for ventilator withdrawal.

Although the patient ultimately has the right to refuse unwanted treatment, we need to assess his capacity to make an informed decision. The quality of his informed consent or refusal hinges on the quality of provided information as well as his ability to assimilate this information. Studies have shown that quadriplegic patients are often given overly pessimistic information about their prognosis and future prospects in acute care settings where their treatment is begun. This pessimism can be compounded by the depression and cognitive impairment that can accompany acute quadriplegia—and associated head injuries—for months.

These factors warrant caution and suggest the need to engage in a careful process of patient assessment and counseling. A rush to judgment could compromise the quality of disclosure as well as preclude the mobilization of rehabilitation specialists who might be best equipped to advise the patient about his future. Many patients experience a desire to die after sustaining this sort of injury only to lead productive and happy lives. Christopher Reeve's experience is a notable example of how an individual can courageously change life plans while still pursuing important goals. And beyond anecdote, the literature demonstrates that quadriplegic survivors lead productive lives in school or the workplace and have marriages that are as stable as the national average.

While this information is necessary to make a rational decision, how it is communicated can determine whether it will be fully integrated into the decision-making process. Care must be taken to develop a therapeutic alliance with the patient while avoiding an adversarial dynamic which pits his right to self-determination against a clinician's felt beneficence. To avoid further conflict, the clinician should clearly state his reservations about a precipitous ventilator withdrawal while simultaneously demonstrating his desire to better appreciate the patient's motivations, fears, and concerns.

The clinician should also explicitly acknowledge that the patient has the legal and ethical right to refuse life-sustaining treatment once certain criteria are met. Disclosing the patient's prerogative will help to balance the power dynamics in the doctor-patient relationship, build trust, and promote a healing alliance. Perhaps most critically, it relieves the patient of the fear of indefinitely being locked into a situation that he might find untenable.

Giving this patient time to become informed and engaged in reflection is key to the clinical management of this case. Although time can not guarantee a particular outcome, it can provide an opportunity to engage in a deliberative process that will help ensure that the patient's decision is well considered and well informed.

OUTCOME: Despite his consistent refusal of treatment, the patient continued to be treated with mechanical ventilation, based on the irrationality of his decision. At two weeks after his injury he was medically stable and was transferred to a rehabilitation facility out of state. No further follow-up is available.

FURTHER READING

Patterson DR, Miller-Perrin C, McCormick TF, Hudson LD. When life support is questioned early in the care of patients with cervical-level quadriplegia. *N Engl J Med* 1993;328:506–9.

☰ ☷ ☷ ☰

PAUL S. APPELBAUM, MD

Let My Wife Bleed to Death

QUESTION: A 69-year-old woman was admitted to the emergency department with two self-inflicted knife wounds to the neck. She was hypotensive, but not actively bleeding. She was intubated, given intravenous fluids, and was about to be sent to the operating room when her family arrived.

Her husband, the appropriate surrogate decision maker, demanded she be extubated and all treatment stopped. He said his wife suffered decades of depression, often expressed the wish to die, and had not responded to treatment with multiple antidepressants and electroshock therapy. The patient's psychiatrist, who was called, said the woman presented the worst case of depression he had seen in 20 years of practice. Observers were impressed by the family's sincerity and good intentions. How would you advise the emergency room surgeon?

REPLY: Refusal of life-saving treatment is an everyday occurrence in our hospitals. So commonplace is this choice that one is almost surprised to see the question raised here as to whether to honor the request of the patient's husband to discontinue treatment, a request that seems consonant with the choice of the patient herself. Yet, I will suggest, whatever the superficial similarities to the usual case, there is a difference here, one that the emergency room surgeon would do well to heed.

The principle that persons have the right to determine what is done to their bodies is derived in our society from well-worn traditions in Anglo-American ethical and legal thought.[1] This ethical precept of personal autonomy has been reflected since the middle of this century in the doctrine of informed consent, and more recently, in the explicit acceptance of patients' (or appropriate surrogates') decisions to terminate treatment, even when that would result in death.

In what way does this situation differ from the ordinary request of a family member for termination of life support for a critically ill patient whose continued existence promises nothing more than unendurable pain?

To recognize the difference, we need to backtrack to the principle with which we began—personal autonomy—and add a caveat. Not every person has the right to determine what will be done to their bodies. Adults who lack decision making competence will have the choice made for them.[2] Parents make decisions for young children. For some classes of decisions—e.g., sterilization—more formal decision procedures may be required, and all involved will have recourse to the courts.

When someone has suffered from decades of depression, as the patient in this instance, and then elects to end her life, one is forced to ponder the competence of her choice. Depression is frequently associated with convictions of hopelessness and despair, and sometimes with guilt of delusional proportions. Patients' abilities to understand relevant information, appreciate its implications, reason with it, and in the extreme, even communicate a choice—the criteria on which determinations of competence are based—may well be impaired. Moreover, though many depressed people truly desire to die, their will to live often revives when the symptoms of their depression are brought under control. We do not know from the brief description of the case precisely what motivated this patient's actions, but the presumption that her depressive state played a critical role is a reasonable one. Strong concerns, therefore, exist about the patient's competence to make the choice to die.

Even granting this argument, what of the husband's role here? When a patient is incompetent, we turn to a surrogate. In this case, her husband is present and requesting that treatment be withheld. Insofar as he is giving voice to his wife's expressed wishes, however, he may be basing his decision on her incompetent choice. And yet another factor must be considered. Every state's mental health law permits hospitalization of mentally ill, suicidal persons, usually without inquiry into the competence of their decisions. This embodies society's interest in the preservation of the lives of its citizens.

We do not, of course, know that the patient made an incompetent choice to die. Nor can we, given her current state. (Neither can we be certain that her depression is truly untreatable; perhaps it has just been poorly managed to date.) A careful assessment of her decision making abilities can only occur after she is stabilized, by which time the immediate decision will be moot. Whatever choice we make in the bustle of the emergency service runs the risk of error. We may sustain the life of a competent patient, who has elected to die, or allow an incompetent patient to terminate her life, despite her impaired decision making. If an error is made, however, it seems preferable to err on the side of saving life. That seems to be the intent of the involuntary commitment statutes.

I would advise the ER surgeon to contact the hospital attorney for assistance in reaching an appropriate judge, who can authorize surgery, on the grounds that the patient's choice (as expressed by her husband) is quite likely to have been so influenced by her depression as to be incompetent. If the patient's condition is such that she is likely to suffer serious harm before judicial approval can be obtained, the surgeon should take whatever steps are necessary in the interim to sustain her life.

OUTCOME: The patient remained in the emergency department while the situation was discussed with the family. Before a final decision was made, the neck wound began to bleed forcefully and the patient bled to death.

NOTES

1. Appelbaum PS, Lidz CW, Meisel A. *Informed consent: legal theory and clinical practice.* New York: Oxford University Press, 1987.

2. Grisso T, Appelbaum PS. *Assessing competence to consent to treatment: a guide for physicians and other healthcare professionals.* New York: Oxford University Press, 1998.

☷ ☵ ☵ ☷

NUALA P. KENNY, MD, FRCP(C)

A Teenager's Refusal of Assent for Treatment

QUESTION: A 14-year-old boy was diagnosed with early-stage Hodgkin's disease. Two pediatric oncologists recommended aggressive treatment with chemotherapy and radiation therapy, offering a 90 percent probability of complete cure. But the boy obstinately refused to undergo treatment. Counseling sessions with the general pediatrician, pediatric oncologists, and nurses failed to convince him to undergo treatment. His parents very much wanted him to be treated but his pediatric oncologists were reluctant to begin treatment without the boy's assent. How would you advise the pediatric oncologists?

RESPONSE: Caring for adolescent patients can present serious ethical challenges for physicians especially, as in this case, in determining their appropriate role in difficult and life-threatening decisions. Over the last 30 years, professional groups, national commissions, and judges have expanded the role for adolescents in healthcare decisions.[1] The oncologists in this case are understandably concerned about the significance of this boy's refusal of treatment. Does this teen have the capacity to refuse this potentially life-saving intervention? What is the moral authority of the parents here? What is the doctor's duty? How can the physician help identify the proper balance between parental authority and respect for developing autonomy in a serious medical situation?

The law allows exceptional categories for adolescent health decision making for "emancipated minors" and "mature minors" and under "minor treatment statutes" (typically limited to pregnancy, sexually transmitted diseases, and alcohol and drug abuse). "Emancipated minor" is a legal term that refers to an adolescent who lives apart from parents because of marriage, military experience, or parenthood and often because of the neglect or abuse of parents. "Mature minors" are still dependent on families but have decision making capacity for particular medical conditions. So, both law and ethics focus on the teen's context and competence for autonomous decisions.

Parents are primarily responsible for protecting and promoting their children's interests.[2] They are granted wide discretion in making decisions for their children. While the literature demonstrates that adults and older adolescents do not differ significantly in their cognitive capacities and decision making skills,[3] there are still good reasons for parents to limit the autonomy of adolescents, especially in a situation with life-saving potential. These include the need to promote the lifetime autonomy of the teen; the reality that the teen's decisions are based on a limited life experience; the importance of family goals and responsibilities, and finally the need for consistency between health decisions and others, such as smoking or playing competitive sports.[4]

Respect for autonomy is a fundamental principle of ethical practice. For adolescents this means respect for their developing autonomy even as they are dependent on parents for care and support.

Physicians encounter adolescent patients in three categories: (1) those younger than 14 years who generally lack decisional capacity; (2) those 14 to 17 who clearly have capacity for making competent decisions; and (3) those 14 to 17 whose capacity is unclear.[5] Where does this teen fit?

The physician has a primary role in assessing the teen's competence for decisions.[6] This competence requires three elements: (1) *information*—Does this patient have sufficient information about the condition and treatments to understand them? (2) *capacity*—Can he communicate and respond to information? Does he demonstrate reasoning and deliberation, especially regarding the risks and consequences of this decision? Does he show a conception of "the good," i.e., enduring values, with some degree of stability as a basis for the decision? (3) *freedom*—Is he free from undue influence, fear, guilt, and coercion regarding the decision and able to make choices that are meaningful for him?

Is this adolescent capable of making an "authentic choice" and giving an informed refusal? Refusal of a potentially life-saving intervention requires a high degree of certainty regarding competence. If not capable of that degree of decisional maturation yet, can and should he give assent to the treatments?

The concept of assent was developed to respect that intermediate stage in which the parents give permission for the procedure and the not-yet-competent teen gives assent.[7] While there is a certain comfort when the adolescent assents to their parents' and caregivers' decisions, there is great distress when the adolescent refuses or dissents as this boy does. Do both competent refusal and not-yet fully competent dissent mean the treatments cannot be initiated?

More information about this boy's emotional and decisional maturity is essential. What are the real reasons for the refusal? His participation with treatment is essential to its success, so forcing him against his will can be difficult and dangerous. However, the case portrays a refusal that is difficult to take as competent. His best interests seem to be dependent on treatment. The task for the general pediatrician and parents is to find a way forward that has his best interests always in focus and, if possible, gradually allows the teen to actively participate.

OUTCOME: With further intervention by family members, the patient accepted treatment.

NOTES

1. *American Academy of Pediatrics Committee on Bioethics.* Informed consent, parental permission and assent in pediatric practice. *Pediatrics* 1995;95:314–7.

2. Buchanan A, Brock D. *Deciding for Others: The Ethics of Surrogate Decision Making.* New York: Cambridge University Press, 1989.

3. Grochowski E, Bach S. The ethics of decision making with adolescents: what a physician ought to know. *Adolescent Medicine* 1994; 5:485–95.

4. Ross L. Health care decision making by children. Is it in their best interest? *Hastings Cent Rep* 1997;27(6):41–5.

5. Weir R, Peters C. Affirming the decisions adolescents make about life and death. *Hastings Cent Rep* 1997;27(6):29–40

6. Kenny N P, Skinner LE. Skills for Assessing the Appropriate Role for Children in Health Decisions. *Pediatric Clinical Skills.* Philadelphia: Harcourt Health Sciences, 2002:349–59.

7. Bartholome W. A new understanding of consent in pediatric practice: consent, parental permission, and child assent. *Pediatric Annals* 1989;18:262–5.

MANDY GARBER, MD, SUSAN C. HUNT, MD, AND ROBERT M. ARNOLD, MD

Can an HIV-positive Woman Be Forced to Take Medicine to Protect Her Fetus?

QUESTION: An ethics consultation was requested when Ms. D., a 28-year-old HIV-positive pregnant woman, refused to take highly active antiretroviral therapy (HAART). She was five months' pregnant and was known to have had HIV for four years that had not progressed to AIDS despite taking no antiretroviral medication. When she became pregnant, her physician strongly urged her to begin HAART and not to nurse the baby because both actions have been shown to significantly lower the incidence of maternal-to-fetal transmission of HIV. She read extensively about this issue and consulted Web sites and friends. She concluded that HAART had a greater chance of hurting her baby than helping it so she refused to start it. She also planned to nurse the baby. The presentation of objective data of treatment outcomes was unsuccessful in persuading her because she believed that the medical-pharmaceutical establishment was behind the official treatment recommendations and she simply did not believe them. What would you suggest?

REPLY: This 28-year-old HIV-infected pregnant woman refuses to take HAART and insists on breastfeeding upon delivery, actions that are known to increase maternal-fetal transmission of HIV. When faced with patients who oppose medical advice, clinicians routinely request psychiatry and ethics consultations. The psychiatrist's role is to help the clinicians access decision-making capacity; the ethics consultant's role is to help identify and analyze the underlying values at stake and facilitate a decision that respects the values of the parties involved. We assume for the rest of this discussion that despite optimal communication and mediation, the conflict is irreconcilable.[1]

Can a competent, pregnant woman refuse medical therapy aimed at improving the health outcomes of her fetus? Decision making in health care is guided by the ethical principle of autonomy, the individual's right to self-governance, to make choices about if and when to accept medical treatment and to govern the course of that treatment. Beauchamp and Childress note that respect for a patient's autonomy, however, can be overridden by competing moral considerations: if an individual's choices endanger the public health or potentially harm those who are innocent, others can justifiably restrict the exercise of that individual's autonomy. Some argue that the case turns on whether the fetus has moral rights. Some conservatives argue that the fetus claims moral rights from the moment of conception; others argue that it is not until after birth that the fetus has moral rights. We believe, however, that the critical issue is whether one can force unwanted treatment on a competent, pregnant woman.

The law takes this view. In a famous legal case in 1987, *In re A.C.*, Angela Carder, a pregnant woman with end-stage cancer was forced by a court order to undergo an immediate caesarian delivery to save her fetus's life. Both she and the premature baby died shortly after surgery. Advocates for the surgery argued that since Ms. Carder faced imminent death, all efforts should focus on at least saving one life, that of the fetus. A subsequent appeal was lodged by the American Civil Liberties Union Reproductive Freedom project to the District of Columbia Court of Appeals which vacated the prior court decision, "concluding that in virtually all circumstances, the pregnant woman—not doctors or judges—should make medical decisions on behalf of herself and her fetus."[2] In the current scenario, Ms. D. remains in excellent health despite her diagnosis of HIV infection. HAART often causes a variety of unpleasant side effects, and compelling Ms. D. to take HAART for the remainder of her pregnancy might impose significantly on her liberty. We believe that any attempts to force her to take HAART are unethical.

Upon delivery, the newborn is a separate and viable human being with moral, constitutional, and legal rights. The principle of beneficence urges physicians "to prevent harm from occurring to others," to prevent this newborn from acquiring HIV infection. Administration of zidovudine within 48 hours after birth lowers the risk of maternal fetal transmission of HIV; nevirapine reduces the risk of HIV transmission during the first 14 to 16 weeks of life by nearly 50 percent. Therefore administering a zidovudine-nevirapine regimen to the newborn is the logical next step in his or her clinical care. Most important, giving the newborn HAART does not infringe on Ms. D.'s autonomy. It, however, infringes on Ms. D.'s parental rights.

In general, the medical and legal establishments recognize the rights of parents to make medical decisions on behalf of their children. However, when a parent's medical decision on behalf of her child is clearly not in the best interest of that child, parental authority may be suspended. In such cases, an independent, temporary guardian is sought to make medical decisions for the child. If a physician can show that a parent is endangering her child's life either by denying medical care or engaging in dubious health practices, the courts may rule in favor of the physician.

Our analysis of this case allows us to conclude that: (1) respect for this 28-year-old, competent, pregnant woman's autonomy dictates that her physicians recognize her refusal to take HAART; and (2) after delivery, the pediatrician may seek judicial intervention to determine the best course of treatment for the newborn.

OUTCOME: HAART treatment was not forced on the pregnant woman. The patient did not take HAART and had a Caesarian delivery of an apparently healthy infant. She decided not to breastfeed the infant or have him tested for HIV.

NOTES

1. Stone D, Patton B, Heen S, Fisher R. *Difficult conversations: How to Discuss what Matters Most.* New York: Penguin Books, 2000. Given the irreconcilable nature of this conflict, the consultant's job will be to lay out to both parties what she or he believes the societal-ethical consensus is regarding these matters and to lay out for them what the societally acceptable mechanisms are for resolving the conflict.

2. http://www.aclu.org/ReproductiveRights/ReproductiveRights.cfm?ID=9054&c=30

☰ ☷ ☷ ☰

WALTER M. ROBINSON, MD, MPH

Ethics for Astronauts

The exploration of space is an uncertain enterprise. Fictional accounts of space exploration are at great odds with the dangerous reality of space flight; the recent tragic deaths of shuttle astronauts are an important corrective to the common view of space flight as a routine undertaking. From a medical standpoint, our fantasies often encourage us to believe that we know more about space flight than we actually do. Despite more than three decades of experience in space, there is a paucity of information about the normal consequences of prolonged low gravity or radiation exposure. Since the majority of US space flights have been of short duration, our accrued knowledge has had little impact. In planning for longer duration flights, our lack of knowledge could be ruinous.

My interest in this topic arises from my work as a member of the Institute of Medicine's Committee on Creating a Vision for Space Medicine During Travel Beyond Earth Orbit.[1] I had the pleasure of reviewing the existing plans for medical care and research for a long-duration space mission, such as a trip to Mars, and the greater pleasure of meeting with current and former astronauts and flight surgeons. What was clear is the remarkable dedication and skill of the astronaut corps and the ground staff in charge of their medical care; my remarks should not be construed as criticism of their expertise. However, I believe that NASA's attempt to apply existing clinical and research tenets to what is essentially a unique experience has failed to meet the needs of the space exploration program.

In planning for long-duration flights, ethical issues arise in three related areas: the privacy of astronaut medical data, the participation of astronauts in clinical research, and the in-flight clinical care for astronauts. Given the small number of astronauts and the small number of flights, there is a reasonable concern that the medical data from any individual astronaut may be identifiable. The legal mandates to protect an astronaut's medical privacy were repeatedly cited by NASA as a barrier to collecting data on the human response to spaceflight. The concern is not only a matter of principle, as astronauts evidently fear that identifiable information gathered about their experience before, during, or after a mission might have a very undesirable consequence: it might be used to bar them from future missions.

To understand this concern for privacy it is important to understand the relationship between astronauts and flight surgeons. The astronaut corps, like pilots before them, may come to view the flight surgeon as less an advocate than an adversary who has the power to prevent them from flying. The flight surgeon's ability to certify individuals as flight ready may motivate an astronaut to conceal or minimize symptoms. The wariness inherent in this flight surgeon–astronaut relationship is intensified by both the lifelong preparation of the astronauts corps and the intense competition for a small number of missions. The result is that clinical events in spaceflight may not be disclosed to the flight surgeon, and if information is disclosed, the flight surgeon may be prevented by privacy concerns from passing such data on to those responsible for making spaceflight safe.

Let us take as an example the relatively common occurrence of an ileus-like syndrome, a paralysis of the intestine, during the first few days in microgravity. This can be discomforting and may cause astronauts to restrict their food intake or to use inappropriate medications such as laxatives. Astronauts might not report these symptoms to their flight surgeons or they might not permit the flight surgeon to report such symptoms, for fear that they indicate an idiosyncratic response to microgravity which might limit their ability to return to space. In this way a "normal" physiological response to microgravity might go unreported and thus inappropriately treated.

How might this systematic pressure to underreport symptoms related to space travel be addressed? In part, the answer lies in reconfiguring the medical privacy laws as they apply to astronauts, perhaps in the form of an administrative structure that better balances the need for confidentiality with the need to create a safe environment for spaceflight. It may be necessary, given the small number of flights and crew, for the astronauts to cede some medical privacy rights in return for the chance to participate in missions; any changes in the privacy rules should take place after careful consultation with the astronaut corps and the flight surgeons. An additional part of the answer lies in adjustments to the flight surgeon–astronaut relationship, which may not be easy. Shifting the flight readiness aspect of medical care away from the flight surgeon simply passes the buck.

A second and related ethical issue is the participation of astronauts in clinical research. In the current practice, all clinical protocols in which astronauts might participate are reviewed by an institutional review board (IRB) at Johnson Space Center and the Common Rule principles of voluntary informed consent are followed. In my view, application of the Common Rule, the federal regulations that set out the ethical precepts for federally funded research in the US, fails to recognize astronauts, and space exploration, as unique.

It is reasonable to propose that astronauts have an obligation to participate in clinical data gathering that facilitates the design and maintenance of a safe spaceflight environment. To apply the standard informed consent procedures to this sort of data gathering implies that astronauts could opt out of activities designed to make spaceflight safe by declining consent. NASA recognizes this as a problem, and includes a provision in the IRB handbook allowing for astronauts to be taken off missions if they decline participation in protocols deemed important to the mission. The fact that astronauts always consent to participate in all the offered protocols strongly suggests a problem: An IRB should question the effectiveness of a voluntary consent process in which no one ever declines consent. In applying the earthly standards, one of two problems has occurred: either there has been inappropriate pressure, in the form of mission selection, brought to bear on potential research participants, or there has been a category error in calling this sort of data gathering activity research in the usual regulatory sense of the word.

An earthbound example may help suggest a solution. Imagine that the first nuclear power plants are being built and operated. Workers in the plant may have to provide clinical data and clinical samples such as urine and blood in order to monitor their radiation exposure, in order to see if the expected safety precautions are effective, and in order to detect unexpected consequences of their exposure. As more plants are built, and more knowledge is gained about their safety, less monitoring will be needed.

Astronauts are like those workers in the very early plants. Little is known about the risks of the work, and understanding their physiologic responses to the work environment is necessary to protect them from both expected and unexpected risks. Is every activity that leads to such understanding, research in the usual regulatory meaning of the word, such that it should trigger the use of informed consent? I think it is not, in that astronauts ought not decline to participate and still go on the flights, just as the plant workers ought not refuse to participate and still work in the early plants. Instead, I think that an occupational model of health best describes this activity, and that occupation models of data gathering should be used instead of invoking the Common Rule. If the Common Rule procedures continue to be used, and mission selection pressure is applied, then the voluntary nature of the informed consent is in serious doubt.

On the other hand, there will be research protocols designed for astronauts that closely approximate clinical research done in an earthbound setting. Such protocols will involve research on medications or devices that would not be used to make subsequent spaceflights safer or even possible. The purpose of this research would be to examine physiologic variables or to test pharmacologic therapies that would have terrestrial commercial or industrial uses. In this type of research, it is completely appropriate to use the standard informed consent procedures and IRB review, but inappropriate to apply mission selection pressure in order to encourage participation.

The last set of ethical issues raised by long-term spaceflight is clinical. On long-duration flights such as that to Mars, communication with the ground will be limited and delayed, and there is likely to be no possibility of returning mid-flight due to illness. The crew will be on its own in resolving some difficult ethical issues. How should they decide when to use, and when to withhold, advanced medical treatment?

While there is understandable pressure to include the capacity for technologically advanced medical support on any long-term flight, normative guidelines for the use of such equipment should be developed prior to leaving the ground. For example, should mechanical ventilators be included on long-duration flights? What would be the criteria for initiating or discontinuing ventilation? How might the crew balance mission needs against medical needs? Traditional wartime triage rules, which distribute medical care based on the ability to return the patient to active duty, might form the basis of a policy, but to adopt such rules requires a prior agreement of the sender and the sent, of the spaceflight agencies and the astronauts. Might it be better to limit which types of equipment are sent, so that the options are clearer? Given these issues and the likelihood of an international crew with a variety of ethical perspectives on triage, careful attention should be paid to these issues in setting up clinical protocols.

In summary, space exploration and space explorers have unique characteristics that do not easily fit into the existing ethical templates for medical privacy, medical research, and clinical decision making. This is not to say that a new ethics must be devised, but that in this new situation, care must be taken to devise a set of ethical standards that are appropriate to a new environment.

NOTE

1. Ball JR, Evans CH Jr. (eds). Committee on Creating a Vision for Space Medicine During Travel Beyond Earth Orbit. *Safe Passage: Astronaut Care for Exploration Missions.* Washington, DC: National Academy Press, 2001.

☷ ☶ ☵ ☴

PAUL ROOT WOLPE, PHD

Bioethics in Space

Outer space is inimical to human life, and constructing subenvironments that preserve life in a cold vacuum far from earth is no easy task. Along with other harsh environments—Antarctica, the Himalayas, the deep sea—the need to sustain and repair the body in hostile territory has led to the development of a specialty known as "Medicine in Extreme Environments"[1] and journals such as *Human Performance in Extreme Environment.*[2] As long as human beings insist on colonizing these inhospitable places, they will be faced with an ongoing set of medical and bioethical dilemmas.

Walter Robinson's thoughtful article, "Ethics for astronauts," correctly identifies three of the thorniest current bioethical issues facing the space program: (1) astronauts' rights as research subjects versus our need for data on the physiological and psychological impacts of spaceflight; (2) astronauts' right to privacy versus the need to disseminate such data to the scientific community; and (3) the difficult decisions facing clinical care for astronauts on long-duration spaceflights. All three evoke much debate and handwringing at the National Aeronautics and Space Administration (NASA), which is one of the reasons that NASA asked the Institute of Medicine (IOM) to create the Committee on Creating a Vision for Space Medicine During Travel Beyond Earth Orbit, on which Dr. Robinson served. The Committee produced a report, Safe Passage: Astronaut Care for Exploration Missions,[3] which was a thoughtful and probing study of the medical needs of long-duration flight, and NASA is incorporating many of its insights into its planning for such missions. In such a new and difficult area, there will be differences and debates, and so I welcome an opportunity not only to respond to Dr. Robinson's article, but also to the broader set of recommendations made in the Safe Passage report.

Dr. Robinson is correct that the participation of astronauts in clinical research and the related issue of astronaut privacy are problematic. However, Dr. Robinson claims, "The fact that astronauts always consent to participate in all the offered protocols strongly suggests a problem: An Institutional Review Board (IRB) should question the effectiveness of a voluntary consent process in which no one ever declines consent." But it is simply not so that astronauts never decline protocols. In the Life Sciences Spacelab Missions, for example, there was about 20 percent non-participation in planned protocols.[4] (In a post-flight exercise test asked of astronauts in five separate missions, only 30 percent participated.) Of course, that very fact presents the exact opposite dilemma—if the data collected are crucial to understanding the health and treatment of astronauts in future flights, and the number of subjects in any space-based protocol is of necessity severely limited, how can we permit astronauts to refuse to participate in protocols at all?

Similarly, Dr. Robinson and Safe Passage both make the claim that astronaut privacy concerns have impeded the collection of important data; Dr. Robinson suggests that issues of astronaut privacy were "repeatedly cited by NASA" as a barrier to collecting data, and Safe Passage similarly states, "The possibility that an astronaut could be identified is seen as an inescapable barrier to the collection and interpretation of astronaut health data." However, the incidence of refusing to release medical information is actually quite low; in Skylab, for example, all nine astronauts concurred, and six out of seven in Spacelab Life Sciences Mission 1.[5]

In other words, two problems are postulated by Dr. Robinson and IOM: the first has to do with astronaut consent (either Dr. Robinson's contention that it is coerced and so is never declined, or the opposite problem that astronauts refuse to participate and so important data are not gathered), and the second is data lost to astronaut insistence on the privacy of their medical information. Establishing the validity of these claims is important because they are the hook on which both Dr. Robinson and the IOM committee hang their policy recommendations. Yet in neither Dr. Robinson's article nor in the close to 300 pages of Safe Passage are any data brought forth to support either claim. They are simply asserted as true.

The truth of the claims would not be of much concern, except they are being used to justify a modification of the Common Rule,[6] our single most important regulatory standard of subject protection.

For example, Safe Passage states it explicitly:

NASA should pursue . . . a longterm, focused health care research strategy to capture all necessary data on health risks and their amelioration . . . [which would require] a modification of the interpretation of the Common Rule (45 C.F.R., Part 46, Subpart A) for human research participants.

The reality is that the astronaut is, in most cases, the only individual from whom clinical information relevant to space travel can be collected. Therefore, reliance on the voluntary participation of astronauts in clinical research to the same extent as reliance on volunteer participants on the ground may not be appropriate. This is especially true when the information gained is potentially critical to the lives and well-beings of both the individual astronaut and the astronaut corps.

It is true that astronauts are in a unique position to gather certain kinds of information on human functioning in space, and that the data are important for the future of spaceflight. And here Dr. Robinson's suggestion, if not the reasons he gives, seems right to me: We should consider some kinds of data collection in an occupational health model (and, in fact, already do; but the kinds of data included should be expanded). I also agree with Dr. Robinson that other kinds of research, not related to the safety of flight but with terrestrial commercial or industrial uses, clearly falls within the Common Rule and should never be forced upon astronauts.

However, space research does not fall so neatly into those two categories. Space-based medical research can be invasive or uncomfortable and yet still be directly related to future medical or life science needs. Drugs metabolize differently in microgravity, and we must understand that process to accurately prescribe in space, and so drug trials are necessary. Space research can involve blood draws, muscle biopsies, the wearing of harnesses (which can actually be hazardous during some space-based activities), sleep studies that require waking up periodically (sleeping in space is very difficult as it is, many astronauts are severely sleep deprived, and such studies can exacerbate the problem), and so on. In which of Dr. Robinson's categories do invasive or hazardous studies that are precisely for the health and well-being of future astronauts fall? Calling those "occupational health data gathering" is incorrect, and if the astronauts decide to assert their right to refuse consent for these studies, I suspect the Office of Human Research Protections will agree with their right to do so.

It seems to me that NASA should pursue a different strategy, one it has begun but must fully implement. Much astronaut refusal to consent in the past was due to lack of astronaut buy in, coupled with poor central planning. For example, astronauts might be asked to participate in multiple drug studies, which confounded each other, or they would be involved in a number of studies, each requiring a blood sample, and instead of a single stick and shared blood, there would be multiple, separate blood draws. More recently, these problems have been addressed. Astronauts are now involved in the science of NASA from the top down (Shannon Lucid, who has spent more hours in orbit than any other American, has served as Chief Scientist of NASA). Astronauts work in the medical corps at NASA, act as principle investigators on studies, and sit on the IRB. The solution is not to replace coercion with new or modified regulation (simply another form of coercion), but to include astronauts in every aspect of scientific research at NASA, to reinforce participation in the life sciences as an integral part of astronaut responsibility.

The issue of clinical care is of a different nature, and here I fully agree with Dr. Robinson. The ethical issues of clinical care in long-duration spaceflight beyond earth orbit are tricky. In the shuttle and space station platforms, the assumption has been that we can get an injured or ill astronaut back to earth fairly quickly, and so the goal was maintenance until the person could get full care terrestrially. The strategy breaks down on a trip to Mars where the ship is a year away from any possible rendezvous with earth. Before the mission leaves, careful thought must be given to what kinds of medical training to give the crew and what kinds of equipment should and should not be included on the ship. On such long-duration flights, every ounce of weight must be carefully considered; higher likelihood injuries and illnesses must be served before rare or unlikely ones. Even so, the inevitable may occur; an astronaut may have an injury or illness that the available resources are ill-suited to treat. All involved—astronauts, their families, the NASA medical personnel—must be ready for such an eventuality.

Which brings us, finally, to clinical bioethics in space. What is the right thing to do if an astronaut suffers from a traumatic head injury and gets violent in a small craft millions of miles from earth, or becomes clinically depressed? What do we tell or not tell an astronaut, isolated in a way no human has ever been before, if his or her spouse develops cancer, or their child dies tragically? As Dr. Robinson suggests, these issues cannot be left to chance. NASA is already gathering together committees to discuss the medical needs of long-duration flight, to establish protocols and procedures, and to try and grapple with some of these seemingly intractable problems. Do we now need the *Journal of Extreme Bioethics*?

NOTES

1. Palinkas LA, Gunderson EK, Holland AW, Miller C, Johnson JC. Predictors of behavior and performance in extreme environments: the antarctic space analogue program. *Aviation Space & Environmental Medicine.* 2000;71(6): 619–625.

2. http://www.hpee.org/aboutjournal.html

3. Ball JR, Evans CH Jr. (eds). Committee on Creating a Vision for Space Medicine During Travel Beyond Earth Orbit. *Safe Passage: Astronaut Care for Exploration Missions.* Washington DC: National Academy Press, 2001

4. Personal Communication: Charles Sawin, Director of research Johnson Space Center and Chair, Committee for the Protection of Human Subjects (JSC's IRB), November, 2001.

5. Personal Communication: Charles Sawin, November, 2001.

6. The Common Rule is Title 45, the Code of Federal regulations that provides protection of human research subjects. It can be accessed at http://www.hhs.gov/ohrp/humansubjects/guidance/45cfr46.htm

☰ ☷ ☷ ☰

STUART J. YOUNGNER, MD

When the School Bus Driver Is a Drinker

QUESTION: A 47-year-old man has been seen intermittently by a psychiatrist for anxiety and excessive use of alcohol. He completed detoxification programs several times but has been erratic in keeping his office appointments. At the time of his most recent visit to his psychiatrist, he admitted to drinking three liters of wine every evening, often supplementing this with a few beers. He told the psychiatrist that he is currently working as a school bus driver, doing the early morning shift. He says he never drinks in the morning and does not believe his driving is impaired. He has had no accidents and has never been charged with driving while intoxicated. The psychiatrist is reluctant to violate his patient's confidentiality but would be unable to forgive himself if children on the school bus were killed or grievously injured because he did not notify the school that one of their drivers was drinking excessively. How would you advise the psychiatrist?

REPLY: Patient confidentiality may not be what it used to be, but physicians in general, and psychiatrists in particular, continue to take it seriously. Only when a third party's interest is seriously at stake should a physician consider violating confidentiality. The case of the 47-year-old alcoholic man should certainly make his psychiatrist consider breaching confidentiality by notifying the school about the risk posed by his patient's drinking. But how does the psychiatrist decide whether or not to actually violate the confidentiality of his or her patient?

Generally speaking, if the sacredness of confidentiality is put on one side of the scales, then the seriousness, specificity, and likelihood of the danger to the third party must be placed on the other side. In this case, the potential consequences of drunk driving are extremely serious. A driving accident could kill or maim innocent children riding the bus as well as other drivers or pedestrians. And, is a specific, clearly identifiable third party at risk? You bet—a school bus full of children.

How likely it is that a tragedy will occur is a tougher issue, because it involves speculation and judgment. First, is the patient telling the truth? The patient admits to heavy drinking, but denies driving while drunk. He says he has no arrests for drunk driving and is accident free. But substance abusers are known to minimize the extent of their problem, especially when something dear like a job or relationship is at stake. The judgment of likelihood, then, rests with a decision on whether or not to trust the patient. I wouldn't.

At best, the bus driver admits to a serious drinking problem. He has failed detoxification several times. He misses appointments. Maybe he isn't drunk in the morning. Maybe he doesn't have withdrawal symptoms or a horrible hangover while he is driving the kids to school. Maybe. But that's not good enough. Either the patient resigns his job or the school authorities must be told. But there are a few other questions that should be answered.

Why is the patient seeing a psychiatrist anyway? If he is seeking help voluntarily for his anxiety and excessive use of alcohol, I would explain to him that those conditions cannot be successfully treated while he is actively drinking. No psychiatric treatment is possible without detoxification and abstinence. The patient has already started missing appointments. I doubt there is anything therapeutic going on here. I would offer the patient the option of telling the school officials himself and voluntarily entering a detoxification program. If he were willing to do so, I would go to bat for him with the system as best I could and continue to be his physician. If he were not willing, I would call the school and tell the patient to come back to see me when he was ready to quit drinking.

OUTCOME: Neither the school nor the bus company was notified that the patient was drinking excessively.

≣ ⁞⁞ ⁞⁞ ≣

HOWARD BRODY, MD, PHD

Should a Clinical Trial Coordinator Blow the Whistle?

QUESTION: A 34-year-old pharmacist entered a multiinstitutional, blinded, placebo controlled clinical trial for amyotrophic lateral sclerosis (ALS) in which a drug available by prescription was the active agent. At no time was the patient explicitly told that an attempt to ascertain the contents of the pills that she was taking could be considered a violation of the integrity of the study. During one study visit, she confided to a study technician that she had given one of the pills to a friend to be analyzed. That friend had in turn placed the results of the analysis in a sealed envelope and given it to the patient who stated that she had not opened the envelope. With ambivalence, the study technician informed the principal investigator, torn between respecting the perceived confidence that the patient shared, and the apparent violation of the integrity of the study. How should the principal investigator respond?

REPLY: Failure to maintain blinded conditions is a common flaw in randomized clinical trials, and a serious criticism of a great many such trials is that the investigators fail to determine how well the blinding is preserved. In many cases, the experimental drug has common, minor side effects, and unless the comparison drug mimics those side effects, it is relatively easy for subjects to guess if they are getting the experimental or the control drug. Indeed some critics have claimed that the entire case for the efficacy of antidepressants rests on this failure to maintain blinded conditions; if one looks only at studies where the investigators documented that double-blind conditions were scrupulously maintained, then antidepressants cannot be shown to be much better than placebo.[1] I mention this merely to show that one does not have to analyze one's own pills, for the problem of breaking the blind to arise.

Breaking the blind does indeed challenge the integrity of the research study. Fortunately it does so only for this one subject. Therefore, if at the end of the trial, data have to be discarded, they would involve only this one person and one hopes that would not threaten the successful completion of the trial. But that assumes that the blind has been broken, and according to the facts as stated, this has not yet occurred.

If the subject has not yet actually found out what medicine she is receiving, the blind has been preserved. But she must be told that if she wishes to remain in the trial, she must not "open the envelope," and if she does, she is obligated to inform the study team.

I see no reason why the study technician should feel "torn" in this case when one analyzes the ethical duties of all parties. She presumably has no relationship with this person except for her role in the study. She has appeared at this person's doorstep, as it were, solely in her role as a member of the study team. She has no right to any "private" confidences with this woman where matters that impact upon the study integrity are concerned.

The reason the study technician might inappropriately *feel a sense* of being "torn" points out a common ethical misperception about randomized controlled trials of innovative medications. This misperception has been fueled by a schism within the bioethics literature itself. A portion of that literature takes the view that the clinical practice of medicine and the conduct of clinical research trials are two distinct types of activities, and therefore the ethical principles governing them are also distinct. Another portion of the literature takes the view that all of medicine ought to be governed by the ethical principles of therapeutic practice, and that clinical research is really a subset of practice and so should fall under those same principles.

My position is that the first view is correct.[2] The investigator-subject relationship in a research trial is a fundamentally different ethical relationship from the physician-patient relationship in a therapeutic context. The goal of the research enterprise is fundamentally that of discovering new knowledge that will help future patients. The goal of the therapeutic enterprise is fundamentally that of helping each individual patient with the best available remedies.

This example highlights why these goals and relationships are ethically distinct. We presume today that it is virtually never in the best interests of a patient to be denied the knowledge of what medicine she is receiving. The withholding of that information serves the goal of research, not any reasonable goal of therapy. But a person in a clinical trial is not being treated as a patient at all; she is being treated as a research subject. This role is quite appropriate assuming that the conditions of the study, including voluntary informed consent, are not exploitive.

The study technician might assume that she had a therapeutic relationship with this patient and that therefore there was a duty of confidentiality. But no such relationship exists and the technician can report her concerns to the principal investigator with a clear conscience.

It sometimes happens that real-world circumstances cause a blurring of the roles that I have described here as ethically distinct. A neurologist, for instance, may be both the patient's attending physician, and the principal investigator of a study in which the patient is enrolled. I would argue that it is usually desirable to avoid this role conflict, but for various reasons avoidance is not always possible or desirable. When the same physician (and perhaps the office staff) are forced to cross role boundaries, I would argue that it is still highly desirable to think about each encounter with the patient as falling within one role or the other. That is, the technician should remind herself that in this situation the "patient" is really a research subject and not truly a patient, even though in another setting this same individual might be a patient. Some difficulties and gray areas will inevitably arise, but trying to maintain role clarity in one's mind will go a good way toward resolving many ethical problems.[3]

OUTCOME: The technician and the principal investigator explained their dilemma to the patient. She stated that she had not opened the envelope, and she was allowed to continue in the study with the caveat that she would be dropped if there was an additional violation. The patient remains enrolled in the trial.

NOTES

1. Greenberg RP, Bornstein RF, Greenberg MD, Fisher S. A meta-analysis of antidepressant outcome under "blinder" conditions. *J Consult Clin Psychol* 1992;60:664–9.

2. Miller FG, Brody H. A critique of clinical equipoise. Therapeutic misconception in the ethics of clinical trials. *Hastings Cent Rep* 2003;33(3):19–28.

3. Brody H, Miller FG. The clinician-investigator: unavoidable but manageable tension. *Kennedy Inst Ethics J* 2003;13:329–46.

☷ ☶ ☵ ☳

JAMES L. BERNAT, MD

Do Physicians Overtreat the Seriously Ill?

During the final quarter of the twentieth century, American society has reached consensus that patients have both an ethical and legal right to refuse unwanted life-sustaining therapy. American society also has increasingly recognized that palliative care is the most appropriate form of medical treatment for hopelessly ill and dying patients, particularly for those who refuse life-sustaining therapy. Enshrining these achievements, the "death with dignity" movement has gained momentum as a positive social force. Implicit in this movement is the concept that it is the physician who refuses to grant a patient these rights, not the terminal disease that becomes the adversary in the patient's struggle to die with dignity.

Everyone knows of instances in which ostensibly well-meaning physicians have continued to aggressively treat dying patients with life-sustaining therapies, thereby inappropriately prolonging their dying. Numerous studies have shown that many physicians do not communicate adequately with dying patients to elicit their treatment preferences, nor do they seek or follow their advance directives for medical care. The adversarial attitude exhibited by some dying patients toward such physicians has spawned another movement best described as "antitherapy." Here, the patient's goal becomes to receive less medical treatment, not more. This movement has been inadvertently advanced by some scholars who, arguing from concepts of distributive justice, have wisely urged physicians to "set limits" on medical treatments.

It was within this social context that a recent publication of the SUPPORT study was received. The Study to Understand Prognoses and Preferences for Outcomes and Risks of Treatment (SUPPORT) was a carefully planned and executed four-year, two-phase study of over 9,000 hospitalized, seriously ill patients. The goals were to measure the quality of end-of-life decision making and the frequency of unnecessarily painful or prolonged deaths in the hospital and to attempt to improve terminal care.[1]

With publication of the findings that many dying patients did not receive do-not-resuscitate (DNR) orders until two days before death, that half of the conscious dying patients suffered pain before death, and that physicians failed to incorporate prognostic data into their treatment behaviors, both the academic community and the popular press excoriated the medical community for their insensitivity and arrogance. Even the usually temperate and pragmatic medicolegal scholar George Annas fumed: "Physicians simply have never taken the rights of hospitalized patients seriously.... the only realistic way to improve the care of dying patients in the short run is to get them out of the hospital ..."

Professor Annas suggested that a reasonable corrective would be for our society to establish a system of law firms, connected to hospitals by a hotline, whose sole purpose would be to routinely sue physicians who refused to grant patients their right to refuse life-prolonging therapy.[2]

But what else did SUPPORT show? Many of the popular press and non-clinical academic responses showed a failure to appreciate the important distinction between critical and terminal illness, and to understand the reality of the clinical context in which sick patients must make treatment choices. Patients were enrolled in SUPPORT who were in the advanced stages of one or more of nine serious illnesses and most were admitted to intensive care units (ICU) for treatment. SUPPORT was a study of physicians' treatment of critically ill but not necessarily terminally ill patients. Indeed, three-fourths of the study patients later were discharged from the hospital and two-thirds of those discharged were alive six months later.

That a critically ill patient also is terminally ill is a determination often made more accurately in retrospect. Despite the fact that trained nurses provided the study physicians with prognostic data from computerized models, a serious and possibly insurmountable barrier prevented both physicians and patients from incorporating these statistical data into their life-or-death treatment decisions.

To illustrate this barrier, consider the case, described by Dr. Bernard Lo, of a 63-year-old woman admitted with urospesis and respiratory failure.[3] She would be a typical SUPPORT patient because the prognostic model would provide a 40 percent probability that she would die in the hospital and a 50 percent chance that she would survive for six months. Because there is nothing necessarily irreversible or terminal about her presenting condition, most such patients, their families, and their physicians would choose ICU admission and mechanical ventilation with the intent of cure. But if her ICU course were to become complicated by gastrointestinal bleeding and continued respiratory failure, subsequently she may refuse further ventilatory therapy because she clearly had become terminally ill. In such a case, as was found commonly in SUPPORT, her physician may have written a DNR order only two days before her death because only then had the therapeutic intent been converted from cure to palliation. In practice, it is exactly this group of critically ill patients with intermediate prognoses for survival for whom decision making is most vexing. Would most patients with a critical illness who are given a 60 percent chance of cure and a 50 percent chance of surviving an additional six months choose life-sustaining treatment or palliative care? I believe that most patients and families given those odds would, as in the Lo case, choose an initial trial of life-sustaining treatment, at least until it became clear that the patient's prognosis was poor.

The decision whether to choose curative or palliative care in the face of intermediate statistical prognoses is hellish and cannot be simplified. Critics, like George Annas, who concluded that the SUPPORT study showed that physicians were systematically overtreating such patients, must answer the thorny question of at what threshold of survival would ICU care count as proper treatment? Would Professor Annas refuse treatment in an ICU if, as was true in the mean of the SUPPORT patients, he was given a 75 percent chance of leaving the hospital? What odds would he find acceptable?

The SUPPORT study revealed serious inadequacies about the contemporary medical treatment of critically ill patients. Clearly many physicians practice within a hospital subculture whose values and behaviors automatically encourage treatment and discourage nontreatment. Many physicians do not listen adequately to their patients or follow their advance directives. Many physicians do not pay sufficient attention to providing optimal palliation of pain and suffering. But it is a serious oversimplification to conclude that these deficiencies are caused solely by intransigent physicians unwilling to afford patients their proper rights and that what is needed is a hospital lawsuit hotline.

Rather, the principal problem is caused by the unpleasant biological reality that patients, families, and physicians must make life-or-death treatment decisions on critically ill patients in the face of a continuum of changing statistical outcome probabilities. It does not contribute to this important debate, in effect, to conclude in retrospect that when critically ill patients who opted for intensive treatment survived they were treated appropriately, but when they died they were overtreated.

NOTES

1. SUPPORT Principal Investigators. A controlled trial to improve care for seriously ill hospitalized patients. The Study to Understand Prognoses and Preferences for Outcomes and Risks of Treatment (SUPPORT). *JAMA* 1995:274:1591–1598.

2. Annas GJ. How we lie. *Hastings Cent Rep* 1995; 25 (6 suppl):S12–S14.

3. Lo B. Improving care near the end of life. Why is it so hard? *JAMA* 1995; 274; 1634–1636.

Dr. James L. Bernat uses the lead article in the June Newsletter to criticize my own criticism of the way medical care is delivered in ICUs, as this care was described in the SUPPORT study. He is quite correct in noting that I recommend what most physicians see as harsh and unnecessary action to change the way patients are mistreated in ICUs (and hospitals generally) at the end of life. My recommendations include encouraging lawsuits against physicians who ignore patient wishes, and moving palliative care out of the hospital setting altogether. This is because the SUPPORT study is consistent with the conclusion that "physicians simply have never taken the rights of hospitalized patients seriously," and under managed care regimes may be even less likely to (as evidenced at the other end of life by increasing insurance mandates to limit hospital stays for childbirth).

Dr. Bernat asks the right question of me (or any patient) when he asks, "Would Professor Annas refuse treatment in an ICU if, as was true of the mean of the SUPPORT patients, he was given a 75 percent chance of leaving the hospital? What odds would he find acceptable?" The problem is not with these questions; the problem is that many (if not most) ICU physicians don't care what the answer is for the individual patient: they have, as the SUPPORT study documents, already made up their own minds as to what the appropriate care is for whole categories of patients, and will deliver that care without discussing the patient's wishes at all (44 percent of the physicians in the SUPPORT study didn't even bother to read the report that special nurses had put in the patient's chart about the patient's wishes, let alone discuss this issue with the patient). Dr. Bernat may really care about what I or other individual patients want, but his comments on this point are at best unclear. Instead of using an individual consent standard, for example, he assumes he already knows the answer for almost everyone by proclaiming, "I believe that most patients and families given those odds [50 percent chance of surviving six months] would . . . choose an initial trial of life-sustaining treatment . . ." I think the question is much more complicated than this, and cannot be answered by probabilistic prognosis information alone. The patient will need to know what will be done in the ICU, what his quality of life is likely to be, and how his pain will (or won't) be managed, and how all these things change without ICU intervention. Perhaps most important, the patient should be assured that care WILL be discontinued and palliation provided when the patient concludes that "treatment" for a cure is no longer serving the patient's goals. Such assurance will remain hollow if ICU physicians do not discuss the care and goals of ICU treatment with patients and their families on a daily basis, and do not take patient wishes as their guide in continued treatment. ICU physicians know how they feel about the value of ICU care; isn't it time to involve the patients and the public in this discussion? We really do have a long way to go to make informed consent the rule, rather than the exception, in ICU care.

REPLY BY JAMES L. BERNAT, MD

I have no disagreement with the points raised by Professor Annas in his response to my article. I fully subscribe to the informed consent rule that he advocates. My article simply pointed out that many people, including Professor Annas, overreacted to the findings of the SUPPORT study. I do not believe that a hospital lawsuit hotline will improve the care of dying patients any more than has the current profusion of malpractice suits improved the practice of medicine. A better solution is to educate physicians about proper standards of decision making and the principles of palliative care.

⁝ ‖‖ ‖‖ ⁝

ROBERT M. TAYLOR, MD

Is Terminal Sedation Really Euthanasia?

QUESTION: A 51-year-old man suffered intractable pain from widespread bony metastases of lung cancer. Pain management required over 3000 mg per day of controlled-release oxycodone, high-dose daily fentanyl patches, high-dose glucocorticoid therapy, and large dosages of benzodiazepines. He had declined placement of an intraspinal opiate pump because of fatigue, cachexia, and the wish to avoid invasive procedures. One weekend evening, his physician received a desperate call from the patient's wife that he was frantic with pain. On admission, he was writhing, moaning, and restless. After discussing treatment options with his wife, the physician ordered intravenous midazolam (Versed). Impressively large doses were required to sedate him adequately but adequate sedation and pain palliation was accomplished without obvious respiratory depression. No hydration was given other than that necessary for pain palliation. The physician was concerned that sedating him in this way would accelerate the moment of death and therefore might be construed as euthanasia. How would you advise the physician?

REPLY: Despite widespread ethical and legal support for terminal sedation (TS), concern persists that this is a form of euthanasia. Furthermore, a few prominent proponents of the legalization of physician-assisted suicide (PAS) and voluntary active euthanasia have intentionally minimized the distinctions between TS and euthanasia and have argued that the similarities are strong reasons to legalize PAS.[1,2]

Nevertheless, there are important ethical and legal distinctions between TS and euthanasia that justify permitting the former in appropriate circumstances while prohibiting the latter. Indeed, the U.S. Supreme Court, in its landmark decision stating that there is no constitutional right to PAS, explicitly endorsed TS as an acceptable legal alternative to PAS for patients with intractable suffering.[2]

Before discussing the ethical issues, it is important to comment on two medical issues. First, although it is not clear from this vignette whether a hospice referral had been made prior to his admission, this patient with widespread bony metastases from lung cancer, severe pain, fatigue, and cachexia appears to have been very appropriate for hospice support. Second, it should be emphasized that, when such a patient is terminally sedated, opiates should be continued at doses equianalgesic to those previously used (usually given intravenously) to avoid worsening of pain as well as opiate withdrawal symptoms.

Terminal sedation—perhaps more properly called palliative sedation—consists of sedating a patient to the point of unconsciousness to relieve one or more symptoms that are intractable and unrelieved despite aggressive symptom-specific treatments, and maintaining this condition until the patient dies. Typically, artificial hydration and nutrition are withheld, as they no longer offer any benefit to the patient and may cause adverse effects, such as pulmonary edema. In rare cases, terminal sedation may be initiated in patients who are alert and cognitively intact but suffer from one or more severe and intractable symptoms. In such cases, because TS is likely to significantly shorten the patient's life, its use remains controversial. However, in most instances of TS, patients are suffering from terminal delirium in combination with other symptoms, such as pain or dyspnea, and are imminently dying. In these cases, because it is very unlikely that TS shortens the patient's life significantly (indeed there is some evidence is may slightly prolong it) the use of TS is much less controversial.[3-5]

This patient appears to fall into the latter category. Whether sedated or not, it is unlikely that this patient will ever again take food or fluid orally or survive more than a few days to a week or two. As in most cases of TS, it is difficult to imagine an alternative method of keeping this patient comfortable for whatever time he has left. To assure that comfort cannot be achieved otherwise, once he is sedated and receiving appropriate intravenous opiates, it might be reasonable to cautiously lighten his level of sedation to determine whether he can be comfortable and awake. However, it is unlikely that this will be possible and therefore, to assure his comfort, resuming aggressive sedation will be necessary. Furthermore, because he appears to be imminently dying of his advanced cancer and has already suffered greatly, and because such an "experiment" is most likely only to increase his suffering, it is by no means obligatory.

The principle of double effect is often used to justify TS, on the assumption that it may hasten death. According to this principle, an action which may have both a good effect and a bad effect is ethical if it fulfills the following criteria: (1) the act itself is not unethical; (2) the good effect is the intended effect whereas the bad effect, though foreseeable, is not intended and there is no alternative of achieving the good effect while avoiding the bad effect; (3) the good effect is not achieved by means of the bad effect; and (4) the good effect is sufficiently desirable to compensate for the allowing of the bad effect.[6] Thus, TS is ethical because: (1) sedation itself is not unethical; (2) although TS may hasten death, death is not intended and comfort cannot be achieved without this risk; (3) comfort is achieved as a direct result of sedation and not by means of death; and (4) for a terminally ill patient, comfort is more important than slightly prolonging life. In contrast, euthanasia is unethical because: (1) killing itself is generally unethical; (2) death is intended and comfort could be achieved by other means (e.g., TS); (3) comfort is only achieved by means of death; even though (4) for a terminally ill patient, comfort is more important than prolonging life.

Therefore, even if TS does shorten the patient's life, it is not equivalent to euthanasia and is an appropriate and ethical form of palliative care for this patient.

OUTCOME: The patient was admitted and sedated with intravenous midazolam (Versed) to produce comfort. He died on the third hospital day.

NOTES

1. Quill TE, Lo B, Brock DW. Palliative options of last resort: a comparison of voluntary stopping eating and drinking, terminal sedation, physician-assisted suicide, and voluntary active euthanasia. *JAMA* 1997;278:2099–104.

2. Orentlicher D. The Supreme Court and physician-assisted suicide: rejecting assisted suicide but embracing euthanasia. *N Engl J Med* 1997;337:1236–9.

3. Lynn J. Terminal sedation (letter). *N Engl J Med* 1998;338:1230.

4. Quill TE, Byock IR. Responding to intractable suffering: the role of terminal sedation and voluntary refusal of food and fluids. *Ann Intern Med* 2000;132:408–14; (see also letters: *Ann Intern Med* 2000;133:560–2).

5. Rousseau PC. Palliative sedation. *Am J Hosp Palliat Care* 2002;19(5):295–7.

6. Sulmasy DP, Pellegrino ED. The rule of double effect: clearing up the double talk. *Arch Intern Med* 1999;159:545–50.

☰ ☲ ☲ ☰

GARY FISCHER, MD AND ROBERT M. ARNOLD, MD

My Mother Was a Fighter

QUESTION: A 90-year-old widow with advanced Alzheimer's disease was admitted in coma to the ICU (Intensive Care Unit) for treatment of urosepsis and respiratory failure. She had lived in a nursing home and had become bedbound, mute, and incontinent. She was fed by a gastronomy tube. Her only child, a daughter aged 62, was her Durable Power of Attorney for Health Care. The daughter insisted on all possible life-sustaining treatments, including a ventilator and dialysis, if necessary. The patient had been a nurse and the daughter argued that the patient "was a fighter" and wished to continue living as long as possible, irrespective of the quality of her life. There were no religious reasons offered for this decision. The medical and nursing staff were unanimous in their belief that such treatment was inappropriate and that palliative care was appropriate medical treatment. The staff argued that the patient's "mind had died several years ago and now her body was trying to die, too" but the daughter was unmovable. How would you advise the ethics committee?

REPLY: Often when patients appear to be asking for something that healthcare providers believe is irrational, careful inquiry can disclose a reason for the request that can then be addressed.[1] By applying the same approach to surrogate decision makers, the ethics committee can better understand why the family is demanding treatment. This may change the situation from a conflict in which one party feels that its values are overridden, to one in which both parties find a satisfactory resolution.

Why might the family be demanding aggressive treatment? The surrogates may (1) misunderstand the prognosis; (2) be answering the wrong question; (3) not be aware of the alternatives to life-sustaining treatment; (4) lack decision-making capacity; (5) act from ulterior motives; or (6) order values differently than the health-care team.

Let us examine each of these. There are a number of reasons why the family might not understand or believe the prognosis. Physicians' beliefs about prognosis are often not communicated clearly. Family members may not have had time to accept a change in prognosis. Furthermore, they may be suspicious of the motives of the healthcare team, especially if they have had trouble accessing the healthcare system for social or economic reasons, or if they have been misinformed in the past. To explore these possibilities, the ethics committee should ask the family questions like: "What have you been told is going on with your mother?" to evaluate understanding of what the physicians have said. Questions like: "What do you think will happen if treatment is continued?" will help get at family members' beliefs. "Why do you think the doctors want you to do that?" gets at issues of trust.

The committee should ensure that the family is answering the right question. Too often physicians ask surrogates, "Do you want us to withhold dialysis?" rather than asking "Would your mother want to continue dialysis in this situation?" In this case, the committee should get more information about why the daughter believes that her mother would want *curative* treatment. Committee members might ask: "What did your mother say about patients she encountered when she was a nurse who were in a similar situation?" or "Did your mother ever say that she would want to live no matter what state she was in?" Focusing on the family's role to reflect their mother's wishes may relieve any guilt felt over not doing *everything* for their mother.

It is crucial that family members understand that their loved one will not be abandoned. The team should explain what will occur if life-sustaining treatment is forgone and describe the type of comfort care that they will provide. The family must not be abandoned either. Dealing explicitly with emotions like anger, fear, and grief may allow them to work through the reality of their loved one's impending death.

The fourth and fifth possibilities are, in our experience, fortunately rare. Convincing demonstration of these factors will raise serious questions about the suitability of the family to be the decision maker. Legal intervention may then be appropriate.

Approaching family members in this manner will resolve most conflicts. However, there will still be some cases in which the family continues to insist on treatment which the healthcare team deems inappropriate. Although some may argue that healthcare providers are not obligated to provide futile care, in this case the care requested by the daughter may prolong the patient's life, and even restore her to her previous state of health. The question turns on whether it is worthwhile to use intensive medical care to achieve these aims. Who should make this decision is very controversial and space does not permit a full discussion. We believe that since healthcare providers have no claim to special expertise regarding what makes life worth living, they should not unilaterally override a family's desire to continue treatment in this case.

OUTCOME: Despite intervention from the ethics committee, the daughter would not alter her insistence about the necessity of ICU treatment. The patient was intubated and ventilated in the ICU. Renal failure ensued but dialysis was not performed because the dialysis physicians declared the patient not to be a dialysis candidate. The patient died on ICU day seven.

☷ ☶ ☵ ☳

SUSAN D. BLOCK, MD

Rational Suicide and the Terminally Ill

While many mental health clinicians believe that rational suicide does not exist and that contemplating suicide is inherently a manifestation of a psychiatric disorder, consideration of suicide by patients with terminal illness is often viewed differently. In the context of terminal illness, suicide may be seen as a rational choice in response to a life-threatening illness; the desire to die is seen as a "reasonable" response to impending death and expected physical suffering.

While this construct has many advocates, including the Hemlock Society and other right-to-die organizations, it is critical that we examine the values and assumptions inherent in the notions of reasonableness, rationality, and choice.

The vast majority of patients with terminal illness, even those who are close to death and suffering from devastating symptoms, do not want to die. Instead, they seek to live as long as possible, even when living is accompanied by severe physical distress.

Overwhelmingly, patients desiring assisted suicide suffer from unrelieved, but potentially ameliorable problems, including physical symptoms, psychological distress, communication problems with the care team, family dysfunction, spiritual distress, fear of abandonment, vulnerability due to illness, and/or lack of a vision of a "good dying." Addressing these issues usually enhances the subjective sense of choice and control and reduces the patient's desire for assisted suicide.

PHYSICAL SUFFERING

The notion that extreme physical suffering is an inevitable feature of terminal illness is directly challenged by recent advances in palliative medicine, which has pioneered clinical approaches to treat symptoms, including pain, and to maintain quality of life. Patients' fears about physical suffering are often mediated by past experiences with friends and relatives, and are often worse than reality. Meticulous attention to pain relief and control of other distressing symptoms reassures the patient that symptoms can be managed, improves quality of life, and often reverses the patient's feeling that suicide is the only "way out" of suffering.

Effective communication about end-of-life care options and the feasibility of relieving symptoms, as well as aggressive efforts at symptom control, provide reassurance that makes the dying process less frightening and more manageable. Their absence supports unrealistic fears that preclude a rational decision about suicide. Unfortunately, many patients in our country still lack access to state-of-the-art palliative care.

PSYCHOLOGICAL DISTRESS

Among the common psychological factors that contribute to patient desires for assisted suicide are painful grieving with inadequate support, personality characteristics including a tendency to overvalue perfection and control, anxiety about uncertainty and the process of dying, and organic mental disorders associated with difficulty with impulse control. Depression, in particular, contributes to desires for hastened death, and limits the individual's ability to perceive all but the most negative of possible futures. An individual who can only conjure up terrible scenarios for the future because of the presence of a major depression is incapable of making a fully informed choice about suicide. Depression is a highly treatable illness, even among the terminally ill; treatment dramatically changes the individual's ability to be hopeful about comfort and connection in the dying process.

COMMUNICATION PROBLEMS WITH THE CARE TEAM

Patients who do not feel confident that their professional caregivers will listen to and respect their wishes for care may feel that assisted suicide is a way of asserting control over the dying process and reducing the risk of receiving unwanted medical interventions. In addition, physicians' concerns about upsetting or frightening patients in the course of discussions about wishes for care at the end of life may lead to euphemistic or incomplete discussions. Other communication problems—physician withdrawal due to feelings of failure, over-identification with well-liked long-term patients, difficulty addressing the ambivalence which is a universal feature of thinking about suicide—may also contribute to desires for hastened death and to the subjective diminution of choices about how the end of life can be managed.

FAMILY DYSFUNCTION

Difficulties in interpersonal relationships—anger, disappointment, abandonment—may also contribute to desires for early death. When patients have the opportunity to address these seemingly insoluble interpersonal dilemmas, they often feel a restored sense of connection, meaning, and self-worth, reducing the desire for accelerated death. Additionally, difficulty in communicating key concerns and inner experiences to family, friends, and professional care providers may lead to isolation and a sense of attenuated options. Opportunities to explore these issues often permit an expanded sense of positive possibilities in continuing to live.

SPIRITUAL DISTRESS

Patients who are facing death confront questions of meaning that may give rise to unbearable existential/spiritual suffering. Common themes are guilt over past actions, anger at God, fear of punishment, and despair about lack of meaning. Exploration of the patient's current and past religious and spiritual identity, affiliations, and beliefs are an important first step in understanding such concerns. Further discussion of the patient's feelings about the sources of meaning in her/his life, beliefs about why s/he became ill, and expectations about what happens after death provide critical data about how the patient might be able to restore his/her sense of meaning and purpose, even during the dying process. The help of a pastoral counselor is invaluable.

FEAR OF ABANDONMENT

One of the most disturbing fears expressed by dying patients is that they will be abandoned—by family, friends, and professional caregivers. The expectation of abandonment may lead some patients to "prefer" a self-controlled exit, before they are left alone to die. In reality, our healthcare system does abandon many patients. Through lack of information, lack of appropriate treatment, inadequate services in the home, and lack of professional attention, the system does not engender a sense of security about the availability of help and support for the patient or family. Terminally ill patients may consider suicide when they feel that there is no alternative to abandonment.

THE VULNERABILITY OF THE SICK

The subjective experience of choice is attenuated, too, by the experience of being seriously ill, which tends to make even the most strong and forceful healthy persons regress into more childlike modes of relating. These inner experiences are reinforced by the healthcare system and the power dynamics of professional relationships, which tend to engender physician activity and control and patient passivity and acquiescence. Lack of a sense of efficacy and control reinforces feelings of helplessness and hopelessness, cardinal features of suicidal thinking.

LACK OF A VISION OF "GOOD DYING"

Next, inherent in the idea that suicide is a rational response to the awareness of impending death is a notion that nothing good can happen in the dying process, and that dying is fraught only with suffering and misery. This assumption, too, deserves to be challenged. Many patients find a sense of meaning, closure, and reconciliation in the processes of remembering, reckoning, and saying good-bye that take place as they confront impending death. These processes can be immeasurably valuable for the patient who is dying, as well as for his/her family members and other survivors. While some patients might choose to forego these potential growth experiences, because of our cultural aversion to death, and the pervasive notion that death is an evil to be conquered, few individuals have the opportunity to learn what is possible in the dying process. Unless a person has a vision of a potentially good or meaningful dying process, can a choice to foreshorten the dying process through suicide be truly rational and informed?

Thus, there are many factors attenuating or limiting the ability of individuals in this society to make fully rational and informed choices about suicide in the context of terminal illness. Only when all of these concerns have been addressed can an individual begin to make a "rational choice."

While expressing skepticism about the notion that the desire for suicide among terminally ill patients is always or usually fully "rational," it is critical to recognize that not all symptoms and distress are ameliorable, and that for some patients, late in the difficult disease process, the benefits of continued existence may not be worth the travails caused by the illness. Even state-of-the-art care with meticulous attention to each of the above-mentioned issues may not allow the individual to maintain a subjectively acceptable quality of life. Who else is to judge quality of life but the person whose life it is? If a competent terminally ill person is receiving care that maximally enhances a sense of options and possibilities for comfort, support, and meaning in the dying process and still finds existence intolerable, a decision to commit suicide, either alone or with the physician's help, may be fully rational.

REFERENCE

Block SD, Billings JA. Patient requests for euthanasia and assisted suicide in terminal illness: the role of the psychiatrist. *Psychosomatics* 1995;36:445–457.

☰ ䷀ ䷁ ☰

HERBERT HENDIN, MD

Rational but Wrong

In "Rational Suicide and the Terminally Ill," Susan Block, MD, concludes an otherwise admirable article on the care of terminally ill patients by stating that at least in some situations, a "patient's desire to commit suicide, either alone or with the physician's help, may be fully rational," particularly if other options have been tried and failed. My own experience in this country and the Netherlands, in studying cases where patients request euthanasia, is that when doctors practice euthanasia the options described by Dr. Block are not, in fact, adequately explored.[1]

In this short piece, Dr. Block was probably not able to present case illustrations. In a longer article on the same subject,[2] she presents as a model example an AIDS patient who was assisted in suicide by his doctor after consultation with a psychiatrist who declared the patient to be rational and not depressed. But the case description is of a man in no pain but weakened by illness and no longer eager for the companionship of his friends. He is strongly influenced in his desire to control his own death by having witnessed the painful death from AIDS of his lover. There is no indication of an attempt by the psychiatrist to deal with any of these concerns. Instead, a decision was made by the physicians regarding the importance of honoring the patient's request. The case, which conveys no sense of meaningful communication between doctor and patient, seems less than persuasive.

The fact that doctor and patient are in agreement and both are rational does not assure that their judgment is sound. Recently, I saw a vivid example of how knowledge and experience affect decisions concerning rationality and autonomy with regard to euthanasia. At a small, international workshop that addressed problems in the care of the terminally ill, two American cases were presented in which terminally ill patients requested assisted suicide.

In one case, a man was confined to a wheelchair with advanced symptoms of AIDS that included cystic lung infection, severe pain due to inflammation of the nerves in his limbs, and marked weight loss. By the appropriate use of steroids, antidepressants, and psychological sensitivity in dealing with his fears of abandonment, he was enabled to gain weight, be free of his pain and his wheelchair, and to live an additional ten months, for which he was grateful.[3]

In another case, a woman with great pain due to lung cancer that was invading her chest wall wished assisted suicide. A nerve block relieved her pain, and she was happy to be able to leave the hospital and live her remaining months at home.[4]

I presented these cases to several euthanasia advocates in the Netherlands and in this country. They agreed that the first patient had a right to have euthanasia performed but were not so sure after they heard the actual outcome. In the second case, aware that a nerve block could provide relief, most would not perform euthanasia.

Believing they could not help the first patient, the physicians felt he was rational in his request and that respect for patient autonomy required them to proceed. They felt free to ignore patient autonomy when they knew how to help the patient, and might not have considered rational a patient who refused relief. Patient rationality and autonomy were in essence the justification for euthanasia when doctors felt helpless and did not know what else to do.

Rational people disagree all the time because they operate on the basis of different premises, knowledge, and values. For some doctors, a concern with patient rationality and autonomy is paramount. But that concern may interfere with their ability to understand and relieve the desperation that underlies the request for death. Medical practice means more than simply following patients' requests.

Euthanasia advocates believe that if they can persuade us that, at least in some cases, euthanasia is rational and justified, we will be obliged to concede that legalization of assisted suicide and euthanasia is necessary, if only to help such patients. Although it is probably true that no one who is suffering while confronted with death can be fully rational, the real question is not whether individual decisions are fully rational but whether it is rational for society to sanction them.

My experience has persuaded me that it is not in society's interest to legalize assisted suicide and euthanasia. In the Netherlands, euthanasia intended originally for exceptional cases has become an almost routine way of dealing with serious and terminal illness. Patient ambivalence about wanting to die is frequently ignored; viable options are often not presented. Palliative care has become one of the casualties of euthanasia. Rationality and autonomy are the justification. "Rational suicide," like the "right to die," is a catchy, but misleading, slogan designed to promote euthanasia while obscuring its complexities.

NOTES

1. Hendin H. *Seduced by death: doctors, patients and the Dutch cure.* New York: W. W. Norton, 1997.

2. Block S. Patient requests for euthanasia and assisted suicide in terminal illness: the role of the psychiatrist. *Psychosomatics* 1995;36:445–457.

3. Case presented by C. Gomez. Workshop on care of the terminally ill, Bellagio, Italy, 1997.

4. Case presented by K. Foley. Workshop on care of the terminally ill, Bellagio, Italy, 1997.

☲ ☶ ☷ ☳

G. K. KIMSMA, MD, MPH

Euthanasia for Existential Reasons

Euthanasia for existential reasons is an issue of public debate in the Netherlands. Advocates of voluntary active euthanasia (VAE) and physician-assisted suicide (PAS) believe that individuals should have the right to choose the time and manner of their death. Both VAE and PAS represent a conflict between the physician's duty to protect life and to alleviate unbearable suffering.

Existential suffering occurs in the absence of severe physical or mental illness. Requests for existential euthanasia come mostly from elderly people who suffer from age-related physical ailments and have lost the appetite for living because they experience life as meaningless and empty. For example, in a recent and typical case, a 69-year-old man who lost his wife said that he was lonely and wanted to join her in the afterlife. A psychiatric consultation found him competent and not depressed. He asked me for euthanasia.

In a philosophical sense, the terminology of existential suffering requires clarification, because all suffering, mental or physical, presupposes a mind and an existence capable of perceiving suffering and is existential. For pragmatic reasons, we adopt the distinction of suffering as physical, mental, or existential. People who request VAE for existential reasons are usually not adherents of the philosophy of existentialism as expressed by Jean Paul Sartre, Albert Camus, or Sören Kierkegaard.

In a recent publication of representative interviews, 410 physicians (GPs, specialists, and nursing home physicians) reported about 400 requests yearly to end a life from patients who did not have serious disease. These were mainly from patients over 80 years old, a minority of whom had ailments but no serious medical disease, and almost all after losing a spouse or being single with social problems. In this sample, only 3% of the physicians said they had ever complied with such requests; most had refused, suggesting alternatives to VAE or PAS.[1] If legalized, VAE for existential reasons could become an option for anyone, because these existential motives are entirely subjective and not amenable to objective evaluation.

VAE AND PAS IN THE NETHERLANDS

VAE is legally practiced in the Netherlands, Columbia, and Belgium, and PAS is legally practiced in those countries as well as the state of Oregon. PAS is not a crime in Germany nor Switzerland, which allows it if accomplices have no personal interest. The position of the Dutch arose from legal cases involving seriously ill patients and was not based on a public discussion of the principles of VAE/PAS.[2] The first prominent court case dates from 1974 when a physician ended the life of her ailing mother after repeated requests and was found guilty on technical charges and sentenced to a week of probation. This case was soon applauded as a landmark case in favor of VAE because the verdict outlined, for the first time, the requisite conditions to help someone die.

The Dutch legal definition of euthanasia is ending the life of a person, at his or her voluntary request, who suffers unbearably without hope of improvement. Contrary to popular belief, VAE and PAS are technically a crime in the Netherlands, even though the Dutch Voluntary Euthanasia Society[3] attempts to decriminalize assisted suicide. A law called the *Law Review Procedures for Termination of Life on Request,* active since April 1, 2002, defines the conditions a physician must follow to help a patient die without being prosecuted. The physician (1) must be convinced of the presence of a voluntary and carefully considered request, (2) must be convinced that the patient's suffering is unbearable without prospect for improvement, (3) must have informed the patient of their medical situation and future prospects, (4) must have concluded with the patient that reasonable alternatives are absent, (5) must have consulted with at least one other physician not otherwise connected to the case, and (6) must end the life of a patient effectively and carefully.

Each case of VAE or PAS must be reported as a case of unnatural death to a civil servant, comparable to a local medical coroner, who conducts an immediate investigation, consults with prosecutors about the case, and allows burial or cremation, or refers the case to the local prosecutor. The most formal evaluation is conducted afterward by one of five regional Euthanasia Evaluation Committees that determines whether the law has been upheld. These Committees have three members: a judicial expert, a physician, and an ethicist. I am a physician member in one of these committees.

VAE and PAS are performed primarily by family physicians with long-term patient relationships; most patients suffer from a terminal malignancy. VAE and PAS were performed on 2.7% (3,600 cases) of patient deaths in 2001. Of the 1,886 cases in 2004 for which data are available, 1,647 persons suffered from an end-stage malignancy; 81% of the VAE/PAS acts took place in private homes with family physicians, and 3.5% of the cases took place in nursing homes. The dominant age bracket in cases of VAE/PAS is between 65 and 79, conforming with cancer statistics on age.

Ninety percent of the Dutch population supports the option of VAE and PAS. Eighty-eight percent of Dutch physicians approve of VAE/PAS, while 8% are personally opposed but support the option for others, and 4% oppose it under all circumstances. For American readers, these figures may seem surprising, but keep in mind that the Dutch Courts have allowed the option of VAE/PAS since the early 1970s and the number of supporters has risen steadily since that time.

VAE/PAS are not just interventions to end a life at a particular moment, but more the end of a long process with an intensely emotional culmination.[4] Patients usually cite several reasons for ending their life: unbearable and hopeless pain and suffering, avoidance of further deterioration and meaningless suffering, death without dignity, dependence, fatigue, fear of suffocation, and being a burden to their family. In most cases that pass the Euthanasia Evaluation Committees, the descriptions of suffering are focused on medical symptoms such as unbearable pain despite treatment, nausea despite antiemetics, extreme fatigue, and breathing difficulty. Additional problems include insomnia, poor concentration, and impaired communication.

RELEVANT COURT CASES

Two important cases are relevant to the discussion of euthanasia for existential reasons. In 1994 the Supreme Court acquitted psychiatrist Dr. Boudewijn Chabot for assisting a woman in suicide who did not suffer from a terminal somatic or bodily disease. The woman wanted to end her life after she was alone following a divorce and both of her sons had died. The Court argued that unbearable suffering could be due to life experiences in the absence of physically debilitating diseases, ending the discussion that terminal illness should be conditional for euthanasia.

UNBEARABLE SUFFERING

What complicates an assessment of unbearable suffering is the complexity and intricate nature of human experience. What people experience and what they find unbearable is not "simply pain" but pain as shaped by their character and biography. The difficulty for a physician is to grasp this complexity and understand why the patient's experience leads to a request for assistance with dying. Each assessment becomes a delicate journey to respect and explore the thoughts of an individual, to understand why the totality of symptoms result in a patient's conviction that life is meaningless and prolonging it undesirable. Meaninglessness tends to become a final personal assessment, leading to a decision that "enough is enough."

CONCLUSION

VAE or PAS for existential reasons is not formally possible in the Netherlands, nor do physicians in general see a justification for it at this time. However, there are attempts to politicize the issue by demanding the decriminalization of assistance in suicide through a change of law in Parliament, which will not be successful in the present climate. As a physician, I support the present limitations on VAE/PAS and find these realistic and justified. As a philosopher, I support the position that euthanasia for existential reasons may be acceptable. But I find it difficult to justify the professional participation of physicians—these decisions are beyond the expertise of the medical profession.

In the instance of the 69-year-old man who asked me for existential euthanasia, although I was sympathetic, I told him that his case fell beyond the scope of the law. He decided to commit suicide with sleeping pills and a bag that would cause him to suffocate. I gave him my advice on the effectiveness of his choice, and days later he ended his life. I supported his sons afterwards. If Dutch society chooses euthanasia for existential reasons, though it would pain me, I would refuse to participate.

I would, however, consider it my professional duty as a family physician to help and support the patient during the process, and the family afterwards.

NOTES

1. Rurup M, Muller MT, Onwuteaka-Philipsen BD, Van derHeide A, Van derWal G, Van der Maas PJ. Requests for euthanasia or physician-assisted suicide from older persons who do not have a severe disease: an interview study. *Psychol Med.* 2005;345: 665–71.

2. Kimsma GK, van Leeuwen E. Euthanasia and assisted suicide in the Netherlands and the USA. Comparing practices, justifications and key concepts in bioethics and law. In: Thomasma D et al, eds. *Asking to Die. Inside the Dutch Debate about Euthanasia.* Dordrecht/ Boston/London: Kluwer Academic Publishers; 1998:35–71.

3. http://www.nvve.nl/nvve/pagina.asp?pagnaam=english

4. Norwood F. Euthanasia Discourse, General Practice and End-of-Life Care in the Netherlands. Dissertation presented at: University of California; July 2005; San Francisco, Calif.

ADDITIONAL READING

Van derWal G, van der Mass PJ. Clinical problems with the performance of euthanasia and physician-assisted suicide in the Netherlands. *N Eng J Med.* February 24, 2000;342:551–556.

☱ ☲ ☲ ☱

TIMOTHY QUILL, MD

How Much Suffering Is Enough?

In his article "Euthanasia for Existential Reasons," Gerrit Kimsma, a physician, philosopher, and end-of-life activist from the Netherlands, addresses the question of whether voluntary active euthanasia (VAE) or physician-assisted suicide (PAS) might ever be justified on the basis of pure existential suffering. As a philosopher, he can make a strong argument for its justification, but as a physician he is inclined to draw a line and say that such assessments are beyond his province and expertise, and therefore, he could not justify his participation and assistance.

Just how bright are the lines between physical, psychological, and existential suffering? Callahan has argued that physicians should restrict themselves to physical suffering and that psychological, spiritual, and/or existential suffering should be left to others with more expertise.[1] On the other hand, Cassel persuasively suggests that suffering is an inherently integrated experience that cannot be so easily objectified or dissected, and can only be understood by exploring the inherently human experience of the patient.[2] For some patients, there is a direct easily comprehensible connection between physical symptoms, debility, and suffering. Others, however, with seemingly overwhelming symptoms and debility are able to adapt and experience relatively low levels of suffering. And still others experience overwhelming suffering with seemingly little physical discomfort or debility. Frankl has taught us that suffering has as much or more to do with the meaning attached to one's experience than to its physical dimensions.[3]

Thus, understanding an individual's suffering requires full exploration of both its physical and non-physical dimensions. In fact, this exploration is at the core of the humanistic practice of medicine. To reduce the physician's role exclusively to the physical realm would reduce them to technocrats, not humanists, and would ultimately deprive them and their patients of many opportunities to address and potentially alleviate non-physical suffering. On the other hand, considering only the psychological and existential dimensions of suffering without contextualizing them within the physical concomitants would severely restrict our potential understanding of the totality of a person's experience. Furthermore, without the centrality of a disease process, it would not make sense to have physicians involved in assessing or responding.

So how should a physician address a patient's suffering that he reports to be "unbearable"? What if the ante is upped by the patient sharing that he is considering ending his life and asking for the physician's assistance?[4] (If you want to take the VAE or PAS controversy out of this discussion, consider a patient with chronic renal failure who wants to discuss stopping dialysis.) The first step in this inquiry would be to fully explore with the patient what makes his situation so "unbearable" and to make sure the underlying issues are fully understood. Before any decisions are made about how to respond, use a patient-centered interview that includes a: (1) bio- *(Are you having any pain, shortness of breath, nausea . . .?),* (2) psycho- *(Are you depressed, anxious, terrified . . .?),* (3) social *(How are things going at home? Have you talked with your family about this?)*, (4) spiritual *(Do you have a sense of why this is happening? Are there any religious parts of this decision in your tradition?)* and (5) existential *(Are there things that still make life worth living for you?)* exploration.

Restricting this exploration to the physical domains would lead to an incomplete understanding of the underlying issues beneath such requests and would also severely restrict the physician's opportunity to be responsive. We know from both Dutch data on VAE and PAS[5] as well as the Oregon data on PAS[6] that the main reasons patients give for requesting PAS/VAE are often a mix of physical, psychological, and existential dimensions. The recently reported 2005 data from Oregon, for example, cite that terminally ill patients report psychological, existential, and physical reasons that cannot be easily dissected, including loss of autonomy (79%), loss of dignity (89%), unable to engage in enjoyable activities (89%), losing control of bodily functions (45%), burden on family/caregivers (42%), inadequate pain control (24%).

Existential issues are often central to such descriptions of suffering. But there must be a direct relationship between the degree of disease-related physical suffering and the existential distress as well as a reasonable effort to find acceptable alternative approaches before considering any last resort response by a physician (be it stopping a life support or PAS).[7] The request for a hastened death by a patient who is already near death from lung cancer and whose severe shortness of breath cannot be adequately relieved is relatively easy to understand, and may require a relatively fast-paced, but nonetheless thorough, exploration before there is a response. The patient with ALS who is dependent on a respirator, who feels his life has lost meaning and wants to stop the respirator and die, should receive a multidimensional exploration of potentially reversible aspects of his suffering, but should ultimately be listened to and assisted if no acceptable alternatives can be found. Philosophical and ethical issues that justify such actions include respect for patient autonomy, the right to bodily integrity, compassion, mercy, and nonabandonment.[8]

The bereaved patient cited in Dr. Kimsma's article who no longer finds life worth living would be much more problematic. The patient's suffering is certainly severe, but the wish to die can be a central feature of severe depression, which clearly warrants aggressive, multidimensional assessment and treatment before being assisted in this manner. The elderly patient who is simply tired of living also would be problematic, in part because the desire to die may be part of an underlying depression, but also because there is no physical illness to anchor a physician's involvement.

In Oregon, the presence of a terminal illness is an absolute requirement to receive legalized physician-assisted suicide (along with a voluntary request, an evaluation by a second physician, and a mandatory two-week waiting period). There have been no reported cases of PAS for pure existential suffering, and, in fact, such patients would not qualify for PAS under the law. The numbers of cases of PAS in Oregon has remained very low and stable over the first 8 years, accounting for under 0.1% of deaths each year. But 1 out of 50 patients talk to their physicians about PAS, and 1 out of 6 talk to their families, so the main impact of legalization has probably been more open conversation between terminally patients and their doctors and families about these challenging issues.[9]

In the Netherlands, where both PAS and voluntary active euthanasia are openly practiced, there is no absolute requirement for a terminal prognosis.[10] Instead, a patient who requests such assistance must be experiencing unbearable suffering with no prospect for improvement, and that situation must be verified by two physicians. The Netherlands only recently legalized the practices of PAS and VAE, but they had studied the extralegal practice for over 20 years before making this public policy decision. (Previously, physicians would predictably not be prosecuted for breaking the law provided they met agreed upon criteria prior to this time.) The Netherlands is a much more legally permissive and socially tolerant society than the United States, and they wanted to have data about the practice's safety before legalization. In the Netherlands, there have been a few well-publicized cases of euthanasia for existential reasons, and such cases remain very controversial both legally and in public opinion because of the absence of an incurable terminal disease. The overall number of PAS and VAE cases have remained remarkably stable in the Netherlands over the last 15 years. The Dutch seem to rely heavily on the good clinical judgment of their physicians to work with patients to decide how much suffering is too much. (Unlike the US, the Netherlands has universal health care and a stable corps of family physicians who have long-standing relationships with their patients and their families, creating a much more conducive context for these difficult decisions.)

With regard to hastened death for existential suffering, I personally draw a line close to where Dr. Kimsma does. There needs to be some direct relationship between the severity of unrelievable, illness-related physical distress and the existential suffering for me to potentially provide any last resort option as a physician. The more uncertain the relationship between the two, the more I would require involvement of others with more expertise in the non-physical domains. Sometimes that might be a psychiatrist or other psychological counselor with experience with seriously ill patients, other times, a spiritual counselor or a family therapist. Although I would empathize with, explore and do my best to help alleviate pure existential suffering, without the anchor of proportionate physical suffering, it would be beyond my expertise (and comfort level) to assist as a physician.

NOTES

1. Callahan D. *The Troubled Dream of Life: In Search of a Peaceful Death*. Washington DC: Georgetown University Press, 2000.

2. Cassell EJ. *The Nature of Suffering and the Goals of Medicine*. New York: Oxford University Press, 1991.

3. Frankl VE. *Man's Search for Meaning*. Boston: Beacon Press, 1959.

4. Quill TE. Doctor, I want to die. Will you help me? *JAMA*. 1993; 270:870–873.

5. van der Maas PJ, van der Wal G, Haverkate I, de Graaff CL, Kester JG, Onwuteaka- Philipsen BD et al. Euthanasia, physician-assisted suicide, and other medical practices involving the end of life in the Netherlands, 1990–1995. *N Engl J Med*. 1996; 335:1699– 1705.

6. http:www.oregon.gov/DHS/ph/pas/index. shtml

7. Quill TE, Lo B, Brock DW. Palliative options of last resort: A comparison of voluntarily stopping eating and drinking, terminal sedation, physician-assisted suicide, and voluntary active euthanasia. *JAMA*. 1997; 278:1099–2104.

8. Quill TE, Cassel CK. Nonabandonment: A central obligation for physicians. *Ann Intern Med*. 1995; 122:368–374.

9. Tolle SW, Tilden VP, Drach LL, Frojje EK, Perrin NA, Hedberg K. Characteristics and proportion of dying Oregonians who personally consider physician-assisted suicide. *J Clin Ethics*. 2004; 15:111–118.

10. Kimsma GK, vanLeeuwen E. Assisted death in the Netherlands: physicians at the bedside when help is requested. In: Quill TE, Battin MP, eds. *Physician-Assisted Dying: The Case for Palliative Care and Patient Choice*. Baltimore, Md: Johns Hopkins University Press; 2004:221–244.

☱ ☲ ☳ ☴

ROBERT A. PEARLMAN, MD, MPH

Managing Cross-cultural Conflicts in the Doctor-Patient Relationship

QUESTION: A 59-year-old Chinese man was found to have a cancer in his left kidney. The cancer was resected by a urologic surgeon. During the postoperative period, before the pathology reports were available, the patient's wife met with the surgeon. She requested that, if the pathology reports indicated an unfavorable prognosis, her husband not be told the truth. She explained that in China it is considered detrimental to a patient's health and even mean-spirited to tell them they have an incurable disease or that they may die.

The urologic surgeon always told his patients the truth and was troubled by the wife's request. How would you advice the surgeon?

REPLY: The cross-cultural conflict raises many ethical issues. First is the nature of the doctor-patient relationship and medical decision making.

Since the 1980s, shared decision making has been recommended to ensure that decisions are targeted to patients' goals and interests.[1,2] Second, the dyadic, doctor-patient relationship often represents an oversimplification of social reality. In many families the emphasis on individual autonomy and control is culturally inappropriate. Thus, family members and community representatives often are involved in medical decisions.[3] Third, the moral foundation for veracity and informed consent is respect for persons, beneficence, and avoiding harm. Sometimes, such as when cultural or religious traditions conflict with secular prescriptions, full disclosure may need to be modified to respect the underlying principles.[4] Lastly, there are situations when cultural traditions or sensitivities should not trump standard medical practices. When requested behavior is illegal, breaches professional integrity, or represents an offensive moral belief, accommodation to culture-related requests is probably not ethically justifiable.[5]

THREE SETS OF QUESTIONS NEED TO BE ANSWERED BEFORE ADVISING THE SURGEON

· How long have the patient and wife lived in the United States? How are they employed? Do they live in a closed community? These questions help to characterize their degree of acculturation. A married couple may not share the same opinion about a cultural belief.

· How were medical decisions made previously? What was communicated in the informed consent process for surgery, and with whom? These questions may help characterize the patient's style of decision making and the role of family members.

· What was the nature of the patient's symptoms and concerns that led to identification of a cancerous kidney? This question may illuminate the patient's expectations.

The surgeon should develop a deeper understanding of the patient's and wife's beliefs. The surgeon should ask the patient, "What do you think caused the symptoms? This would help identify the patient's folk beliefs about the illness.[6] The surgeon should ask the wife, "Why is communication about these topics detrimental or mean-spirited? How is negative information communicated or handled in your culture?" The patient and wife should be asked, "How was advance care planning discussed with your doctor?" The answers to these questions would help explain the meaning and significance of the wife's request, as well as identify family responses to similar situations.

The surgeon should ask the patient if he has any questions that he would like answered, and determine the patient's understanding of the reasons for the surgery. Sincere and repeated invitations to ask questions permit the surgeon to glean how much information the patient wants to hear. The patient's story about the need for surgery should provide insights about his handling of negative information.

If the surgeon discussed the surgical indications and possible complications during the informed consent process, and the patient discussed the possibility of negative outcomes, then the surgeon should proceed with an honest discussion about the pathology report. Prior to this discussion, however, the surgeon should communicate with the wife his rationale—including professional and ethical considerations—and any conversations with the patient that suggest acceptance of a shared decision-making role.

Alternatively, if the patient consented to surgery without understanding the implications, then depending on the patient's postoperative questions, the physician should tailor the amount of information to the questions asked and the wife's concerns. The precise style and content of the communication with the patient would likely benefit from discussions (negotiations) between the surgeon and the wife. This latter approach may undermine the patient's autonomy by not providing him with sufficient information to judiciously decide how to live his remaining life. However, if this approach accurately reflects the patient's values and beliefs, it demonstrates respect for persons, and likely maximizes good outcomes and minimizes harms. Presumably, giving incomplete information in this context does not transgress professional integrity. Therefore, in this case, partial disclosure is ethically permissible.

This type of case suggests the need for preventive strategies. Physicians should explore how their patients envision an ideal doctor-patient relationship and decision making. After learning about proscriptions (e.g., cannot discuss negative information), physicians should inquire how other patients and/or their families should be approached if something untoward is a possibility. Furthermore, incorporating the patient's cultural beliefs into shared decision making can be practiced on more mundane day-to-day decisions. Finally, discussions with cultural leaders in a patient's ethnic or cultural community and institutional ethics committees can facilitate understanding and resolution of cross-cultural ethical conflicts.

OUTCOME: The pathologic findings showed that the tumor had been completely removed. There was no additional bad news to deliver.

NOTES

1. President's Commission for the Study of Ethical Problems in Medicine and Biomedical and Behavioral Research. *Making Health Care Decisions.* Washington, DC: U.S. Government Printing Office, 1982.

2. Emanuel EJ, Emanuel LL. Four models of the physician-patient relationship. *JAMA* 1992;267:2221–6.

3. Blackhall LJ, Murphy ST, Frank G., Michel V, Azen S. Ethnicity and attitudes toward patient autonomy. *JAMA* 1995;274:820–25.

4. Carrese JA, Rhodes LA. Western bioethics on the Navajo reservation. Benefit or harm? *JAMA* 1995;274:826–29.

5. Jecker NS, Carrese JA, Pearlman RA. Caring for patients in cross-cultural settings. *Hastings Cent Rep* 1995;25(1):6–14.

6. Kleinman A, Eisenberg L, Good B. Culture, illness and care: clinical lessons from anthropologic and cross-cultural research. *Ann Intern Med* 1978;88:251–58.

☷ ☶ ☳ ☴

XIUYUN YIN, PHD, BENFU LI, MD, AND YALI CONG, PHD

Should This 96-year-old Woman Be Allowed to Die?

QUESTION: A 96-year-old-woman is on a mechanical ventilator in the intensive care unit (ICU) because of respiratory failure. She has multiple medical problems that include a severe cardiomyopathy and cerebrovascular disease. The patient had previously told her physician she did not want to be placed on a mechanical ventilator or resuscitated. However, her children have insisted that all life supports be continued and have specifically requested the placement of a feeding tube. The healthcare team is distressed, because they believe continued treatment is almost surely futile, the patient is suffering needlessly, and that by honoring the family's wishes they are violating the patient's wishes. How would an ethicist in China advise the healthcare team?

REPLY: Recently, a similar case involved one of our colleagues whose 84-year-old mother was hospitalized in the ICU with multiple organ failure. The healthcare team consulted with the colleague about whether to use a mechanical ventilator because of respiratory failure, since otherwise, her mother would die soon. Having taken care of her mother for many years, the colleague often heard her mother say that she did not want to be placed on a mechanical ventilator or resuscitated at the end of life. But other family members, especially the elder brother, didn't agree with her wish to act in accordance with her mother's will.

Her mother was placed on a mechanical ventilator and given full medical treatment. Several days later, no miracle happened, and all family members agreed unanimously to withdraw the breathing machine and stop treatment. The mother died soon afterward. This may be the most common way such problems are resolved currently in China. First, the key element of clinical decision making is not the will of either the patient or the healthcare team, but that of the patient's family members. The "patient" has a special role in Chinese society and is viewed as someone who deserves care and love and should be free of responsibilities, such as decision making. Although usually a group decision, it may be expressed by the most authoritative family member, such as the patient's spouse or an adult child if the patient doesn't have a spouse. Sometimes it is the elder son; usually it is the one who contributes most to the family.

The healthcare team's advice is very important and usually accepted by the family. The ethical issues here are not only the advice itself, which may be the opinion of the physician in charge (and may be wrong), but also potential conflicts of interest. If there are spare beds in the hospital, the physicians may prefer to accept the patient and administer futile treatment in order to raise the income of the hospital. Conversely, if a patient doesn't pay the hospital, the doctor will be under pressure from his department and the hospital to discharge the patient.

In the case of the 96-year-old mother, in the US healthcare team's view, the treatment is almost surely futile. But a Chinese healthcare team would not inform the family member that it is "surely futile," except in the state of brain death,[1] when the mechanical ventilator cannot prolong life. We can say that the Chinese healthcare team usually views the situation from the standpoint of "quantity" (how long the patient will live), rather than "quality of life." The question the healthcare team usually asks family members is "Do we give up treatment or not?" and the answer of family members at first usually is don't give up, whether or not the patient has expressed his or her wish for continued treatment. But how long treatment lasts depends on the cost, whether the cost can be covered by patient's insurance, and the economic condition of the family. If the economic condition is not good, the treatment will be stopped after a short period. The cost for one day on a mechanical ventilator is 500 yuan ($60.39) or 15,000 yuan ($1,812) a month; the average monthly income in China is 1,022.62 yuan ($123.50).[2] Therefore, these expenses can be a large amount for a family.

To properly analyze this question, we need to clarify several cultural differences:

1. In the US, the ethical issue is whether to withdraw treatment. This is not the issue in China, where the decision to "give up" treatment is, in fact, commonly made for economic reasons.
2. There are differences in the role of family members. In Chinese tradition each member of the family is not an isolated person but part of the

family; family members usually share a similar mindset with the patient, which reflects the family members' emotions and the effects of external pressure from other people who may judge them to be lacking in filial piety if they don't treat the patient. The treatment, even if futile, may last for a time during which the family can adjust psychologically. Otherwise, they will feel guilty.

3. Another significant difference is in the US, the healthcare team is distressed by having to administer futile treatment and violate the patient's wishes. Whereas, in China, it is uncommon for the healthcare team to raise such questions, for they will not regard the interests between patient and family members as in conflict. Only if the whole family has made a decision will the healthcare team act according to the family's requirement. When the healthcare team is distressed, usually it is because they think the patient should be treated and believe there would be a good outcome, but the family members don't agree due to the lack of financial support or other reasons.

Theoretically speaking, the ethical issue in such a case is who can represent the best interest of the patient. The US healthcare team's distress relates to issues of autonomy, both their autonomy and the patient's. But in China, the healthcare team and whole family share similar values, that is, for the best interest of the patient. Here the "best interest of the patient" is not seen from the view of the patient, but of the healthcare team and all the family members.

The autonomy and voice of the patient in China has begun to emerge (but not strongly enough) with more attention paid to the patient; however, decisions are still usually made by the family. The patient is not regarded as a person who has the capacity to make decisions, so the healthcare team will not be troubled by the patient's wish for termination of treatment or by any violation of patient autonomy. Informed consent is obtained mainly from the family, not the patient, and the family's decision is accepted even if the patient would have chosen differently.

NOTES

1. The concept of brain death as equivalent to death has not been widely accepted by the average Chinese person.

2. Income is higher in cities like Beijing (1,500 yuan or $181.16/month) and Shanghai (2,000 yuan or $241.55/month).

☰ ☷ ☷ ☰

FRANK A. CHERVENAK, MD
LAURENCE B. MCCULLOUGH, PHD

I Can't Watch this Baby Die Inside Me

QUESTION: A 23-year-old woman was found to be carrying twins during a routine ultrasound at 20 weeks' gestation. One of the twins appeared to have significantly compromised growth. A follow-up ultrasound at 24 weeks showed the smaller twin to be growth retarded and in extremis. The patient says she believes in the sanctity of all life and would be unable to bear losing one of the twins, particularly if the baby were to die in her womb.

If the mother is taken for immediate cesarean section, in an effort to "save" the growth-retarded fetus, there is a strong possibility that the normal baby would not survive intact or would require prolonged mechanical ventilation with multiple potential complications.

A neonatologist states the likelihood of survival for the smaller twin is negligible. The father fears that his wife will choose immediate cesarean section if offered this option. How would you advise the obstetrician?

REPLY: This case illustrates that ethics is an essential dimension of modern obstetric practice. At the heart of this case is the question, "When is the fetus a patient?"

We have argued elsewhere the fetus is a patient when a human being is presented to the physician and there exist clinical interventions that are reliably expected to be efficacious in that they are reliably expected to result in a greater balance of goods over harms in the future of the human being in question.[1] For both fetuses in this case, both conditions are clearly satisfied. In a recent excellent review, Rennie reports survival at 24 weeks to be 35 percent and of the survivors, 48 percent are normal.[2]

Both fetuses in this case are patients in that both the pregnant woman and her obstetrician have beneficence-based obligations to them. These obligations, of course, should be balanced by the obstetrician against beneficence-based and autonomy-based obligations to the pregnant woman. A complicating factor here is that the obstetrician must also balance competing beneficence-based obligations to the two fetal patients. We emphasize that our approach does not depend on—indeed, it rejects—the language of fetal rights and the concept of the fetus as a potential person.[1]

In our approach to obstetric ethics, these are just viable fetal patients. If the distressed fetus were a singleton, we would recommend cesarean delivery because it would appreciably benefit outcome and not performing a cesarean delivery would not guarantee death and might result in survival with a significant likelihood of brain disease. After discussion with the pregnant woman, her wishes should be respected because cesarean delivery at 24 weeks represents a real, but marginal, benefit to the fetal patient.

In the case of twins, however, performance of cesarean delivery would subject the larger twin to a high probability of death or damage when expectant management would likely lead to a normal outcome. Given the borderline benefits to the distressed twin and overwhelming harms to the larger twin, we would view cesarean delivery in this case as inconsistent with beneficence-based clinical judgment. The clinical implication of this position is that cesarean delivery should not be offered as an option and a request by the woman for cesarean delivery should be met with respectful, but firm, refusal.

In this case, such a request was made by the woman, based on "sanctity of life." In the Judeo-Christian tradition, this concept does not mean that preservation of life at all cost is ethically obligatory.[3] Instead, the obligation to preserve life, under the principle of sanctity of life, is properly limited when the chance of saving life is low, as it is for the distressed twin, and the chance of causing death or damage is very high, as it is for the large twin.

The preventative ethics approach, in this case, should have been to not offer cesarean delivery and to have counseled the woman about the ethical limits of the principle of sanctity of life. We describe this approach as respectful persuasion, i.e., recommending alternatives because they support and advance the patient's values.[1] When a principle such as sanctity of life is invoked by the woman, involvement of trusted religious advisors in the process of respectful persuasion is appropriate. In addition, the woman should be offered and provided ongoing psychosocial and spiritual support so that she can cope well with the loss of the distressed twin by understanding that this loss would be consistent with respect on her part for the principle of sanctity of life.

OUTCOME: At the mother's strong insistence, she was taken to C-section. The growth-impaired neonate died shortly after delivery and the normal premature newborn did not survive a stormy course. The mother remains emotionally devastated by her decision.

NOTES

1. McCullough LB, Chervenak FA. *Ethics in obstetrics and gynecology.* New York: Oxford University Press 1994.

2. Rennie JM. Perinatal management of the lower margin of viability. *Archives of Diseases of Childhood* 1996;74:F214–F218.

3. McCormick RA. To save or let die: the dilemma of modern medicine. *JAMA* 1974;229:172–176.

☰ ☷ ☷ ☱

LAWRENCE J. SCHNEIDERMAN, MD

Family Demand for Futile Treatment

QUESTION: JB, a 53-year-old man, had progressive liver failure associated with hepatitis C. During evaluation for a liver transplant, a biopsy disclosed liver cancer. Consequently, he was no longer considered a candidate. He developed pulmonary failure and renal failure and is now in the intensive care unit (ICU), comatose, ventilator dependent, and requiring vasopressor medications to sustain his blood pressure. His physicians agreed that treatments aimed at life prolongation were futile and that comfort care should be the goal. However, members of his family repeatedly voiced their strong opposition to withdrawal of life support. They also refused to agree to a Do Not Attempt Resuscitation order, insisting that cardiopulmonary resuscitation be attempted if his heart stopped and dialysis be provided if necessary.

When the physicians suggested that the family might wish to obtain their own outside consultation or involve religious counseling, they refused. When asked what the patient himself would want, one son stated that JB had once demanded life support for an infant who the doctors allegedly claimed was dying and the baby miraculously recovered. Therefore, he was sure his father would want aggressive measures in hope of a similar miracle. What would you do if you were the physician?

REPLY: The right of patients capable of decision making (or, when appropriate, their authorized surrogates) to refuse unwanted treatment is now clearly established in ethics and the law. But what about the reciprocal situation? Do patients (or their surrogates) have a right to demand any treatment? Specifically, do they have the right to demand a treatment judged by physicians to be futile? What if the goal of the patient or family is a miracle, or life confined to the ICU, or even permanently unconscious life? Are there patient goals that do not comport with medical goals, hence should not be considered obligatory for the physician? Exploring these issues has forced us to revisit the doctor-patient relationship in a very fundamental way.[1]

First, we have to consider the problem of uncertainty in medicine. JB's loved ones hope for a miracle and the son claimed that JB was witness to one. "How can you be absolutely certain my father won't miraculously recover?" To this question, JB's physicians must admit they can never be absolutely certain. But based on empirical experience, they have concluded that recovery from his present state is not a realistic possibility. Attempting aggressive, life-prolonging treatments would so likely cause him harms, burdens, and suffering that it would violate both the principles of nonmaleficence (avoiding harm with no benefits) and proportionality (assuring that benefits are not severely overweighed by burdens and harms). Also, it would deter the physicians from pursuing the important obligation of alleviating suffering.[2]

In my view, the family's goal may be a miracle but it cannot be imposed on physicians as a goal of medical practice. Physicians can empathize with their desires and encourage their prayers. But physicians cannot do more than nature allows. Indeed, the very meaning of "miracle" depends on the premise that "the things which are impossible with men are possible with God" (Luke 18:27).

A patient is neither a collection of organs and body parts, nor a customer seeking to satisfy idiosyncratic desires. Rather, a patient (from the phrase "to suffer") is a person who seeks the healing (meaning "to make whole") powers of the physician. The physician's duty is to provide not merely an effect upon some organ, body part, or physiologic function, but a benefit to the patient as a whole.[3] For example, the effect of JB's vasopressor medications is to maintain his blood pressure. But at this stage in the dying man's illness there is no point in keeping his blood pressure up unless it restores his consciousness and grants him, at the very least, the capacity to appreciate the effect as a benefit.

The hospital in which JB was a patient has a policy that defines medically futile treatment and outlines procedures to follow in the event of a dispute. The policy defines futile treatment as "any treatment that has no realistic chance of providing a benefit that the patient has the capacity to appreciate (as distinguished from producing physiologic effects limited to parts of the body), or merely preserves permanent unconsciousness or cannot end permanent dependence on medical care that is available only in an intensive care unit." The policy also distinguishes between "treatment" and "care," emphasizing that "although a particular treatment may be futile, care such as palliative or comfort care is never futile." This hospital policy provides specific definitional grounding and principles for the dispute resolution process involving the patient, his or her family, healthcare providers, and the ethics committee, which includes lay community members. Many hospitals are developing such policies, which offer an approach to asserting a professional standard of care.[4]

The evidence suggests that if physicians request prior permission to discontinue futile treatment the courts will refuse it, but if the futile treatment is withdrawn after careful deliberation and due process, the courts will side with the physicians.[5]

The healthcare team should work with the family to make a reasonable accommodation to their needs to grieve and come to terms with the patient's dying. It is important to emphasize that "doing everything" in this case means doing everything possible to assure that the patient undergoes a peaceful, dignified, pain-free death.

OUTCOME: The family was given a date and time at which anyone who wished could be present with JB when all life support would be withdrawn. This date gave the family sufficient time to seek transfer of the patient or court intervention—which they chose not to do. All treatments and monitors were withdrawn and JB died peacefully in the presence of his family.

NOTES

1. Schneiderman LJ, Jecker NS. *Wrong Medicine: Doctors, Patients and Futile Treatment.* Baltimore, MD: Johns Hopkins University Press, 1995.

2. Schneiderman LJ, Faber-Langendoen K, Jecker NS. Beyond futility to an ethic of care. *Am J Med* 1994;96:110–4.

3. Schneiderman LJ. The futility debate: effective versus beneficial intervention. *JAGS* 1994;42:883–6.

4. Schneiderman LJ, Capron AM. How can hospital futility policies contribute to establishing standards of practice? *Cambridge Q Healthcare Ethics* 2000;9:524–31.

5. Johnson SH, Gibbons VP, Goldner JA, Wiener RL, Eaton D. Legal and institutional policy responses to medical futility. *AHA Journal of Health Law* 1997;30:21–47.

☷ ☶ ☶ ☷

JEFFREY BURNS, MD, MPH

Does Anyone Actually Invoke Their Hospital Futility Policy?

QUESTION: The clinicians in the Intensive Care Unit (ICU) seek to invoke the hospital futility policy over demands for treatment by the parents of a patient in their unit and ask the advice of the hospital ethicist. The ICU clinicians believe that the parents are insisting on interventions that will merely prolong the dying of their child and seek consultation and assistance from the hospital ethicist in overriding the parents' authority to make medical decisions about life-sustaining treatments.

The child is 14 months old, was delivered prematurely at 24 weeks, and now has multiorgan failure. He has MRI findings of extensive hypoxic-ischemic brain injury, dependence on inotropic support for biventricular insufficiency, dependence of mechanical ventilation for chronic respiratory failure from hyaline membrane disease, dependence on parenteral nutrition and a colostomy for short gut syndrome from necrotizing colitis, and dependence on dialysis for chronic renal failure. The clinicians believe the toddler demonstrates evidence of feeling pain and discomfort. However, they have been hampered in their ability to provide complete symptom relief by the parents who believe narcotic analgesics interfere with the child's cognitive development. In multiple family meetings the parents have been told by the ICU attending physician that their baby cannot survive and the interventions he is getting now are simply prolonging his dying. The ICU nursing staff members uniformly support this assessment and have consistently relayed the same prognosis at the bedside. All clinicians agree that the toddler's parents are rational, loving, and very devoted to their son whom they visit for 5 or 6 hours every day. The parents both work in the healthcare field. This is their first child. They remain hopeful and are willing to take their little boy home "in any shape."

REPLY: The late Supreme Court Justice Potter Stewart once remarked of pornography, "I shall not today attempt further to define the kinds of material I understand to be embraced within that shorthand description; and perhaps I could never succeed in intelligibly doing so. But I know it when I see it . . ."[1] So too with futility. It is difficult to define but we know it when we see it. But how should ethics consultants respond when they "see it"?

Helft and colleagues noted that discussions of futility can be grouped into four categories: attempts to define medical futility, attempts to resolve the debate with the use of empirical data, discussions that cast the debate as a struggle between the autonomy of patients and the autonomy of physicians, and attempts to develop a process for resolving disputes over futility.[2] Our Ethics Committee long ago abandoned definitional attempts at futility and instead adopted a procedural approach to futility cases. We agree with others who see attempts to define futility as illusive, for such attempts only expose and exacerbate a clash of values and fail to provide an ethically coherent ground for limiting life-sustaining treatments.[3]

Our institution has adopted process over definitional attempts to address concerns about futility. This approach is backed by our hospital policy on futility that was developed over a yearlong process in 1997, with broad input from the community and with attention to the diversity of individual values and goals. The futility policy is disclosed in the public record and outlines a series of steps in dispute resolution, as well as a mechanism to assist a patient or their family in an appeal process before the court if necessary, and leaves open the possibility of transferring the patient's care to another physician or institution. These features of a futility policy have been deemed essential by other institutions as well.[4] Our futility policy culminates in the institution sanctioning ". . . the unilateral foregoing or removal of life-sustaining treatments" if all previous steps fail to resolve the conflict.

Yet, despite an increasing number of ethics consults on questions of futility we do not invoke our own futility policy. Why? We have concluded that our hospital futility policy is sound in theory but less so in actual practice. First, not placing our futility policy formally in motion on these consults allows a more flexible ad hoc process in dispute resolution. The absence of a formal document that outlines the crescendo in the dispute resolution process when performing a consult on futility, in our experience, paradoxically seems to avoid the aura of an inevitable path to confrontation and thus mitigates a polarization of positions. If the parties are not aware of the trajectory of the formal policy, more room for common ground appears to be preserved. Second, the simple fact is that the mission of a large, academic pediatric medical center does not align with a public confrontation with parents over the benefit of life-sustaining treatments for their child. Third, the low-key, ad hoc process outlined above eventually gets us to a point of mutual acceptance by all parties in the dispute. At the end of the day a consequentialist rather than Kantian approach to ethics case consultation on issues of futility is most effective.

OUTCOME: After more than a dozen meetings with the hospital ethicist and ethics consult team, the parents and caregivers reached agreement on decision making about analgesia, concluding that narcotics would be given if the clinicians or parents felt that the child was experiencing discomfort. The parents and caregivers also reached agreement on an order to withhold specific steps in resuscitation and to withhold further escalation in life-sustaining treatment. The clinicians reported that being able to provide symptom relief to the infant removed enough of their reservations about burdensome treatments to continue to support the parents' medical directives.

NOTES

1. *Jacobellis v. Ohio,* 378 U.S. 184 (1964).

2. Helft PR, Siegler M, Lantos J. The rise and fall of the futility movement. *N Engl J Med* 2000;343:293–296.

3. Truog, RD, Brett AS, Frader J. The problem with futility. *N Engl J Med* 1992;326:1560–1564.

4. Halevy A, Brody BA. A multi-institution collaborative policy on medical futility. *JAMA* 1996;276:571–574.

Posthumous Sperm Retrieval

QUESTION: Mr. Smith died of a narcotics overdose at the age of 36. He had been engaged for three years to a 34-year-old woman, Ms. Jones. When the medical examiner released the body, Ms. Jones indicated a desire to have sperm retrieved from her fiancé's body and frozen so she could later bear his child. The dead man's mother, who had legal custody of the body, supported Ms. Jones' request.

Ms. Jones called several area hospitals until a urologist at one of the hospitals said he could retrieve her fiancé's sperm. The deceased's wishes concerning sperm donation were not known. When the body arrived, the urologist reconsidered and questioned whether he should retrieve sperm from the dead man. How would you advise the urologist?

REPLY: The urologist's misgivings about retrieving sperm from this dead man are as understandable as the fiancée's impulse to want the sperm retrieved so she could bear Mr. Smith's child. The latter is an immediate response to loss: Ms. Jones is trying to put herself back on the life path she had imagined as the mother of children with the man she loved. In her eyes, there is nothing wrong with applying artificial reproductive technologies (ARTs) in a novel fashion to achieve her goal.

The question of whether it would be ethical for Ms. Jones to proceed as she proposes is related to, but not necessarily coincident with, the question of whether it would be ethical for the urologist to retrieve the sperm. This distinction is important because some issues here turn on the relationship of various parties to any children who might be born from this unusual use of ART, with resulting differences in their obligations to these children.

While children benefit greatly in developmental, social, and material terms from being raised in a two-parent family,[1] many who are born to single mothers do well. If a woman decides to become pregnant and then raise the child without involving the father, we may think she is acting foolishly or selfishly, but her offense is hardly so great as to justify invoking any of the extreme measures—such as forced sterilization or abortion—that would be needed to prevent her from carrying out her plan.

The urologist is in a different position precisely because ruling his involvement out-of-bounds does not require any heavy-handed intervention; it merely requires his refraining from using his professional expertise and the available technologies. ARTs are used in a process that has been described as "collaborative reproduction."[2] By signifying that baby-making is no longer a private, intimate matter for a couple engaged in sexual intercourse but now directly involves medical professionals, this term is an attempt to normalize the use of ARTs. But it also reminds us that the professional collaborators have obligations of beneficence and nonmaleficence to the products of their labor. Thus, the question is what effect should those obligations have on the urologist's conduct?

A urologist who refused to aid Ms. Jones because he felt it would be wrong to bring children into the world in this circumstance, would certainly be acting ethically. But would a urologist who did aid her have acted unethically? In other words, is the harm imposed on the unconsenting patient (the future child) so great as to make it wrong for the physician to proceed?

Certainly, being born under these circumstances entails burdens, perhaps grave ones. At the worst, the child may be treated primarily as a means for its mother's ends. She may, on the one hand, treat the child as an icon, the embodiment of her dead fiancé. She may place unusual (and unreasonable) demands on the child in social and psychological terms, as a source of comfort in her grief or as a means of continuing the dead man's life. On the other hand, the child could become the object of Ms. Jones' unresolved anger at this premature death and, more specifically, at Mr. Smith for the behavior that led to his death. Likewise, the woman may use the child as a means to receive psychological or material support from her fiancé's family.

Reasonable people can differ on the likelihood and weight of these burdens and hence on whether the potential harm to a child would make it wrong for any urologist to aid Ms. Jones. That does not end the analysis, however. Suppose an obstetrician diagnosed a woman's pregnancy immediately after her husband had died suddenly. Further suppose that the woman was at risk of miscarrying, and the physician would have to manage the pregnancy very carefully; the woman cannot have the child without the help of a physician. If it would be ethical for the physician to aid the birth of that child, why is it unethical in the present case?

The first of three important differences is that there is already a child-in-being, albeit still unborn. The primary obligation to such patients—namely, to aid its being born healthy, if that is feasible—does not arise in the present case, where no new human being yet exists. No obligations exist to ensure each egg and sperm a chance to be born.[3]

Second, unlike the dead man in the present case, the pregnant woman's dead husband consented (knowingly or at least by his act) to becoming a father. Even if Mr. Smith had clearly stated that he intended to have children with Ms. Jones someday, that would not amount to consent to becoming a posthumous father. Such consent cannot be presumed, as the risks to the potential children, and the benefits to the man, are so different. As Professor Lori Andrews has argued, collecting sperm without explicit consent is perilously close to rape.[4]

Finally, if the obstetrician is successful in bringing the hypothetical pregnancy to term, the resulting child will be recognized as the legitimate offspring of the dead husband, entitled to all the resulting benefits. The legal status of any children born as a result of this posthumous sperm retrieval—and there is nothing to prevent the fiancée from having more than one child or from selling the sperm to others, resulting in additional children—is very unclear.

Hence, the urologist ought not to aid Ms. Jones' project in this case. Instead, the medical profession should concentrate on finding other means of responding to the grief of spouses, parents, or significant others when death occurs rather than developing gamete retrieval and posthumous reproduction as a new form of ART in which dead people are, without their consent, made "parents" of offspring who are half-orphans from the moment of conception.

OUTCOME: Because of legal and ethical uncertainties, the urologist was advised by the hospital's legal counsel not to retrieve sperm from the dead man without a court order. Mr. Smith's mother obtained a court order from a probate court judge and the sperm was retrieved. The director of the recipient sperm bank said he would not release the sperm for use by Ms. Jones without another court order.

NOTES

1. McLanahan S, Booth K. Mother-only families: problems, prospects, and politics. *J Marr & Fam* 1989;51:557–80.

2. Robertson JA. *Children of Choice: Freedom and the New Reproductive Technologies.* Princeton: Princeton University Press, 1994.

3. Steinbock B. Sperm as property. In, Harris J, Holm S (eds): *The Future of Human Reproduction: Ethics, Choice, and Regulation.* Oxford: Clarendon Press, 1998;150–61.

4. Andrews L. The sperminator. *NY Times Magazine,* Mar 28, 1999;62–5.

☷ ☶ ☵ ☳

ROBERT D. ORR, MD, CM

Must Multiorgan Donors Be Brain Dead?

QUESTION: A 37-year-old man was admitted to the intensive care unit because of massive intracranial hemorrhage. He was treated with ventilator support, lowering of intracranial pressure, and neurosurgical decompression. Despite these measures, eight weeks later he was unimproved: he remained unconscious and ventilator dependent. Neurological consultants disclosed he was in a severe form of a persistent vegetative state with brain-stem impairment, and stated that he would never recover awareness nor be weaned from the ventilator.

Given this grim prognosis, his wife convinced the attending physician that, based on his prior statements, the patient would not wish to continue living in this meaningless, hopeless state. Accordingly, she refused further ventilator support on his behalf. However, because he had signed an organ donor card, she hoped that his organs could be procured and transplanted. The attending physician explained that his organs could not be procured because he was not brain dead. Is there any way to accommodate his wife's request that organ donation proceed?

REPLY: This young man is in a persistent vegetative state which, in this case, has a very high likelihood of being permanent, and he is ventilator dependent. Based on his previously stated wishes, his surrogate has asked that measures to postpone his death be stopped. She also asked that his wishes for organ donation be honored, but his caregivers are unwilling to pursue this because he was not yet dead.

When a patient has a very poor prognosis for survival or improvement, it is appropriate for his professional caregivers and his family to consider limitation of treatment. Decisions for or against the use of specific treatment modalities should be based, when possible, on the patient's expressed wishes or known values. When it is expected that a patient will die, it is also appropriate to honor his wishes about the disposition of his body, including such things as organ donation, rituals, and burial.

In this case, the patient's wife clearly understood his values and was convinced that he would not want to survive in his current condition with his current prognosis. It is therefore ethically permissible to withhold or withdraw any treatment that is intended to postpone his death. Her request for organ retrieval is more problematic, however.

Our society has established a consensus that the "dead donor rule" must be followed in multiorgan procurement: a person must be dead before vital tissue or organs are retrieved. In addition, the death must not be caused by the retrieval process, nor may death be induced in order to obtain organs. The concept of death by neurologic criteria was developed, in large part, to follow this rule and yet allow organ retrieval when it is certain that the patient's entire brain, including the brain stem, is totally and irreversibly nonfunctioning. Currently most solid organs are retrieved from patients who have been declared dead using these clearly defined neurologic criteria ("brain death").

Because of the inadequate supply of usable organs, there have been new proposals to attempt to expand the donor pool. One proposal is to further expand the conceptual definition of death to include patients born with anencephaly or those in a permanent vegetative state. While this proposal has serious proponents, the idea of calling someone dead who is still breathing causes sufficient cognitive dissonance to make most unwilling to make this major policy shift.

Another proposal is to abandon the dead donor rule and define special categories as eligible for donation. In 1994, the American Medical Association Council of Ethical and Judicial Affairs reversed its 1988 policy and declared that it was ethically permissible to retrieve organs from still breathing and crying infants born with anencephaly. Public and professional criticism forced them to recant and to reinstate their former adherence to the dead donor rule.

A third proposal is to try to retrieve organs from persons who have been declared dead by cardiopulmonary criteria but have not fulfilled the neurologic criteria for death, often called non-heart beating organ donors (NHBODs). While this approach offers fewer conceptual problems—because the person is, in fact, dead—it does offer major logistic problems due to rapid organ deterioration after death.[1,2,3] In some NHBOD protocols, attempts have been made to retrieve organs from patients declared dead using cardiopulmonary criteria by using organ preservation techniques, such as immediate cold perfusion of the body several minutes after declaration of death.[4] Since this almost always required that perfusion be started without family consent, it was criticized as disrespectful treatment of a dead body and has been abandoned. A second attempt at using NHBODs has been to control the death process by discontinuing life support in the operating room and declaring death after only two minutes of pulselessness.[5] This protocol has been called "gerrymandering," "policy creep," and "an ignoble form of cannibalism."[1,2,3] A third proposal, which has so far been used only in laboratory animals, is to leave the body undisturbed at ambient temperature for up to 30 minutes after cardiac death, and then to retrieve organs.[6]

These proposals highlight the urgent need for organs as our current demand far outstrips our supply. The criticisms highlight the importance of maintaining respect for living patients and for the bodies of recently deceased persons. Our current national organ donor law, the Uniform Anatomical Gift Act, permits adults to consent in advance to donate organs upon death. Although organ donation legally does not require family consent, it is common practice for organ donor nurses to request family consent. Usually, the consent is granted. But occasionally, families may deny permission for organ procurement, thus overruling the patient's wishes as expressed by completing an organ donor card.

In this case I would recommend that it is ethically permissible to discontinue the ventilator in accordance with the patient's prior directives. His wife should be informed that since he has some residual brainstem function, he might survive for minutes, hours, days, or longer. His wife should be educated about the ethical, legal, and logistical constraints on organ retrieval. She should meet with a representative from the local organ procurement organization to discuss possible tissue donation options. In the absence of a hospital program and policy for NHBOD, however, it will be extremely unlikely that any of his organs can be procured.

OUTCOME: The patient died 30 minutes following disconnect from the ventilator. Because the medical center had no existing non-heart-beating organ donor protocol, none of his organs could be procured for transplantation. The patient's corneas were procured.

NOTES

1. Arnold RM, Youngner SJ. The dead donor rule: should we stretch it, bend it, or abandon it? *Kennedy Inst Ethics J* 1993;3:263–78.

2. Caplan AL. The telltale heart: public policy and the utilization of non-heart-beating donors. *Kennedy Inst Ethics J* 1993;3:251–62.

3. Fox RC. "An ignoble form of cannibalism": reflections on the Pittsburgh protocol for procuring organs from non-heart-beating cadavers. *Kennedy Inst Ethics J* 1993;3:231–9.

4. DeVita MA, Snyder JV, Grenvik A. History of organ donation by patients with cardiac death. *Kennedy Inst Ethics J* 1993;3(2):113–29.

5. University of Pittsburgh Medical Center Policy and Procedure Manual. In Management of terminally ill patients who may become organ donors after death. *Kennedy Inst Ethics J* 1993;3 (2):A1–15.

6. Orr RD, Gundry SR, Bailey LL. Reanimation: overcoming objections and obstacles to organ retrieval from non-heart-beating cadaver donors. *J Med Ethics* 1997;23(3):7–11.

☰ ☷ ☷ ☰

LAINIE FRIEDMAN ROSS, MD, PHD

Should a PVS Patient Be a Live Organ Donor?

QUESTION: Mr. P. is a 58-year-old man with end-stage renal disease awaiting a kidney transplant. Because the wait for a deceased donor kidney is long, Mr. P. seeks a living donor. He has two healthy children, both of whom are willing to donate one of their kidneys, but for "emotional reasons," he is reluctant to accept their offers. A third child suffered anoxic brain damage in a drowning accident at age 5. She has been in a persistent vegetative state (PVS) for 21 years and lives in an extended care facility. Mr. P. considers this daughter "essentially dead," but his wife has not agreed to terminate her life-sustaining therapy. Both parents jointly serve as their daughter's guardian and now agree that a kidney should be retrieved from this child. Because she is in a PVS, they believe she cannot be harmed by the donation as much as their healthy children. But she cannot provide consent either. The transplant surgeon requests an ethics consultation before proceeding. What should the ethics consultants advise?

REPLY: The case of Mr. P. represents failures in our healthcare system: the failure to procure enough deceased donor organs, so that we permit, even encourage living donors; and the failure to prevent end-stage renal disease (also known as kidney failure) in the first place.

Mr. P. is lucky because he has two competent adult children who are willing to donate. However, Mr. P. is reluctant and not without reason. It may be that there is a genetic component to his kidney failure. If so, his adult children may want to retain their second kidney to delay kidney failure and their own need for a transplant in the future. It may be that Mr. P's grandchild will suffer kidney failure and need a kidney, but one parent will not have a kidney to spare, having donated to Mr. P. It also may be that he fears the small but real chance of serious perioperative morbidity or even mortality.[1]

Mr. P. has a third child who is incompetent and will never develop competency. Mr. P. would prefer that the surgeons procure her kidney because he considers her "essentially dead," and, therefore, believes that she cannot be harmed by the procurement in contrast with his healthy children. His wife agrees.

Living donation is morally permissible if the benefits to the donor and recipient outweigh the medical and psychological risks of donation for the donor. The physical risk of harm does not differ between the three children, although how both the donor and the family will experience the harms does differ. If a rare but catastrophic event occurred (e.g., stroke) to either healthy adult donor, the donor's quality of life would be significantly diminished, and life itself may be shortened. Mr. P. and his wife would experience sadness, anger, and possible guilt that they asked their child to make this sacrifice. In contrast, if the daughter in PVS were to suffer a stroke, her life may be shortened, although her quality of life might be minimally affected. Moreover, her parents might not suffer any distress.

Regardless of who donates, the transplant offers Mr. P. a large medical benefit. The two healthy adult children may experience great emotional benefit from this opportunity, and the donation may improve family relationships strained by ill health and the demands of caregiving. However, the daughter in PVS cannot benefit psychologically. Her inability to experience psychological benefit, but to be at physical risk, makes her donation immoral, because the benefit/risk must be interpreted from the perspective of the donor.[2]

That the parents cannot authorize their daughter to serve as a living kidney donor but can authorize termination of life-sustaining treatment may seem incoherent. The difference is that the decision to withdraw life-sustaining treatment is only morally permissible if it is based on the belief that is in their daughter's best interest.[3] It is immoral to withdraw to ease the parents' burdens alone. The authorization to procure a kidney from this daughter is not in her best interest, because she cannot experience psychological benefit. Therefore, it is immoral to use her kidney as a living donor graft, now or in the future, merely to benefit a third party, even if the third party is her guardian.

The case would be more challenging if Mr. P.'s wife and two healthy adult children were willing but medically unable to donate because of their own health problems, and the family had turned to the third child as a "donor of last resort." And yet, even in that case, I would argue that it is ethically impermissible to authorize the procurement of her kidney, because it uses her solely as a means. The donation violates her human dignity, because it fails to respect her right to bodily integrity and her right to be valued as an end in herself, even if she cannot demand that these rights be respected.

The ethics consultant should advise Mr. P. that his daughter in PVS cannot morally serve as a living donor. Either of his two competent adult children can morally serve as his living donor, although each would need to undergo a full medical and psychological work-up to ensure that there is no medical contraindication and that the decision is voluntary and informed. Alternatively, Mr. P. can continue on dialysis and wait for a deceased donor organ.

OUTCOME: The ethics committee advised that there was a duty to protect the vulnerable and noted that failure to do so facilitated many of the great crimes of history. Even if done with legal sanction, it said retrieval of the kidney would remain an unjustified assault on a defenseless person who could not benefit from the intervention. The ethics committee's advice was accepted and the daughter's kidney was not retrieved.

NOTES

1. Najarian JS, Chavers BM, McHugh LE, Matas AJ. 20 years or more of follow-up of living kidney donors. *Lancet* 1992;340: 807–810.

2. Glannon W, Ross LF. Motivation, risk, and benefit in living organ donation: a reply to Aaron Spital. *Cambridge Q Healthcare Ethics* 2005;14:191–194.

3. Veatch RM. Limits of guardian treatment refusal: a reasonableness standard. *Am J Law Med* 1984;9:427–468.

PART FIVE

Ethics and the Law

DAVID STEINBERG, MD

Introduction: Ethics and the Law

Although moral persuasion and an uneasy conscience can motivate proper behavior, those influences are often dwarfed by the power of the law which can inflict punishment. The law may express itself in many forms including specific state and federal laws, case law including that established in medical liability suits, judicial interpretation of constitutional rights and responsibilities, the regulations of governmental agencies, and the recommendations of governmental commissions.

The guiding principles of the law and of bioethics are different. The law must protect established rights such as the right of privacy, the right to due process, freedom of religion, and the right of "equal protection." Precedent is important in law. Bioethics is guided by a variety of theories and principles; although ethical justifications often make reference to philosophies that are centuries old they are not necessarily bound by those theories. The guiding principles of both law and bioethics require analysis and interpretation when applied to specific cases.

Annas notes the rubric of the law is patient rights and that is "why American law, not philosophy or medicine, is primarily responsible for the agenda, development and current state of American bioethics."[1] Jonsen disagrees and accords the major influence on bioethics to philosophy and theology.[2] Regardless of which discipline is the dominant influence, both the law and bioethics have been concerned with the protection of patient rights. These rights may pertain to patient autonomy, confidentiality, the doctor-patient relationship, relationships with health insurers, justice in health care, and informed consent in clinical practice and medical research.

Law has a strong influence on bioethics; bioethicists often quote important case law such as the Quinlan case,[*3] the Cruzan case[† 4] and the case of *Quill v.Vacco*.[‡ 5] The law, in turn, has been influenced by the deliberations of bioethics. Debates on major issues typically involve a mix of law and bioethics.[§] Wolf

* In Re Quinlan the court established the right of a patient to refuse medical care, in this case the removal of a mechanical ventilator.

† In *Cruzan v. Director, Missouri Department of Health* the United States Supreme Court established the right to refuse artificial nutrition and hydration; it also permitted the state of Missouri to require clear and convincing evidence of the patient's wish to have nutrition and hydration withdrawn.

‡ In *Quill v. Vacco* the Supreme Court declared the Equal Protection Clause of the Fourteenth Amendment does not guarantee a right to assisted suicide.

§ I have selected their dominant characteristics for purposes of this discussion and should acknowledge that neither law nor bioethics is a homogeneous entity; laws differ in different states and state and federal law may conflict. Bioethics also embraces many points of view.

finds the relationship between law and bioethics sufficiently intimate to describe the two as "married"; but she also believes there are areas in which bioethics and law can learn from each other. Wolf implies the law is not always morally correct and cites as one example Minnesota's "Crack Baby" law, which violates the tenets of medical ethics by compelling physicians to breach patient confidentiality and identify pregnant women using illegal drugs who will then be locked up for the duration of their pregnancy. In turn she notes bioethics could learn "process values" from the law, for example as applied to the procedures of ethics committees.[6]

The law can establish rules to promote fairness. The National Organ and Transplantation Act (NOTA) created the Organ Procurement and Transplant Network (OPTN) to fairly allocate deceased donor organs for transplantation. Recently "donor rights" laws have been passed to ensure that organs are retrieved from people who have expressed the wish to have them donated. Laws that facilitate surrogate decision making and advance directives help promote the wishes of those who can no longer advocate for themselves.

Novel practices that extend the boundaries of what's permissible often provoke the "slippery slope" argument. If we allow physician-assisted suicide for the terminally ill, soon the practice will be applied for less compelling reasons. The law can set boundaries that make certain practices more acceptable. Physician assisted suicide, a practice that is legal in the state of Oregon, probably would not have been acceptable without legal safeguards.[7][8][9]

The law, in common with ethics, may be slow to respond to novel technologies. Adequate legal protections for women who choose to be egg donors are lacking. In an unusual case a scientist tried to patent a human-chimp chimera, "a monstrous concoction" that was part human and part chimpanzee and would be "stronger and hairier than a human with mental qualities of both person and ape." This was done to alert the public to the lack of regulations to contain the "dangers of unrestricted technology." For-profit companies, with relatively few legal restraints, make considerable profit from tissues donated by altruistic citizens who may be unaware that their donation will benefit commercial ventures.

The voice of bioethics has been heard in the criminal arena. Andrea Yates was vilified and jailed for life as a criminal for drowning her five children. Spinelli argues Yates was mentally ill and her sentence a miscarriage of justice. Brain damage can cause a variety of "cognitive, emotional and behavioral" disabilities; Winslade notes in one study all 29 inmates on death row had a history of traumatic brain injury. Insights from medicine can help the law become fair in its judgments. Biotechnology such as DNA analysis has proven the innocence of convicted criminals. Accusations of criminal childhood abuse have been based on recovered memories, some proven false. The discredited science of eugenics which was adopted by the Nazis reached its peak in the United States when the Supreme Court in *Buck v. Bell*,[10] approved sterilization of epileptics and the feeble-minded and Oliver Wendell Holmes issued his famous statement, "Three generations of imbeciles are enough."

In contrast to philosophers and bioethicists who discuss and analyze problems the law can make an ethical position mandatory and enforceable. Before that happens lawyers must define and describe neglected problems and injustices and suggest appropriate legal remedies. That work best describes the legal scholarship in this section.

NOTES

1. Annas G.J. *Standards of Care: The Law of American Bioethics.* Oxford University Press. New York, 1993.

2. Jonsen A.R. *The Birth of Bioethics.* Oxford University Press. New York, 1998.

3. Menikoff Jerry. *Law and Bioethics.* Georgetown University Press. Washington DC, 2001, page 242.

4. Menikoff page 304. (see ref 3)

5. Menikoff, page 327. (see ref 3)

6. Wolf Susan M. Law and Bioethics: From Values To Violence. *Journal of Law, Medicine and Ethics* 2004; 32: 293–306.

7. Oregon Death With Dignity Act, Oregon Revised Statute 127.800–127.897.

8. Chin Arthur E, Hedberg Katrina, Higginson Grant K, Fleming David W. Legalized Physician-Assisted Suicide in Oregon—The First Year's Experience. *N Eng J Med* 1999; 340: 577–583.

9. Sullivan Amy D, Hedberg Katrina, Fleming David W. Legalized Physician Assisted Suicide in Oregon—The Second Year. *N Eng J Med* 2000; 342:598–604.

10. Menikoff, p 40.

☰ ☲ ☲ ☰

LEONARD H. GLANTZ, JD

Keeping Genetic Secrets

On September 16, 2003 the New York Times ran a story in its science section entitled "When a Doctor Stumbles on a Family Secret." The article was about what to do when it is determined that the apparent father of a child is not the child's biological parent. Should one tell the child? The mother?

The "father"? Indeed, unlike the title of this article, this was not a family "secret"; it could well be that no one knew the truth until the biological testing was done.

In the coming era of widespread genetic testing and counseling, many people will discover information about themselves that might have importance for others. Unlike other medical tests, genetic testing provides possible information about families, as well as about the individual. For example, a woman who finds out that she has the BRCA1 gene and therefore is at higher risk for breast cancer than the general population also has information that might be useful to her sister—particularly her identical twin. The question then becomes, is there some obligation to share that information with the untested, but possibly at risk, sister?

Like other good ethical and legal quandaries there are strong arguments on both sides. The two principles involved are the obligation of physicians to keep private patient information secret, and the desire to aid another person to avoid harm. It is also a question that presents the issue of weighing positive long-term social goals against positive short-term benefits. The reason both law and ethics safeguard patient privacy is because it is felt that in order for patients to disclose their most personal and embarrassing health concerns, patients have to feel secure that what their doctor knows about them will remain secret. Both individuals and the general society benefit from this doctrine, as patients will not be discouraged from getting treatment by the fear of gossip. On the other side of the argument is the desire to make disclosures to protect others from possible harm.

Generally the law does not require one person to act for the benefit of another unless there is some relationship between the people that requires such action. It should be obvious that a doctor is obligated to act to attempt to save the life of a patient who has had a sudden heart attack. But a stranger who sees the person having a heart attack is under no legal obligation to perform CPR even if the stranger is well trained to do so. In the law we would say that the doctor has a duty to the patient as a result of the doctor-patient relationship but strangers have no duty to other strangers. How does this pertain to the genetic testing and counseling scenario? If it is determined, for example, that a woman has the BRCA1 gene, is she or the doctor required to inform her sister? In general the legal answer is "no." Neither the tested sister nor the doctor has a legal duty to protect the health or safety of the untested sister. The doctor has no relationship with the untested sister at all, so how could he have such a duty? The untested sister is a "stranger."

Difficult questions generally embody some twists and turns in deriving an answer and this one is no exception. In 1976 the California Supreme Court decided a case entitled *Tarasoff v. The Regents of the University of California*,[1] in which the parents of a college student who had been murdered sued the murderer's therapists and the school that employed them for the therapists' failure to protect their daughter from harm. The murderer had disclosed his intent to kill the young woman, Tatiana Tarasoff, to the school psychologist in the course of treatment, and the psychologist and his psychiatrist colleagues took a few ineffective steps to begin commitment procedures. They asked the campus police to detain their predicted violent patient, and when the campus police released him, the psychiatrists did nothing further to protect the potential victim. At his first opportunity, the patient killed Tarasoff.

The victim's parents sued the psychiatrists arguing they did not do enough to protect their daughter, which might include warning Tarasoff of their patient's murderous intent. The psychiatrists argued that they had no duty to the victim since she was a stranger to them. The Supreme Court of California ruled that, while as a general rule individuals do not have a duty to control the actions of another to protect strangers, there are times when a "special relationship" exists that does create such a duty to strangers. While the court did not say what made the psychiatrist-patient relationship a "special" one, in general one only has a "special relationship" in circumstances where one is in a position to control another person's actions. In this case we can only guess that the California court decided the therapist-patient relationship is a "special relationship" because of the therapist's authority to commit the patient. Indeed, in the Tarasoff case the therapists began the process of exercising this authority.

This can be compared to a case following Tarasoff in which a teenage girl put her newborn child up for adoption. The adoption agency later learned from the adoptive parents that the child was afflicted with and died from severe combined immunodeficiency disease (SCID), a genetically transmitted X-linked disease. A few years later the biological mother of the deceased child married and bore a child who died from this same disorder. She sued the adoption agency arguing it should have warned her of her risk of transmitting this genetic disease to her future children. The same court that decided the Tarasoff case found that the adoption agency had no duty to disclose this fact to the plaintiff because it had no "special relationship" with her. [2] In other words, the fact that the information might have been very important to the woman was not enough to say that the adoption agency was required to inform her. This is much more analogous to the case of a doctor aware of a genetic risk to a sibling of a patient than the Tarasoff case. Furthermore, unlike the Tarasoff case, the adoption agency did not "cause" the genetic injury, which is the result of biology, not the inactions of a physician. If there is an obligation to disclose genetic information to a family member, it comes from societal norms and the moral obligation of family members to care for each other. A family member who has knowledge of genetic risks to other members can, and should, in ordinary circumstances, inform relevant family members that they may be at risk and may wish to be counseled and tested themselves. But the failure of a family member to take such action does not transform that obligation into the physician's obligation.

What flows from this for physicians and others who conduct genetic testing and counseling is the obligation to inform the tested person of the risks to other family members, and to suggest ways to make this information available to them so that the tested person has the opportunity and ability to make this knowledge available to others. Failure to adequately disclose this information to a patient makes it impossible for tested persons to understand or act on their natural desire to help family members. Indeed, there is one case in which a court explicitly adopts this as a doctor's legal obligation.[3]

The second obligation rests on those physicians and counselors who feel they have a responsibility to make these disclosures about genetic risks to family members if the patient does not do so. They must inform the person to be tested that the results will not remain private. Unlike the Tarasoff situation, which presents a relatively rare circumstance, genetic tests will routinely reveal information that is often important to others.

If there are professionals who feel a need to regularly disclose this information without patient consent, they must inform patients that the ordinary rules of confidentiality and privacy will not apply. This is not only the fair thing to do, it will give a potential patient a chance to go elsewhere.

Secrecy in medicine is an ancient and socially beneficial doctrine. The sensitive secrets of patients that will be learned in the new genomic era will present the opportunity and need to apply venerable rules to novel situations.

NOTES

1. 17 Cal. 3d 425; 551 P.2d 334(1976).
2. *Olson v. Children's Home Society of California*, 252 Cal. Rptr. 11, 13 (Cal. App 2 Dist. 1988).
3. *Pate v. Thelkel*, 661 So.2d 278 (Fla 1995).

☷ ☶ ☵ ☳

JANE GREENLAW, JD

Rights and Responsibilities of Gamete Donors

John and Luanne Buzzanca, a California couple, wanted a child but were infertile. Using the resources that modern medicine and science offer, the Buzzancas decided to have a child using a gestational surrogate. They entered into a signed agreement whereby they provided an embryo created from donor gametes (an egg and a sperm), which was implanted into the uterus of a woman who would carry the pregnancy to term and then allow the Buzzancas to adopt the child. The Buzzancas separated shortly before the child was born and Luanne adopted the child, Jaycee. When Luanne then went to court seeking child support from John, he argued that the court had no jurisdiction since Jaycee was not a "child of the marriage." An appellate court rejected this argument, ruling that the signed agreement warranted a finding that John was Jaycee's father. When the case was returned to the lower court, the judge then ruled that neither John nor Luanne was Jaycee's legal parent. This ruling has been overturned by the California Court of Appeals.[1]

The Buzzanca case illustrates the confusing and disparate results reached when there are gaps between technology, medical practice, and the law, and highlights the need for regulation and legislation in this area.

Who are parents and what are their responsibilities to their offspring? These have traditionally been relatively simple and straightforward questions. Historically, disputes about parentage were almost exclusively questions about paternity and involved children born to unmarried women or to married women who were alleged to have had adulterous affairs. Common law provided that a child born to a married woman was presumed to be the child of her husband, a presumption designed to ensure the "legitimacy" of children and said to be "one of the strongest and most persuasive known to the law."[2] Most states allowed the woman's husband to offer proof to overcome the presumption, but this was difficult to do prior to the availability of modern blood tests. Even then, blood tests were conclusive only in ruling out paternity; the availability of DNA testing has only recently allowed for conclusive proof of parentage.

Early treatment for infertility brought about some statutory modification of the common-law presumption of paternity. The oldest form of assisted reproduction, artificial insemination using donor sperm (AID), is a practice that has been used for over one hundred years to treat male factor infertility. The usual practice was for the anonymous donor's semen to be mixed with the semen of the woman's husband and placed near the woman's cervix at a time when conception was most likely to occur. In virtually all US jurisdictions the practice itself was largely unregulated, although many states passed laws designed to prevent or resolve paternity disputes resulting from AID. Most of these laws were based on the Uniform Parentage Act (UPA), a model statute designed to guide the development of state laws, and provided that when a married woman was artificially inseminated by a licensed physician with the written consent of her husband, the resulting child was the legal child of her husband. Although the UPA additionally recommends that the state law should explicitly divest the semen donor of parental rights and responsibilities, some states did not follow the recommendation. The reason for this is unclear; it may have been thought that the donor's rights were implicitly extinguished or it may have been thought unnecessary because of the anonymity of semen donation.

Recent social changes and developments in the treatment of infertility have rendered the presumption of paternity a quaint legalism, obsolete and incomplete. A report by the New York State Task Force on Life and the Law examines the impact of assisted reproductive technologies (ARTs), analyzes the gaps in existing laws, and makes recommendations for appropriate changes.[3] Although its recommendations are for specific changes in New York law, they can be generalized because they address public policy issues not yet systematically addressed.

A major inadequacy of existing laws in most states is that there are no provisions about children born as a result of assisted reproductive technologies other than artificial insemination. The Task Force's simple recommendation is that the statutes be amended to provide that when a married woman undergoes any assisted reproductive procedure, the resulting child is the child of her husband, provided the procedure was performed by a licensed physician with the husband's consent.

Another change is that gamete donation is no longer limited to sperm. Donor eggs are now commonly used in ARTs, and their use has been enhanced by cryopreservation techniques. Typically, state laws address only paternity and have not been amended to address questions of maternity. For parity, the Task Force recommended that state laws should specifically provide that a woman who gives birth to a child conceived with a donor egg is the child's legal mother.

An additional development is that gamete donation can no longer be anonymous because of the risks of transmitting infectious diseases or genetic defects; regulations and standards of practice require record keeping to permit the linking of gamete donors and recipients. The ability to trace donors (and for donors to trace their offspring) highlights the inadequacy of laws that do not explicitly extinguish donors' parental rights and responsibilities—in the absence of such a provision there is uncertainty and ambiguity. A related social development is that women who do not have husbands are becoming pregnant through artificial reproductive technology. Some are fertile and choose artificial insemination because they prefer to achieve a pregnancy through noncoital means, and others are infertile and will accept the full array of assisted reproductive techniques, including in vitro fertilization (IVF). For these women, the presumption that a child is the legal child of its mother's husband clearly does not apply. In these situations, the ability to trace the gamete donor(s) and the ambiguity of the law with regard to parental rights and responsibilities of gamete donors are likely to be even more problematic. Accordingly, to address both of these issues, the Task Force recommended that state law should explicitly allow gamete donors to relinquish, in writing, their parental rights and responsibilities, effective at the time of donation and irrespective of the marital status of the recipient.

Finally, surrogacy agreements and donated embryos make it possible for women to give birth to children not genetically related to them (or their husbands). It is beyond the scope of this article to discuss the complexities of state laws regarding surrogacy agreements. However, it is worthy of note that the Task Force recommendation is for the law to provide that a woman who gives birth to a child is the child's legal mother, and further, to provide for legal procedures and standards that would apply in a dispute.

The Task Force recommendations were guided primarily by the interests of children who will be created by assisted reproductive technologies. To that end, the stability of families, the desirability of eliminating or reducing ambiguity about parentage, and the importance of having safe means of creating families are all factors that led to the Task Force recommendations. The goal is to protect parents and children from claims of parental rights by gamete donors, and to protect gamete donors from unwanted, unexpected parental responsibility.

As is often the case in medicine, it is likely that technology will outpace the development of the law in this area. Furthermore, it is likely that assisted reproductive technologies will continue to be the focus of much public policy debate.

NOTES

1. *Jaycee v. Superior Court*, 61 Cal. App. 4th 1410 (1998).

2. *State ex rel. H. v. P.*, 90 A.D.2d 434, 437, 457 N.Y.S.2d 488, 490 (1st Dep't 1982) (quoting Matter of Findlay, 253 N.Y. 1, 7 (1930)).

3. New York State Task Force on Life and the Law. *Assisted Reproductive Technologies: Analysis and Recommendations for Public Policy*. New York, NY: April 1998.

⠿ ⦀ ⦀ ⠿

JANE GREENLAW, JD ✳

Pregnant Women and Their Fetuses: Legal and Ethical Issues

Should healthcare providers intervene when a pregnant woman's behavior poses a threat to her fetus? This question is not new to physicians and others who provide prenatal care, but it is arising with increasing frequency. Some pregnant women refuse recommended interventions, such as cesarean sections, and some drink alcohol, smoke cigarettes, or fail to conform to prescribed dietary restrictions. While we accept the rights of competent adults to engage in risky behaviors and to refuse medical treatment, and while we recognize that states will intervene on behalf of born children whose parents are acting against their interests, neither of these two approaches seems to fit perfectly in the cases involving pregnant women.

Among the most troubling cases are those of pregnant women who use illegal drugs. Medical, social, and political institutions are struggling to develop appropriate responses to these problems. This fall, the United States Supreme Court will hear arguments in a South Carolina case involving this complex issue.

In the late 1980s, nurses and doctors providing prenatal and obstetrical care to primarily poor, African American women at the obstetrical clinic at the Medical University of South Carolina noticed a high number of babies born with medical problems due to maternal cocaine abuse. To address the problem, a task force was formed, which included a prosecuting attorney who advised that since a viable fetus is considered a person under South Carolina law, a woman who ingested cocaine after the 24th week of pregnancy was guilty of the crime of distributing a controlled substance to a minor.

In the fall of 1989, a policy that had been developed by the task force was instituted. The policy identified a "profile," or list of indicators, of prenatal cocaine use: separation of the placenta from the uterine wall; intrauterine fetal death; no prenatal care; late prenatal care; incomplete prenatal care; preterm labor without an obvious cause; a history of cocaine use; unexplained birth defects; or intrauterine growth retardation without an obvious cause. When any one of these indicators was present, the policy provided that the woman's urine would be tested for cocaine without her knowledge or consent. Women who tested positive for cocaine were informed in writing that they would be arrested if they did not report for free drug treatment.

Some civil rights groups later brought legal action against the clinic on behalf of the women who were arrested, claiming primarily that the involuntary urine tests violated the Fourth Amendment constitutional prohibition against unreasonable searches. A federal District Court ruled in favor of the clinic; in July 1999 the Fourth Circuit Court of Appeals affirmed the decision, ruling that the circumstances fit within the "special needs" exception, which allows a Fourth Amendment intrusion that "serves special governmental needs."[1] This exception explicitly does not apply to searches that result in criminal prosecutions, however the court was persuaded that the primary goal of the clinic's policy was not to prosecute the women, but to encourage them to get treatment, thereby serving a special governmental need.

It is difficult to predict how the US Supreme Court will rule on this issue. However, if the Court affirms that a pregnant woman's constitutional rights are diminished because of the viable fetus she carries, that decision could have important implications. It is worth noting that in the US, nearly half of the state jurisdictions have had cases attempting to prosecute women whose prenatal behavior caused serious harm or death of their fetuses, and virtually all of these attempts have been rejected by the courts, because the criminal statutes proscribe causing harm to persons, not fetuses.[2]

Whatever the Supreme Court's ruling, it is unlikely to change the professional standard that is reflected in the practice guidelines put forth by the American College of Obstetrics and Gynecology (ACOG) and the American Medical Association (AMA).[3,4] Both of these organizations advocate for recognizing the autonomy of the pregnant woman, using the strength of the clinician-patient relationship to persuade the patient to accept recommended treatment and to comply with prenatal instructions that are designed to maximize the likelihood of a good obstetrical outcome for both "patients." Both the AMA and ACOG positions call attention to the long-term negative effects that could result from coercive treatment of pregnant women: turning the clinician-patient relationship into an adversarial one; pitting the interests of the pregnant woman against those of her fetus; reducing the likelihood that the woman will seek postnatal care for herself and her baby; and diminishing the likelihood that the woman will seek prenatal care if she has future pregnancies. These authorities recognize that there could be drastic circumstances, which would warrant resort to the legal system, but recommend that this should be seen as a last resort.

Interestingly, the only comprehensive report on this subject in the medical literature to date shows that obstetricians rarely attempt to use the law to force treatment in situations involving pregnant women, despite the fact that nearly half of those surveyed believed that there could be cases in which forced compliance would be warranted. The survey included responses from most of the US hospitals with obstetrics teaching programs, and found only 14 cases in which court authorization was sought for obstetrical interventions—11 cesarean sections, two hospital detentions, and one intrauterine transfusion. Authorization was granted in 86 percent of the cases.[5]

Most pregnant patients are highly motivated to achieve compliance with the recommendations of their obstetrical care providers; there is ample anecdotal evidence that women who smoke, drink alcohol, and are inattentive to nutritional needs abstain from these behaviors during pregnancy, even if they are unable to continue their healthier habits after giving birth. Indeed, the characteristic compliance of pregnant women may even cause them to accept interventions they do not need. There is much in the literature to support the view that obstetrical interventions, such as cesarean sections, are overutilized and frequently performed unnecessarily, providing evidence that this is a much more common problem than that of pregnant women refusing recommended treatment or failing to comply with directions.[6]

There is little doubt that the best way to achieve optimal maternal and fetal outcomes is to maximize the availability of good prenatal and obstetrical care for all women.

NOTES

1. *Ferguson v. City of Charleston* [No. 97–2512 (4th Cir. Ct. App.)] 1999.

2. *Reproductive Freedom New*s, Vol. 8, No. 11, p. 7 (December 1999).

3. ACOG Committee on Ethics, Committee Opinion Number 55, "Patient Choice: Maternal-Fetal Conflict" (Washington DC: American College of Obstetrics and Gynecology, October 1987).

4. Cole HM. Legal interventions during pregnancy. Court-ordered medical treatments and legal penalties for potentially harmful behavior by pregnant women. *JAMA* 1990;264:2663–70.

5. Kolder VE, Gallagher J, Parsons MT. Court-ordered obstetrical interventions. *N Engl J Med* 1987;316:1192–6.

6. See, e.g., Young D. A new push to reduce cesareans in the United States. *Birth* 1997;24(1):1–3; Luthi JC, Dolan MS, Ballard DJ. Evidence-based healthcare quality management in obstetrics and gynecology. *Clin Obstet Gynecol* 1998;41(2):348–58; Public Citizen's Health Research Group. *Unnecessary Cesarean Sections: Curing a National Epidemic.* Washington, DC, 1994.

☷ ☶ ☵ ☳

STUART A. NEWMAN, PHD

The Human Chimera Patent Initiative

Listening to congressional debate on H.R. 1644, the Human Cloning Prohibition Act of 2001,[1] many people were surprised to learn that the US has no federal laws prohibiting manipulation of human embryos chemically or genetically, or the bringing to term of any such embryo. This situation, which is out of line with that in Europe, Japan, and a growing number of countries throughout the world, was on my mind in 1997 when, with the help of the social critic Jeremy Rifkin, president of the Foundation on Economic Trends in Washington, D.C., I decided to apply for a patent on embryos and animals containing human along with nonhuman cells—so-called chimeras.

I had no intention of producing such creatures, nor does US patent law require that an actual prototype for an invention be supplied, only that feasibility be demonstrated, as well as novelty and utility. But ever since the

1980 Supreme Court decision in *Diamond v. Chakrabarty*,[2] it has been legal in the US to obtain a patent on living organisms and their descendants. Moreover, Congress has drawn no line that would preclude a preterm human embryo, if appropriately modified, from being patented. Nor has it indicated how many human genes or cells an animal would have to contain before it could not be patented by virtue of the constitutional protections pertaining to members of the human community. While a decision as to patentability by the US Patent and Trademark Office (PTO) would not control whether or not it would be legal to produce human-animal chimeras, or other types of biologically manipulated humans, we considered that applying for a chimera patent would raise these issues before the public and the legal system in a particularly dramatic fashion.

In the legal process that ultimately led to the Chakrabarty decision, an appeals court overruled the PTO's original rejection of the General Electric Corporation's application for a patent on oil-eating bacteria in an opinion that stated, absurdly, that bacteria are "more akin to inanimate chemical compositions . . . [than] to horses and honeybees and raspberries and roses." Within a few years, however, the Chakrabarty decision had served as a precedent for the issuing of patents on mice, pigs, and cows, some containing introduced human genes, as well as on naturally occurring human bone marrow cells.

As a research scientist in the field of embryonic development who has been concerned that the fruits of this work not be used to society's detriment, I acted on Rifkin's suggestion to invent something that was useful but also so disquieting that it would alert the public to the consequences of unrestricted technological development in this area. The proposed human-animal chimera, whose production would depend on techniques developed in the 1980s that led to the actual generation of "geeps"—animals that were part goat and part sheep[3,4]—could contain anything from a minuscule proportion to a majority of human cells. Like the geep, a human-chimp chimera would have recognizable resemblances to both originating species, perhaps stronger and hairier than a human, with mental qualities of both person and ape.

The proposed applications of this invention included the use of partly human embryos to test drugs and chemicals for toxicity, and the use of partly human animals as sources of transplantable organs for human patients. It is clear from such examples that biotechnology is capable of producing items that, while legal and eminently useful, could nonetheless conflict with other cultural values, and would therefore be considered immoral and undesirable by many people.

Scientists can make such things, but would they? If so, would anyone market them and would physicians and the public accept their use? At the time our original filing was announced in early 1998, advocates of the patenting of organisms, including the scientist who patented the first mammal (the "Oncomouse," a research animal that developed cancer at 40 times the normal rate) criticized us for scaremongering. They accused us of presenting monstrous concoctions that no responsible scientist would contemplate producing or patenting. Since then, though, the Massachusetts biotechnology company Advanced Cell Technology has obtained a patent on a technique for creating cloned embryos produced from human cell nuclei and cow eggs. And the Geron Corporation of California, which holds licenses on patents for human embryo stem cells, has acquired the Scottish company that holds the patents on the cloning techniques that produced Dolly the sheep.

Indeed, the driving force behind the Congressional Human Cloning Prohibition Act, mentioned above, was concern about the desire of Geron and a number of university-based researchers, as well as patient advocate groups, to produce cloned human embryos to serve as sources of donor-matched human embryo stem cells. Such embryos would be both laboratory materials and potential children for anyone reckless enough to ignore the disastrous biological results of animal cloning experiments. The latter scenario has advocates in the scientific and medical communities, some of whom were afforded the prestigious forum of the National Academy of Sciences this past August. Because H.R. 1644 intended to block the possibility of full-term cloning by prohibiting the production of cloned embryos, it was supported by commentators across the political spectrum, including some prominent abortion rights advocates, and was passed with a bipartisan majority. (It is due to come before the Senate in early 2002). Among the scientific societies and their allies in Congress, however, this position was a minority one.

These developments suggest that, in the absence of binding restrictions—which would represent a societal agreement not to cross certain troubling lines—the public could quickly accommodate itself to fabricated humans and near humans, organisms that previously existed only in the realm of speculative fiction. With commercial interests continually touting the benefits of such "breakthroughs," the production of quasihumans for research or therapy, using our technique or different ones, cannot be too far behind.

As it attempted with the Chakrabarty patent application, the PTO rejected our chimera patent in its initial reviews. Of course, the major difference between the Chakrabarty case and ours is that the PTO no longer opposes patents on organisms. Instead, it would like to draw a line between obviously troublesome inventions of the sort we propose and other life forms they have allowed to be patented, such as human bone marrow cells and pigs containing human genes. Given the common evolutionary heritage and biological continuity of all organisms on earth—we share more than 98 percent of our DNA sequence with chimpanzees, for example—this may be an impossible task. Ultimately, the patentability of part-human organisms may have to be resolved by the courts or Congress. But concealed within the patent issue is the deeper one of how far we as a society will go in permitting technology to blur the lines between human and non-human, person and artifact.[5,6]

NOTES

1. Congressional Record: July 31, 2001 (House) Pages H4916-H4945. http://energycommerce .house.gov/107/action/107–41.pdf

2. 206 U.S.P.Q. 193.

3. Fehilly C B, Willadsen S M, Tucker E M. Interspecific chimaerism between sheep and goat. *Nature* 1984;307:634–6.

4. Meinecke-Tillmann S, Meinecke B. Experimental chimaeras-removal of reproductive barrier between sheep and goat. *Nature* 1984;307:637–8.

5. Magnani TA. The patentability of human-animal chimeras. *Berkeley Tech Law Journal* 1999;14:443–60.

6. Lee K. *The Natural and the Artefactual.* Lanham, MD: Lexington Books, 1999.

☷ ☶ ☶ ☷

LAWRENCE J. NELSON, PHD, JD

The Wendland Case: On Families and Fantasies

In the fall of 1993, an auto accident left Robert Wendland comatose for well over a year. Hoping for his recovery despite the odds, his wife, Rose, wanted him to receive all available treatment. Some 16 months after the accident, Robert regained consciousness, but was left profoundly and permanently physically and mentally disabled. Despite receiving months of therapy, Robert remained paralyzed on his right side; he was aphasic and could not meaningfully communicate even with assistive devices. His wife and children never saw that he recognized them. He could not perform any activities of daily living; he could not swallow and so needed a surgically implanted tube to get food and water. Nevertheless, he could at times follow some simple commands but only with much coaching and then only inconsistently. He could at one point operate an electric wheelchair on his own, although he could not avoid obstacles in his path or reverse course if he bumped into a wall. Clearly, Robert lacked the mental capacity to make contemporaneous decisions about his life and future.

Almost two years after the accident, Rose, whom the attending physicians had always turned to for consent for Robert's continued treatment, decided to stop the administration of food and fluid to him through the feeding tube. This decision came after Robert had pulled this tube out of his body four times and his physicians had told her he would never get any better. Based on previous conversations with him regarding such matters and his values, she and her children (as well as his brother with whom he was close) were convinced that Robert would not want to live under these circumstances and would refuse to be kept alive by medical treatment.

Her decision was challenged in court by Robert's estranged mother ("estranged" because the court heard uncontradicted sworn testimony that his mother had not set foot in Robert's and Rose's home in the 10 years prior to the accident and that their children did not recognize her as their grandmother). The trial judge ruled that Rose could not legally stop his tube feedings. Ultimately, the California Supreme Court ruled that Rose lacked the legal authority to refuse tube feedings on her husband's behalf that would have allowed him to die.[1] Had Robert used a Durable Power of Attorney for Health Care to give Rose his medical decision-making authority or if had he left formal, written instructions about future treatment or about who should make medical decisions on his behalf, the Court stated (albeit somewhat grudgingly) that his choice should have been respected.

In the absence of a durable power of attorney or another formal document, the Court concluded that the incompetent patient's constitutionally protected right to life and right to privacy require that his surrogate prove by "clear and convincing evidence" that either the patient previously had refused the treatment in question under the exact circumstances he now is in or that stopping treatment is in his best interest. (For reasons very hard to understand given that everyone must have the same constitutional rights, the Court exempted conscious, *terminally ill* incompetent patients and *permanently unconscious* patients from the reach of its ruling.) As Rose had not produced evidence sufficient to meet either of these standards, the Court ruled that she could not refuse tube feeding. Consequently, the Court required that all life-sustaining treatment (including, of course, the tube feeding) must continue despite the sincere conviction of Robert's closest family members that he would not want such treatment or to live under the heavy burdens his injuries imposed on him. The extent of this burden was confirmed by the two independent medical experts hired by Robert's own lawyer: both found that he evinced experience of nothing other than frustration, pain and discomfort, irritability, aggressiveness towards others, and unhappiness.

Close family members will find the Court's standard of proof nearly impossible to meet. The patient must have expressed his or her wishes very precisely in order for the family to be able to utilize them. The family must be able to show that its incompetent relative "would desire to have his life-sustaining medical treatment terminated *under the circumstances in which he now finds himself*" (emphasis added). As none of us has a crystal ball, it is purely a fantasy to think that the typical person will be able to predict the future and express his wishes so precisely.

One lesson from *Wendland* is very familiar: every adult ought to formally designate a person who will have clear authority to act as her surrogate to make medical decisions on her behalf when she cannot do so herself. But despite excellent reasons to create a durable power of attorney or another legally recognized form of advance directive, the overwhelming majority of Americans have not done so. Despite serious efforts to educate the public and promote advance directives, only some 10 to15 percent of Americans have one—and many of these cannot be found at the crucial time or are found to be legally invalid. Why this is true is nowhere as important than it simply is true—and will almost surely continue to be so into the future.

Most Americans count on their close family members being able to make medical decisions for them if they cannot do so themselves, but Wendland ignores this reasonable and common expectation. Close family members should presumptively be the ones who decide when it is right to forgo treatment of their incompetent relative. They treat the patient as an individual person because they know her the best, care for her, and have her best interests at heart. The Latin root of "surrogate," *sur-rogare,* can be translated as "to ask near." When we cannot ask the patient herself, we ask someone as close to her as possible.

Although many disability rights advocates urged the Court to be highly suspicious of families who choose to let their loved ones die, close family should not be stripped of medical decision-making authority for their incompetent relatives. To be sure, family members will sometimes act selfishly, precipitously, or otherwise make ethically objectionable decisions for their relatives, but this is likely to be quite rare. In such situations, we should be able to count on the physicians, nurses, and healthcare institutions who are committed to patient well-being to serve as a check on rogue relations who make medical decisions clearly contrary to the patient's wishes or best interests. In the last analysis, no stranger—be she judge, physician, disability activist, or lawyer—is at all likely to be better situated as a surrogate decision maker, choosing in consultation with a conscientious physician, than a close family member who has a demonstrated personal connection to the patient. Physicians have been doing exactly this for centuries and have created one ethical tradition that should not change.

NOTES

1. Conservatorship of Wendland, 26 Cal 4th 519, 28 P 3rd 151 (2002).

꜒ ꜒꜒ ꜒꜒ ꜒

ANNE L. FLAMM, JD

The Texas "Futility" Procedure: No Such Thing as a Fairy-tale Ending

For years, physicians and other clinicians, ethicists, hospital attorneys, and administrators have struggled with a problem characterized as "medical futility."[1] The term typically refers to end-of-life situations in which patients or their representatives demand aggressive medical interventions that caregivers object to providing because they believe that the interventions will not benefit and may even harm patients. In such circumstances, clinicians' professional judgment and fidelity to their traditional role as healers, as well as their duties to allocate healthcare resources responsibly, weigh against providing interventions they view as medically inappropriate. The controversy derives when patients or their representatives perceive clinicians' judgments to conflict with their autonomous right to identify and pursue their healthcare goals. They may also criticize clinicians' judgments for prejudice or inaccuracy in the prognostication of medical outcome. In the absence of direction from courts or legislatures identifying the consequences of withholding or withdrawing life-sustaining treatments sought by patients, many institutions developed policies for dealing with clinical futility disputes.[2,3]

September 1, 1999, marked the effective date of legislation in the state of Texas that bears directly upon clinical management of patient-driven requests for medically inappropriate or futile treatment. Under the Texas Advance Directives Act (the "Act"),[4] failing to honor a patient's "healthcare or treatment decision"[5] (whether that decision is communicated via a living will, by the patient's representative, or by the patient) exposes the health professional to disciplinary action by the appropriate licensing board and any other action available under state law.[6] However, the Act grants immunity from disciplinary action and criminal or civil liability to health professionals who follow a statutorily prescribed procedure for "failing to effectuate" the patient's decision.

Section 166.046 of the Act directs that an attending physician's refusal to honor a patient's treatment decision "shall be reviewed by an ethics or medical committee."[7] The patient shall be given life-sustaining treatment during the review. Other than prohibiting the attending physician from being a member of the review committee, the statute offers no additional detail about either the composition of that committee or the steps of its decision-making process.

Section 166.046 also lists the patient's or representative's rights during the review process. The patient or representative must be given 48 hours' notice of the meeting called to discuss the controversy, "unless the time period is waived by mutual agreement," and is entitled to attend the meeting. Per revisions completed in June 2003, notice to the patient or representative must include a written description of the review process.[8] The recent revisions also created a registry, maintained by the state healthcare information council, "listing the identity of and contact information for healthcare providers and referral groups ... that have voluntarily notified the council they may consider accepting or may assist in locating a provider willing to accept transfer of a patient"[9] under these circumstances. This registry must be provided to the patient or representative upon notice of the meeting. Finally, Section 166.046 states that the patient or representative is entitled to receive a written explanation of the decision reached during the review process.

If the review committee affirms the attending physician's judgment that the requested treatment is inappropriate, life-sustaining treatment must be provided for 10 days following the notification to the patient of the committee's decision in writing. During the 10 days, the patient may transfer to a physician who is willing to provide the controversial treatment. The patient's physician and personnel at the current facility shall make reasonable efforts to assist in arranging the patient's transfer, if transfer is possible. After the 10th day, the physician and facility "are not obligated to provide life-sustaining treatment" unless ordered to do so by a court. The statute instructs that a court may extend the 10-day period "only if the court finds, by a preponderance of the evidence, that there is a reasonable expectation that a physician or healthcare facility that will honor the patient's directive will be found if the time extension is granted."

REFLECTIONS ON THE TEXAS PROCEDURE

The reassurance against civil, criminal, or disciplinary liability given to providers who follow Section 166.046 before withholding or withdrawing life-sustaining treatment is powerful, particularly when the previous ambiguity of legal consequences often prevented clinicians from fulfilling ethical obligations against providing medically inappropriate care. The promise of immunity, of course, is not guaranteed; plaintiffs can challenge a provider's adherence to Section 166.046 or more generally dispute the reasonableness of actions taken. Texas courts have yet to contribute case law addressing Section 166.046 leaving institutions to forge their own policies from its relatively sparse procedural guidance.[10] However, the existence of the legislatively defined process shifts the "futility" controversy out of the state of impasse that existed previously.

The process offers other advantages. Requiring review of a physician's decision inherently affirms that the physician's authority is not absolute and that decisions should be without unfair bias. Mandatory notice and the opening of the review to patients and their representatives suggest the need for reviewers to consider patient values and preferences along with medical factors. The requirement of openness to patients and families also conveys to healthcare professionals the need to make decisions transparently and to communicate effectively. Finally, the 10-day grace period promotes patient choice—or at least its value—since the practical options for dying patients are likely limited. So long as one accepts that futility controversies require balancing competing interests and some compromise of values, the Act offers a pragmatic and cautious approach to resolving futility problems in the clinical setting.

So far, only one Texas medical center has published data concerning their experience with the procedural mechanism.[11] Ethics consultants at Baylor University Medical Center reported generally positive experience after two years of practice with the Act, in which six cases proceeded through the statutory mechanism. In their experience, no family member challenged the hospital's process in court, and many family members expressed their endorsement once "the law" indicated life support should be stopped. They also noted that the explicitness of the process encouraged physicians' willingness to confront futility situations, promoting safeguards and accountability as decisions are reached. Fine and Mayo[11] articulately described that the legally sanctioned process advances futility problems by imposing boundaries: conceptual boundaries on parties who may believe they have authority over controversial decisions, and temporal limitations on how long a disagreement may stall action.

While my observations are anecdotal, as a clinical ethicist at M. D. Anderson, I appreciate the process itself. Futility controversies are upsetting, time-consuming and emotionally draining for clinicians and patients alike, and having procedural guidance that enables the controversy to progress is beneficial. From the perspective of institutional participants, I consider as positive the protection of physician integrity, and in cases in which withholding or withdrawal occurs, clinicians' release from feeling that they are causing pain and suffering. While some might criticize the review board's authority, the process promotes professional responsibility when the conclusion permits the death of a dying patient, a burden of decision making I see as more appropriately placed on the physician than on a family member in crisis.

Shadowing the advantages of the statutory review process, however, is the nature of futility controversies. The very presence of the controversy means that crucial relationships are jeopardized, good intentions are challenged, and sacred values are threatened. All involved in a futility controversy make substantial investments—of time, energy, as well as physical resources—from which the dividend is either the patient's continuation with burdensome illness and treatment, or death. Even within M. D. Anderson's limited experience,[12] the emotional reactions of participants, whether staff, patients, or family members, to the review board's final decisions have varied; within one family or medical team, gratitude, relief, resignation, and anger often co-existed. As one might predict from the outset of a true, end-of-life dilemma, resolution cannot produce a happy ending.

NOTES

1. I adopt the term *futility,* despite its flaws, in this article for the sake of brevity.

2. Halevy A, Brody BA. A multi-institution collaborative policy on medical futility. *JAMA* 1996;281:937–41.

3. Schneiderman LJ, Capron AM. How can hospital futility policies contribute to establishing standards of practice? *Camb Q Healthc Ethics* 2000;9(4):524–31.

4. Texas Health and Safety Code, Subtitle H. Title 2, Chapter 166.

5. Section 166.002(7). 2003 revisions clarify the Chapter applies to decisions on behalf of minors.

6. Section 166.045.

7. Unless otherwise stated, statutory quotes are from Section 166.046 of the Act.

8. Section 166.052. The statute suggests a form for the explanatory information.

9. Section 166.053. The registry, updated online as of February 2, 2004, contained one physician's contact information.

10. One case from the Texas Medical Center reached a hearing stage by a judge, but the case resolved clinically before the court issued any ruling. See Myrphy B. Comatose man dies after battle over life support; Family cited spiritual beliefs. *Houston Chronicle* 23 March 2001.

11. Fine RL, Mayo TM. Resolution of futility by due process: early experience with the Texas Advance Directives Act. *Ann Intern Med* 2003; 138:743–6.

▤ ▥ ▥ ▤

NICOLAS TERRY, LLM

Legal Pitfalls of Cybermedicine

Cybermedicine is an umbrella term describing the transition of key medical services to the Web. A much broader concept than telemedicine, cybermedicine includes marketing, relationship creation, advice, prescribing and selling drugs and devices, and, as with all things in cyberspace, levels of interactivity as yet unknown. The potential benefits of cybermedicine are obvious: creation of a highly efficient national market for health services, instantaneous access to medical services without travel or lines in waiting rooms, and seamless integration of support services such as gatekeeping, patient records, inpatient scheduling, and prescription fulfillment. Less obvious are some of the serious legal issues that arise. As providers shift into cyberspace, the health law system faces challenges to its traditional approaches to regulation, quality assurance, and confidentiality.

Cybermedicine is already a billion dollar industry, even though very few of its products have reached the marketplace. Least visible are companies such as Healtheon that are pioneering heavily integrated "backend" systems for the health industry. Such systems electronically process claims, patient data, and prescription information, exchanging such data among managed care organizations, hospitals, physicians, pharmaceutical companies, and other suppliers. More visible are so-called vertical portals, Web sites structured to appeal to narrow, particular subsets of Web users. Vertical portals aimed at physicians feature clinical information and specialty interaction, while selling advertising, books, and continuing medical education services. Vertical portals aimed at patients marry consumer-oriented health information to online consultations, prescription drug fulfillment, and related services and products. Examples include ADAM, Mayo Clinic's Oasis, and DrKoop. Some portal sites, such as Healtheon's WebMD and the AMA-led consortium's site, feature both patient and physician areas.

For health lawyers, the most immediate concerns are licensure related. Healthcare professionals are regulated by state-based licensing systems. Yet cyberspace is oblivious to such "real world" jurisdictional demarcations or limitations. Current generation cybermedicine sites deliver "advice" in one of three ways: generalized textual content or "frequently asked questions" (FAQs), open forums for discussions, and personalized interactive sessions (by chat or e-mail) with site "experts."

In most states, the question will arise as to which, if any, of these activities involve the practice of medicine and so implicate licensure and, ultimately, unlicensed practice. The answer may be relatively simple in the case of a one-to-one interaction between physician and patient that leads to prescribing a drug. However, more generalized interactions are far harder to characterize. A related issue has arisen regarding the practice of pharmacy across state lines and, specifically, Web-based pharmacies. For example, Illinois and Kansas specifically regulate electronic transactions and are attempting to prosecute out-of-state pharmacies and associated medical professionals. This kind of activity also implicates federal regulation and enforcement by the FDA and DEA. The FDA is working with various state agencies and regulatory bodies to develop more national policies and solutions

For the average physician, the first indication of problems with Web-based information was when a patient arrived for an appointment carrying a pile of printouts and demanding specific treatments or drugs. Now, concern is growing over the quality of advice that is published on the Web.[1] Under federal law, Internet service providers and those who Web-publish content provided by others generally are immune from liability.[2] As a result, cybermedicine sites that merely aggregate or link to the content of others are unlikely to be liable for negligent medical advice. However, cybermedicine sites that create their own content will have liability exposure. No doubt these sites will rely on various tort and constitutional law decisions that traditionally have protected authors and publishers. However, those decisions may not apply in cases where direct relationships between health professionals and patients have been established or where a site delivers highly targeted or personalized content. Overall, cybermedicine sites will confront extremely complex risk management issues. For example, malpractice insurance typically is written on a state-by-state basis suggesting considerable difficulties for physicians practicing in cyberspace.

Health lawyers may also be forced to change their concept of the medical malpractice defendant. In the real world, health law frequently differentiates physicians, institutions, and manufacturers, often applying discrete legal rules to them. However, cyberspace frequently obscures the nature of the underlying business. For example, is the patient's advice coming from a doctor or a drug company? Furthermore the transition to cyberspace may radically change the traditional (and traditionally regulated) health business models. Business models that were once disaggregated (for example, doctor and pharmacy) may be re-formed as integrated on-line cybermedicine suppliers. Equally, services (for example, sale and delivery of a prescription drug) that traditionally have been integrated may be disaggregated.

Already cyberspace activities of healthcare providers and pharmaceutical companies are impacting the liability rules that apply to their real-world activities. Malpractice law typically has viewed physicians as independent contractors for whom health institutions such as hospitals or managed care organizations (MCOs) are not vicariously liable. As a result, it is the doctor not the healthcare institution who is the primary defendant when substandard medical care is practiced on the hospital's patient. However, fiercely competitive MCOs now are filling the Web with increasingly holistic images of their services. Thus, the tightly integrated provider models that are appearing in cyberspace likely will lead to more instances of institutional liability for malpractice.[3]

Second, pharmaceutical companies that traditionally distanced themselves from direct contact with patients now actively promote their products directly to end users using the Web providing increasingly rich data about their products.[4] The application of strict products liability law to prescription drugs has been subject to the so-called learned intermediary doctrine. This rule provides that the manufacturer is under a duty to warn only the physician intermediary, not the patient. It has essentially immunized the pharmaceutical manufacturer in most failure-to-warn cases. The shift to direct-to-consumer marketing and the provision to patients via the Web of vast quantities of information previously only available to physicians appears to be influencing the liability construct. For example, in the recent case of *Perez v. Wyeth Laboratories Inc.*[5] the New Jersey Supreme Court severely restricted the reach of the learned intermediary rule in a case brought against the manufacturer of Norplant.

Fully integrated electronic systems bring great efficiencies, but pose a threat to patient privacy. While communications between doctor and patient must be secure and encrypted, legal implications go far beyond data integrity. The parties to these electronic exchanges must be assured of the identity of the other parties—a concept at odds with the vaunted anonymity of cyberspace communications. The patient must be assured that his advisor is actually a licensed physician, while the physician must be sure that his morphine-seeking patient is a terminal cancer patient and not a recreational user. The first ameliorative step in this context has been the Intel-AMA initiative to provide for digital credentialing that will allow physicians and patients to establish who is at each end of Net connection prior to exchange of confidential health information.

It must be appreciated that cybermedicine technology itself is in its infancy. As E-services and related hardware mature, patients are likely to have home-based cybermedical appliances, networked devices that facilitate remote services such as diagnosis and treatment. The entry into the cybermedicine market of responsible, well-established entities hopefully signals an end to an unregulated period of illegal prescriptions and suspect advice. However, just as health professions must retool to handle the challenges of cybermedicine, so must the legal rules that were designed for the pre-industrialized healthcare industry be re-fashioned for the information age.

NOTES

1. Biermann JS, et al. Evaluation of cancer information on the Internet. *Cancer* 1999;86 (3):381–90.

2. (47 USC § 230(C)(1))

3. See, e.g., *Kashishian v. Port*, 481 N.W.2d 277 (Wis. 1992).

4. FDA/CDER, *Guidance for industry: Consumer-directed broadcast advertisements* www.fda.gov/cder/guidance/1804fnl.htm August 1999.

5. (734 A.2d 1245 (N.J. 1999))

FURTHER READING

Terry NP. Cyber-malpractice: legal exposure for cybermedicine. *Am J Law Med* 1999;25(2–3): 327–66.

☷ ☶ ☵ ☳

FRANCES H. MILLER, JD

Contracting for Healthcare Quality

The Institute of Medicine's high-profile release of *To Err Is Human*,[1] a study of deficiencies in the quality of US health care, focused the nation's attention on the problem of medical error. Its riveting page one statement that "... health care is the eighth-leading cause of death in the US," was enough to generate headlines for weeks. Less visibility was accorded to the book's underlying message: that most iatrogenic injury (injury resulting from treatment) is less spectacular than patient death, but all of it is best analyzed in terms of systems failures, rather than as isolated instances of provider negligence.

John Wennberg's work on practice variations established that similar medical diagnoses give rise to an astonishingly wide range of treatment options throughout the US. By inference, at least some of this treatment is either ineffective or inappropriate, and some actually harms patients.[2,3] President Clinton urged states to require reporting and analysis of all hospital errors resulting in patient death as a first step toward designing and implementing systems improvements to ameliorate the problem of preventable iatrogenic injury.[4]

Healthcare quality is a notoriously slippery and value-laden concept, both in the context of medical error and beyond. Reasonable minds can differ not only about what constitutes quality in the first place, but also about how best to improve the existing quality of health service delivery. Evidence-based medicine has given us powerful tools for accomplishing that task, however, and crude outcome data are now routinely collected for such purposes as National Committee for Quality Assurance accreditation of health insurers,[5] licensing of healthcare facilities,[6] and, in some states, provider report cards for consumers.[7]

Employers, as purchasers of healthcare services, have a critical stake in ensuring that the medical care they contract for is of reasonable quality. Employee/patients obviously care deeply about the quality of the health services they consume too, but their bargaining leverage to insist on value from providers is relatively limited. Moreover, information inequalities cloud their ability to second-guess their providers' treatment decisions. Employers, on the other hand, can have impressive indirect leverage over quality through the insurers with whom they contract for employee health insurance. Moreover, they have more resources to devote to the task of becoming sophisticated buyers of healthcare quality and are gradually beginning to use them.[8]

Relationships among employers, employee/patients, insurers, and providers are structured primarily through a series of interrelated contracts in the US, as a byproduct of our competitive healthcare delivery system. The pivotal agreement, to which all the others relate, is the master contract between employer and insurer setting forth the basic terms of health insurance price and coverage. The insurer's contracts with subscribers and providers alike piggyback on that master contract. (The government functions somewhat similarly to employers when contracting with providers to furnish services for Medicare and Medicaid enrollees, except that Medicare and Medicaid quality issues are addressed primarily by statute and regulation,[9] rather than by agreement among the parties.) In the past, pricing considerations often overshadowed quality concerns in private contracting, but the larger purchasers are increasingly incorporating quality issues into their pricing decisions.

Employers banding together and bargaining for coverage for a critical mass of employee/subscribers within the same geographic area can wield considerable clout to insist on incorporating quality parameters into the master contracts they execute with insurers.[10] Insurers must in turn specify those same quality requirements in their subsidiary agreement with those providers they authorize to render services to plan subscribers. Otherwise, they risk defaulting on the bargain they made with purchasers in the master contracts. Of course in markets with little choice of managed care insurers and/or providers, employers will have less leverage to insist that the plans meet quality parameters, because insurers will have less leverage over the providers with whom they must contract.

The Pacific Business Group for Health (PBGH), now composed of 38 large employers in the San Francisco Bay area, has been the most visible and successful employer purchasing coalition in the country over the past decade.[11] Its members insure almost three million employees throughout the state, and spend more than $3 billion on health care each year. Its basic methodology of benchmarking performance standards (closely attuned to HEDIS [Health Plan Employer Data and Information Set] measures), and then building in financial incentives to meet quality guarantees, has been emulated by many other group purchasing entities all over the country. The Massachusetts Health Care Purchasers Group, for example, relies heavily on the PBGH purchasing blueprint and puts significant sums of insurer premiums at risk for meeting defined performance standards. Its experience is beginning to demonstrate what all of us instinctively know: that money can be a powerful motivator for improving quality.

The performance standards incorporated into master contracts by powerful purchasers thus far deal almost exclusively with patient satisfaction and basic healthcare quality measures, such as meeting target rates for C-sections, mammography, diabetic retinal exams, Pap smears, childhood immunizations, and prenatal care. PBGH's 1996 incentive structure put two percent of roughly $420 million in premiums from 13 participating HMOs at risk for meeting these targets. Although the California plans did quite well overall in meeting most benchmarks, in toto they had to refund nearly $2 million for failing to meet specified standards. The Massachusetts Group Insurance Commission uses a variation of the PBGH method by requiring rebates from those insurers failing to deliver on bench-marked "quality breakthroughs" from provider groups with whom they have subsidiary contracts. Other large purchasers, such as General Motors and the Xerox Corporation, rely on financial rewards for meeting specified targets, rather than on penalties for failing to achieve them.

The successes of these and other purchasers and purchasing coalitions throughout the country demonstrate that healthcare quality can indeed be improved through the contracting process.[12] The process is still fairly rudimentary and limited to fairly crude measures. As evidence-based medicine tells us more about the constituents of good quality care, however, and as better information technology enables us to collect and analyze data on health services in a more sophisticated fashion, purchaser contracting for quality offers a systems-based approach for improving basic health services. To err may indeed be human, as the Institute of Medicine report found, but employers can help to cut down on its incidence through creative use of the health insurance contracting process.

NOTES

1. Kohn LT, Corrigan JM, Donalson MS, eds. *To Err is Human: Building a Safer Health System* Washington, DC: National Academy Press, 2000.

2. Wennberg JE. Understanding geographic variations in health care delivery. *N Engl J Med* 1999;340:52–3.

3. Wennberg JE, Freeman JL, Culp WJ. Are hospital services rationed in New Haven or over-utilized in Boston? *Lancet* 1987;1(8543):1185–9.

4. Clinton to Order Steps to Reduce Medical Mistakes. *NY Times* Feb. 22, 2000;1.

5. National Committee for Quality Assurance. *Healthcare providers.* www.ncqa.org.

6. New York State Department of Health. *Info for Consumers: Heart Disease.* www.health.state.ny.us/nysdoh/consumer/heart/homehear.htm.

7. See, e.g., Marshall MN, et al. The public release of performance data: what do we expect to gain? A review of the evidence. *JAMA* 2000;283(14):1866–74.

8. Commonwealth of Massachusetts Board of Registration in Medicine. Physician profile system. www.docboard.org/ma/df/masearch.htm.

9. 42 USC 1320c to 1320c Cornell Legal Information Institute. www4.law.cornell.edu/uscode/42/ch7.html.

10. Fraser I, et al. The pursuit of quality by business coalitions: a national survey. *Health Aff (Millwood)* 1999;18(6):158–65.

11. Schauffler HH, Brown C, Milstein A. Raising the bar: the use of performance guarantees by the Pacific Business Group on Health. *Health Aff (Millwood)* 1999;18(2):134–42.

12. Bodenheimer T, Sullivan K. How large employers are shaping the health care market-place. First of two parts. *N Engl J Med* 1998;338(14):1003–7.

☷ ☶ ☵ ☴

ROBERT A. KATZ, JD

Who Should Capture the Value of Donated Tissue?

When implanted into another person, human organs and tissues can significantly enhance or even save a recipient's life. Yet unlike solid organs, most tissues undergo substantial change in their journey from donor to recipient. In recent years, scientists have increased their ability to manipulate or "process" tissues to increase their therapeutic value. Bones can now be demineralized and made into a putty or gel; when packed or injected into bone voids, this material can stimulate the formation of new bone.[1] Skin can be decelluralized while preserving its biological framework; then it can be absorbed by the body without rejection and promote the regeneration of new skin.[2] These and other technologies have been pioneered by several for-profit, publicly-traded corporations that sell tissue products and related services. In 2004, the four leading for-profit tissue processors had combined revenues of over $300 million.[3]

Tissue processors obtain raw tissue from nonprofit tissue procurement organizations or "tissue banks." Some tissue banks are also organ procurement organizations (OPOs), while others recover only tissues. As with organs, tissues are voluntarily supplied by altruistic donors and next-of-kin. Most tissue banks do not inform potential donors that for-profit firms may process donated tissue. The concern is that such information may discourage donations, as in "I'm not donating my loved one's tissues in order to make money for some corporation's investors." It is also feared that such disclosures might spur donors to restrict for-profit entities from processing their donations. Accordingly, many leaders in the tissue industry oppose a federal proposal to require tissue-procuring OPOs to tell potential donors whether for-profit firms will be involved.[4]

Public relations aside, is anything wrong with involving for-profit firms in tissue processing? In theory, no, as federal law bans the commodification of donated tissue as such. The National Organ Transplant Act of 1984 (NOTA) prohibits the purchase or sale of body parts for use in transplantation.[5] At the same time, NOTA recognizes that participants in the transplantation process must be compensated for their expenses and efforts. To this end, NOTA permits "reasonable payments" for goods and services rendered in connection with transplantation.[6] Under NOTA, industry participants wouldn't actually sell donated tissue; they would simply ask a fair price for the value they add to the tissue.

In practice, however, NOTA does not and likely cannot achieve its aims. Although federal law bans the transfer of tissue for "valuable consideration," it does not render such tissue valueless.[7] The economic value of donated tissue originates in the willingness and ability of would-be recipients to pay for it. Under NOTA, recipients should pay nothing for the tissue itself—only the value added by tissue banks, tissue processors, and other intermediaries. This is precisely what would happen if the tissue industry was perfectly competitive: Intermediaries would earn at most a market rate of return (a.k.a. "normal profits") for the value they add, and recipients would enjoy all the value embodied in the tissue itself.

Among the various intermediaries in the tissue industry, tissue banks follow NOTA's commands most closely: They generally sell tissue for no more than the cost to procure, handle, inspect, and ship it, plus normal profits (5–10%) for overhead, capital improvements, etc.[8] For-profit processors are not as scrupulous. By design, such enterprises aim to maximize their net profits and so price their products accordingly. This profit imperative weakens the link between what processors charge for tissue and the value they add to it. If the market will bear it, processors will seek "super-normal profits," i.e., more profit than necessary to keep them in the processing business. Moreover, some processors earn super-normal profits, either because their name recognition and brand loyalty enable them to charge more or because their lowered production costs enable them to earn more profit with each sale. These processors appropriate some of the tissue's inherent economic value for themselves, instead of passing it along to recipients. They then distribute the value of donated tissue—a charitable resource—for the private benefit of their investors.

If not processors, who should capture the economic value of donated tissue? If the free market prevailed, donors and their next-of-kin would do so, but society is not ready to let this happen. If NOTA were effectively enforced, recipients would obtain this economic value. But how to make that happen? One way might be to appoint regulators to set reasonable rates of return for for-profit processors and restrict prices to keep firms from exceeding these rates.

Another approach requires a modification in NOTA. Under the current regime, tissue banks generally earn no more than normal profits, even if processors are willing to pay more. This arrangement enables—if not invites—processors to appropriate the tissue's economic value and so earn super-normal profits. This appropriation can be stopped, however, by letting tissue banks earn super-normal profits. The change would effectively redistribute the tissue's economic value from processors to tissue banks. Because the market for processed tissue still functions reasonably well, these processors might settle for smaller profits (but not less than normal profits), rather than pass on their increased costs to recipients.

Transferring tissue's economic value to tissue banks could have significant and beneficial consequences. Because tissue banks are organized on a nonprofit basis, they must use any new income to advance their charitable missions and to finance their services, rather than enrich private parties. They would thus have more resources to educate the public about donation and transplantation, provide counseling and bereavement for donor families, improve the quality of their facilities, and subsidize transplants for people who need but cannot otherwise afford them. They could also direct the development and production of tissue-based products based on medical need and social concerns, rather than profit. Granted, donors might prefer recipients to capture the tissue's value. If this option is not feasible, however, donors would likely prefer that it go to nonprofit tissue banks rather than for-profit tissue processors, a result more consistent with the altruism that motivated their decision to donate.

Before making any changes, however, we should consider the advantages of the current arrangement. By letting processors capture the economic value of donated tissue, they have more incentive and resources to develop new therapeutic uses for it. And though the status quo does not stop the commodification of donated tissue, it partly conceals it from public view by interposing a nonprofit entity between altruistic donors and profit-maximizing processors. If tissue banks could earn super-normal profits from their activities, the commodification inherent in the tissue industry would become harder to hide. This might deter people from becoming donors. On the other hand, a conscious policy of concealing commodification from donors may itself raise ethical problems.

NOTES

1. See, for example, the Grafton® line of demineralized bone matrix (DBM) products made by Osteotech, Inc. (http://www.osteotech.com/prodgrafton.htm).

2. See, for example, AlloDerm, an acellular dermal matrix made by LifeCell Corp. (http://www.lifecell.com/products/95/).

3. For 2004, Osteotech and CryoLife, Inc., reported revenues of $89 million and $62 million, respectively. LifeCell reported "product revenue" of $59 million, and Regeneration Technologies, Inc. (RTI) reported "net revenues" of $93 million.

4. This proposed rule, written by the Department of Health and Human Services (HHS), sets forth conditions for tissue-procuring OPOs to participate in Medicare and Medicaid programs. See 70 Federal Register 6086 (February 4, 2005) (discussing section 486.342).

5. 42 USC § 274e (a).

6. Id. § 274e (c) (2).

7. Pinkdyck RS, Rubinfeld DL. *Microeconomics*. 4th ed. Upper Saddle River, NJ: Prentice Hall; 1998:298.

8. Anderson MW, Schapiro R. From donor to recipient: the pathway and business of donated tissues. In: Youngner SJ et al., eds. *Transplanting Human Tissue: Ethics, Policy, and Practice*. Oxford: Oxford University Press; 2003:12–13.

☷ ☶ ☵ ☳

THOMAS GUTHEIL, MD

The Controversy over Recovered Memories

> "I did this," says my Memory.
> "I could not have done this," says my
> Pride and remains inexorable.
> Eventually, Memory yields.
> —NIETZSCHE

Sandra Koski began seeing a therapist because she was getting inappropriately angry at her son. The therapist told Koski her symptoms were commonly seen in people who had experienced childhood sexual abuse and referred her to a women's resource group. While in this group, she recovered memories of brutal sexual abuse by her now 70-year-old father. She took him to court because she believed "there has got to be some accountability." Her father, Martin Koski, denied the charges and blamed them on suggestive group therapy sessions. Mr. Koski's lawyer compared the charges to the Salem witch trials.

The malleability and subjectivity of human memory have been known for a long time, but recent curious developments at the medical-legal interface, such as the Koski case, have added a distinct new wrinkle to the subject. This new wrinkle is yet another illustration of the fact that when pendulums swing, they often swing too far both ways. The pendulum in question is the awareness of childhood sexual abuse. The society at large originally was relatively unaware of the scope of childhood sexual abuse, but as a result of a number of sociocultural trends, awareness of childhood sexual abuse and its psychologically harmful effects has dramatically increased. The pendulum counter swing resulted from unsupported conclusions by mental health professionals that most psychological problems in adults originated from childhood sexual abuse.

By directing attention to the past, all expressive-exploratory therapies may bring back forgotten, neglected or unavailable memories. In individual cases, such as the Koski case, forensic psychiatrists, judges, and juries may be placed in the impossible position of having to determine which memories of sexual abuse are true and which memories are false. In fact, only corroboration by external sources can establish this distinction. Memory alone will not serve. Although there are controversial and conflicting data indicating that distorted or wholly false memories can arise through suggestion in therapeutic settings, there is also evidence that some recovered memories are historically true. In one study, after 17 years had elapsed from a documented episode of child abuse, 38 percent of subjects did not recall the incident.[1] Other studies indicate that from 18 to 59 percent of victims of childhood sexual abuse report periods when they had no memory of the abuse. Scientific scrutiny has failed to define any distinct mechanism to explain temporary memory loss, repression, dissociation, or avoidance, or to distinguish clearly amongst them. The American Psychiatric Association has pointed out that the possibility of false accusations should "not discredit the reports of patients who have indeed been traumatized by actual previous abuse."

Some recovered memories are accurate but there is also documentation of recovered memories that are false. False memories can be spontaneous, or they may be suggested through hypnosis, by hearing someone lie, by a trusted family member, and by therapists. Genuinely experienced memories can have inaccurate details: false memories may be strikingly precise in detail. Memory can also be affected by guilt, rage, post-treatment suggestions and influence, competitiveness, litigation, and expectations.[2] Hypnotic transactions are known to distort memory, often with such conviction that it becomes convincing to third parties and resistant to cross-examination. For these reasons post-hypnotic testimony is excluded from evidence by many courts and is repudiated by the American Medical Association Council on Scientific Affairs.

In 1993, Stephen Cook filed a $10 million lawsuit against the late Cardinal Joseph Bernardin of Chicago claiming that the Cardinal sexually abused him from 1975 to 1977. Bernardin denied the charges. Subsequently, Cook became convinced his memories were unreliable and dropped the lawsuit.

There is certainly reason to doubt the veracity of recovered memories that describe extraterrestrial alien abduction and past lives.

In the clinical setting, a "therapeutic presumption" usually favors a patient over significant others. In law, by contrast, the presumption of innocence favors the defendant unless proven otherwise. Many therapists, in response to the patient's quest for understanding of distress, supply a too ready answer—childhood abuse. This explanation provides a resolution to the patient's effort to understand symptoms; it also seems to absolve the patient of responsibility for his or her own life. Unsophisticated therapists often portray litigation as the root of healing, empowerment, and closure for patients with recovered memories. They suggest that the patient must sue to heal. But the law is a blunt instrument, and litigation can have many destructive effects. These harms include arrest of therapeutic development at the point of suit; prolongation of closure while litigation is pending; entrenchment, at least partially, for legal purposes; and revictimization as a result of the stresses of litigation.

To mitigate injustice in cases of recovered memory, the forensic evaluator should be a separate professional from the treating clinician. Information from third parties is crucial and can include journals, diaries, social service agency records, hospitalization and other treatment records, and police reports. Interviews with siblings and friends may yield useful information. Memory is never fully reliable. The only way to protect the presumption of innocence is to require tangible evidence. The damage to those accused because of recovered memories can be significant. An engineer was sued by his daughter in 1993 on the basis of recovered memory. She claimed her father raped her 3,000 times over a ten-year period. Although he denied the charges the verdict against him amounted to an $800,000 judgment. "These actions have destroyed my career," he wrote. "I stand witness to the fact that a psychoanalytic medical practice, which is not based upon controlled repeatable experiment, and hence whose validity is uncertain, has a profound capacity for evil."

Until 1988, in most states, the statute of limitations for sexual abuse in civil cases was three years after the child reached maturity, usually at age 21. In 1988, Washington state allowed victims to bring suit for up to three years after their memory returned. Now nearly half of the states allow the statute of limitations for sexual abuse victims to begin, not at the time of the incident, but at its first recall.

In addition to lawsuits by patients against family members because of recovered memory of childhood abuse, families have brought many suits involving recovered memory against clinicians. Although therapists may not be treating parents, the therapists' alleged support for the validity of patients' memories, as well as the suggestions about abuse allegedly provided by therapists, have provided the basis for lawsuits. This is predicated on the parents being foreseeably harmed participants in the treatment. One legal scholar has quipped that additional responsibility exists when the "therapist" reaches out and touches "someone," as when the therapist arranges a confrontation between a patient and the patient's family.

A child who complained of parental ritual abuse took back the complaint and the court found for the child and the child's parents against the therapist. In another case, parents successfully sued their daughter's therapist for slander after claims of abuse had arisen in therapy.[3] Clinicians should encourage patients to avoid major life changes, such as suing parents or cutting all ties with their family, until these changes have been therapeutically explored. Causes of action against therapists include claims of libel and defamation, malpractice, and civil rights actions.

At present, the best insurance for therapists against falling into trouble in this rapidly changing area derives from familiar standbys: documentation, consultation, and attention to the boundaries of therapeutic intervention.

NOTES

1. Williams LM. Recall of childhood trauma: a prospective study of women's memories of child sexual abuse. *J Consult Clin Psychol* 1994;62:1167–75.

2. Binder RL, McNeil DE, Goldstone RL. Patterns of recall of childhood sexual abuse as described by adult survivors. *Bull Am Acad Psychiatry Law* 1994;22(3):357–66.

3. Gutheil TG, Simon RI. Clinically based risk management principles for recovered memory cases. *Psychiatr Serv* 1997 Nov;48:1403–7.

▦ ▥▐ ▐▥ ▦

MAXWELL J. MEHLMAN, JD

Behavioral Genetics: Can We Prevent Crimes Before They Are Committed?

Scientists have long sought to explain human behavior in terms of inherited factors. Traits ranging from homosexuality to perfect pitch have been attributed to genes. Particular interest has focused on traits that lead to antisocial behaviors, such as committing crimes. If criminal tendencies were due, at least in part, to a person's genetic endowment, then genetic testing might identify potential criminals before they caused trouble, treatments might be devised to correct the biochemical errors that were responsible, and, perhaps, germ line engineering could be employed to eliminate the offending genes from the gene pool. The search for an inherited basis for criminal and other socially undesirable behavior has led from phrenology to reports in the mid-1960s that an unusually high percentage of males institutionalized with violent or criminal tendencies possessed an extra Y chromosome. Most of these claims have been discredited. Identifying genes associated with behavioral traits is difficult because the traits are likely to be caused by the interaction of multiple genes and between genes and the environment, and because the traits themselves are not well defined and cannot be identified consistently by different observers. But the search continues. "Mounting evidence from animal and human studies shows that genetics has a role in human behavior," writes Charles Mann.[1]

One stimulus for the hunt is the criminal defense bar, which is interested in raising "genetic defenses" on behalf of its clients in order to have them found not guilty or to reduce their punishment. The first genetic defense was asserted in the early 1970s, based on the XYY chromosomal abnormality.[2] The courts so far have rejected the XYY defense, but have indicated their general willingness to accept genetic defenses if the genetic condition meets various standards, such as that it "interferes substantially with the defendant's cognitive capacity or with his ability to understand or appreciate the basic moral code of his society."[3]

Occasionally the defense works. In one bizarre decision, a woman who murdered her son and tried to kill her daughter was declared not guilty by reason of insanity when she began to experience symptoms of Huntington's disease, even though the symptoms did not manifest themselves until seven years after the crime.[4] Unfortunately, this case illustrates one of the pitfalls in this area: Judges and jurors typically have a poor understanding of genetic science, and might be led to accept a weak defense.

Apart from being asserted as a defense to culpability, associations between genes and undesirable behavior could make it possible to take preventive measures. For example, criminals could be tested for the offending genes and offered treatment to reduce their antisocial tendencies. Convicted criminals might be eager to volunteer, especially if treatment led to a reduction in their sentence or to early parole. An analogy is the use of the synthetic hormone Depo-Provera in sex offenders. Four states, including California, have enacted laws authorizing the use of this form of "chemical castration" as a condition of parole.[5]

But if geneticists discovered genes that actually caused people to engage in antisocial behavior, particularly violent crimes or sexual crimes against children, lawmakers might go even further. They might screen the population to detect potential offenders and treat them long before they committed crimes. This even could be incorporated into newborn screening programs. Or, we might test the children of convicted criminals and treat those who tested positive. If this proved too expensive or administratively difficult, legislatures simply might order that individuals with these heritable genes be prevented from having children in the first place.

Ironically, we have been down this road once before. We tend to think that we are in the midst of a revolution in human genetics that began with the discovery of the double-helix configuration of DNA in 1953, or perhaps with the advent of the Human Genome Project in 1991, but the real beginning of the genetic revolution was the eugenics movement of 1870 to 1950. Modern geneticists are understandably reluctant to associate themselves with this earlier foray into genetics and social engineering. As Allen Buchanan and his colleagues wrote in their book *From*

Chance to Choice: Genetics and Justice, "the history of eugenics is not a proud one. It is largely remembered for its shoddy science, the blatant race and class biases of many of its leading advocates, and its cruel program of segregation and, later, sterilization of hundreds of thousands of vulnerable people who were judged to have substandard genes. Even worse, eugenics, in the form of 'racial hygiene,' formed part of the core of Nazi doctrine."[6]

What many people don't realize, however, is that eugenics was not the brainchild of Hitler and his cronies. The idea originated in Victorian England. Interest quickly spread across the Atlantic, where the movement received substantial financial support from leading citizens, including the Harriman, Carnegie, and Rockefeller families. Far from being the brainchild of the Nazis, Hitler's eugenics program, which included compulsory sterilization, was heavily influenced by the eugenics movement in the United States.

The zenith of the eugenics movement in the United States was the 1927 Supreme Court case of *Buck v. Bell,* in which the Court, with only one justice dissenting, upheld the constitutionality of a Virginia law authorizing the state to sterilize inmates at the State Colony for Epileptics and Feeble Minded. The opinion, written by Chief Justice Oliver Wendell Holmes Jr. for the majority, culminated in the now infamous exhortation: "Three generations of imbeciles are enough."[7]

Against this grim historical background, modern interest in behavioral genetics understandably has sparked controversy. In 1993, a psychologist named David Wasserman obtained a grant from the NIH to hold a conference on genetics and criminal behavior. The plan drew protests from individuals who claimed that it was a thinly veiled effort to attribute innate criminal tendencies to certain racial groups, particularly, African Americans. The NIH took the unprecedented step of withdrawing the grant at the last minute, causing the conference to be cancelled. This led to the belief in academic circles that behavioral genetics, at least the focus on the association between genes and crime, was taboo. But Wasserman revised his proposal, received a larger grant from the NIH, and finally held the conference in 1995. Since then, there has been a flurry of books and articles exploring the new field.

The shadow cast by eugenics still lies over behavioral genetics. But the allure of crime prevention remains as well: identify persons with inherited antisocial disorders before they misbehave, and modify their behavior prophylatically. If continued genetic research makes this feasible, the question is whether behavioral modification can be conducted in a fashion that comports with the individual rights guaranteed under the Constitution, such as the right of equal protection of the laws and the rights to be free from unreasonable search and seizure and from cruel and unusual punishment.

NOTES

1. Mann CC. Behavioral genetics in transition. *Science* 1994;264:1686.

2. *People v. Tanner,* 91 Cal. Rptr. 656 (Cal. Ct. App. 1970).

3. *People v. Yukl,* 372 N.Y.S.2d 313 (N.Y. Sup. Ct. 1975).

4. Associated Press. Disease cited in murder acquittal. *Cleveland Plain Dealer* 1994; Sept. 29:A6.

5. See Stadler A. Comment, California injects new life into an old idea: taking a shot at re-cidivism, chemical castration, and the constitution. *Emory Law J* 1997:46;1285.

6. Buchanan A, Brock DW, Daniels N, Wikler D. *From Chance to Choice: Genetics and Justice.* Cambridge: Cambridge University Press, 2000:27.

7. *Buck v. Bell,* 274 U.S. 200 (1927).

⌗ ⦀ ⦀ ⌗

WILLIAM J. WINSLADE, PHD, JD

Traumatic Brain Injury and Criminal Responsibility

Traumatic brain injury for decades has been, and continues to be, a major public health problem in the United States. Car crashes, gunshot wounds, falls, and sports injuries account for two million brain injuries a year, nearly 400,000 hospital admissions, and at least 60,000 deaths. Approximately 90,000 people suffer a severe brain injury and survive but require extended, expensive rehabilitation. Some 2,000 people a year lapse into permanent unconsciousness lasting for months or years before they die.

Some survivors of traumatic brain injury fully recover, but many others experience a multitude of cognitive, emotional, and behavioral disabilities. For example, attention deficit and memory loss may affect cognitive functioning. People with brain injuries often deny their disabilities; yet they are extremely frustrated by their inability to think clearly or perform tasks that came easily before their injury. Personality changes are common. Those who were calm and controlled may become quick-tempered and impulsive. In some people anger erupts into aggressive attacks on others. Many with severe brain injuries lack the ability to control their thoughts, emotions, impulses, and their conduct. They may become uninhibited, promiscuous, anxious, paranoid or violent.[1]

People with severe brain injury may require close supervision in a controlled environment to prevent violent outbursts and other impulsive behavior. It is because such people lack the ability to control their impulses and conduct, that they may pose a threat to others and themselves. Although not all people with severe brain injury are dangerous, a history of traumatic brain injury is more common among prisoners than the general population. In two classic studies of 15 adults and 14 juveniles on death row in the mid-1980s, psychiatrist Dorothy Otnow Lewis found all 29 inmates had a history of traumatic brain injury. One might assume that their brain injuries would have been discovered and taken into consideration during their trials or at sentencing. Yet Lewis reported that evidence of brain injury was not uncovered at all, much less presented in the legal proceedings.[2,3]

When I was invited in 2000—15 years after Lewis' studies were published—to speak to the National Public Defenders Association about traumatic brain injury and criminal responsibility, I discovered that only a few of the 800 public defenders were familiar with Lewis' research. This provoked me to explore further the relevance of brain injury to criminal responsibility. It also raises questions about the roles of psychiatrists, psychologists, and other healthcare professionals in evaluating the impact of brain injury on behavior.

Criminal responsibility presumes that people have the capacity to control their conduct and to choose whether to commit crimes. Those whose mental capacity is severely impaired may be found not guilty by reason of insanity for an act they committed that would otherwise be a crime. Although disagreement exists about the tests for insanity, it is sometimes clear that traumatic brain injury can cause cognitive and behavioral changes in a person who meets the test for insanity.

One dramatic example is that of a 20-year-old man severely brain damaged from a near fatal car crash. Although before his accident he was a responsible, polite, nonviolent young adult, afterward he became increasingly suspicious and delusional. He formed an overwhelming paranoid delusion that his mother, with whom he had previously had a good relationship, had become part of a conspiracy to kill his father. One day he was at the drugstore with his mother when she was picking up some cardiac medication (coumadin) for his father. The pharmacist said to her jokingly, "What are you going to do with all this rat poison?" The young man's paranoid delusion about the conspiracy intensified and he felt compelled to kill his mother to protect his father. When he and his mother got home, he shot her to death. The psychiatrists who evaluated the young man all agreed, as did the attorneys, that he was insane because they thought he was a paranoid schizophrenic. Although it was clear that he was legally insane, after he was committed to a mental institution, it was discovered he was not suffering from schizophrenia. Only later did his physicians realize that his traumatic brain injury rather than schizophrenia caused his paranoia.[4]

For purposes of criminal responsibility it is always relevant, as the Lewis research demonstrates, to evaluate psychiatric, neurological, and neuropsychological factors that may have influenced the behavior of a person accused of a crime. When a person seems to have undergone a sudden personality change or acted wholly out of character in a strange manner, possible links to brain injury should be assessed. A history of traumatic brain injury may shed light on an accused person's conduct as well as their cognitive and emotional capacities. Although brain injury—even severe brain injury—may not provide sufficient evidence for insanity, it may help to explain criminal behavior, even if it does not excuse it. Evidence of brain injury may, however, be a factor that affects whether an alleged crime is classified as a serious felony or a lesser offense. If a person is convicted of a crime, evidence of brain injury may be considered as a mitigating factor with regard to severity of punishment. In view of the relevance of brain injury to criminal responsibility, attorneys have a responsibility to consider whether brain injury may have influenced a defendant's behavior. Appropriate health professionals, especially neuroscientists, neurologists, and neuropsychologists, can conduct evaluations to diagnose brain injury. Recent refinements in neuroimaging techniques—such as CT scans, MRIs, or PET scans—and psychological testing for impulse control disorders may help explain a defendant's behavior. As diagnostic techniques become more precise and our understanding of how brain injuries may influence behavior increases, the legal system should take new knowledge into consideration in assessing criminal responsibility.

As health professionals, we must be cautious to avoid making premature claims about our knowledge of how brain function affects behavior. At the same time evidence of brain injury is relevant to judgments about the degree to which a behavior is subject to a person's control. Health professionals should present reliably obtained relevant evidence. Judges and juries must decide how much credibility and weight to assign to the evidence. We know enough already to know that our brains influence our behavior and that damaged brains impair control of behavior. The scientific community should give closer scrutiny to the connections between brain injury and behavior, not only to assist the legal system in assigning criminal responsibility, but also to help discover better ways to help persons with brain injuries to regain control of their impulses and their conduct.

NOTES

1. Winslade WJ. *Confronting Traumatic Brain Injury: Devastation, Hope and Healing,* New Haven and London: Yale University Press, 1998.

2. Lewis DO, Pincus JH, Feldman M, Jackson L, Bard B. Psychiatric, neurological, and psychoeducational characteristics of 15 death row inmates in the United States. *Am J Psychiatry* 1986;143:838–45.

3. Lewis DO, Pincus JH, Bard B, Richardson E, Prichep LS, Feldman M, Yeager C. Neuropsychiatric, psychoeducational, and family characteristics of 14 juveniles condemned to death in the United States. *Am J Psychiatry* 1988;145:584–9.

4. Winslade WJ. Traumatic brain injury and legal responsibility. In Marcus SJ (ed). *Neuroethics: Mapping the Field Conference Proceedings, May 13–14, 2002, San Francisco, California*. Dana Press: New York, 2002;74–82. Available in PDF format at (http://www.dana.org /books/ press/neuroethics/).

☷ ☶ ☵ ☳

MARGARET SPINELLI, MD

Maternal Infanticide and the Insanity Defense

In June 2001, the public was riveted by the news that Andrea Yates had drowned her five children in the bathtub of her Houston, Texas, home.[1–4] Mrs. Yates, an exemplary nurse and mother, was an honor student, a jogger, and a champion swimmer. She also had a history of mood swings. Andrea Yates was persistently pregnant or lactating from 1994 to 2001 and spiraled down into mental illness with the birth of each child. Mood states of high energy and a hyper-religious focus on Satan switched to worsening depression, psychosis, suicide attempts, and four psychiatric hospitalizations in the years preceding the tragedy of the Yates children.[5–6]

Mrs. Yates's fluctuating affect and disorganized, labile clinical picture lend support to the contemporary theory that women with postpartum psychosis have an underlying bipolar disorder diathesis.[7]

In the weeks before the tragedy, Mrs. Yates claimed she was directed by Satan to kill her children to save them from the fires of hell. Both the state and the defense agreed that she was floridly psychotic at the time of the crime.

Mrs. Yates was charged with capital murder with a possible penalty of death. After only three and one-half hours, the jury returned a guilty verdict. The prosecution sought the death penalty; the jury elected a prison sentence for life.[3]

The United Kingdom and 29 other European countries have laws that make infanticide a less severe crime with mandated sentences of probation and psychiatric treatment for mentally ill women who are found guilty. In contrast, in the United States, a woman convicted of infanticide may face a long prison sentence or even the death penalty. And yet, the prevalence of infanticide in countries where treatment is mandated is no different than that in countries where punishment is mandated.[8] If the purpose of punishment is deterrence, then it is not working.

In Texas, the M'Naghten Test, or the "right and wrong test," is used to determine the legal state of insanity.[9] Derived from a landmark 1843 English case, it focuses on the cognitive aspects of behavior.

The M'Naghton formulation has inherent problems. The role of the expert psychiatric witness is to opine whether the mentally ill defendant "knew right from wrong" at the time of the crime. Cognitive capacity during most psychotic states remains unclear. The contemporary literature is filled with ongoing clinical research that queries the effect of psychoses on executive function, memory, cognitive capacity, and attention. In fact, Wisner's group, using objective neuropsychiatric testing, demonstrated cognitive impairment in women with childbearing-associated psychosis compared to those with non-child-bearing psychosis.[10-11] This places into question the appropriateness of using a law based on cognition.

In light of 21st century neuroscience, it is questionable that a 160-year-old legal case can be applied for accurate determination of the state of insanity. Yet, we in psychiatry continue fruitless attempts to adapt our contemporary scientific knowledge to antiquated legislation. We endeavor to fit our current "square peg" into the obsolete "round hole" of the law.[1]

Andrea Yates pled innocent by reason of insanity to capital murder. But the prosecution's expert asserted that she knew right from wrong at the time of the killings, because she knew Satan, who urged her to drown her children, only encourages evil.[5]

Such psychiatric testimony made the difference between this case and that of another mother who killed her children in Tyler, Texas.[12] In 2002, Deanna Laney killed two of her children and tried to kill a third by bashing them with rocks because, she said, God ordered it. Andrea Yates and Deanna Laney both were loving mothers whose severe mental illness led them to kill their children. While Andrea Yates was found not legally insane, guilty of murder and sentenced to life imprisonment, Deanna Laney was acquitted by reason of insanity and remanded to a psychiatric facility.

The outcome and the difference in the expert testimony suggest that we can distinguish right from wrong based on the nature of the perceived authority directing one's actions. Defendants with mental illness who face the criminal justice system have the right to a defense based on scientific fact, not whether God or Satan is a more appropriate moral authority. Such a defense is essential for equal representation under the law.[1]

The fact that the insanity defense is nonexistent in some states and extremely limited in others speaks to our society's disregard for equal protection under the law for persons with mental illness.[1] Until persons with mental illness are afforded the same legal and moral dignity given to other illnesses, the course will remain unchanged.

NOTES

1. Spinelli MG. Maternal infanticide associated with mental illness: prevention and the promise of saved lives. *Am J Psych.* 2004;161:1548–1557.

2. Spinelli M. *Infanticide: Psychosocial and Legal Perspectives on Mothers Who Kill.* Washington, DC: American Psychiatric Press; 2002.

3. CourtTV: Texas mom drowns kids. http://www.courttv.com/trials/yates

4. Grinfield MJ. Mother's murder conviction turns insanity defense suspect. *Psychiatr Times.* June 2002;1–5.

5. Denno D. Who is Andrea Yates? A short story about insanity. *Duke J Gend Law Policy.* 2003; 10:61–75.

6. O'Malley S. *Are You There Alone? The Unspeakable Crime of Andrea Yates.* New York: Simon and Schuster; 2004:1–41.

7. Oosthuizen P, Russouw H, Roberts M: Is puerperal psychosis bipolar mood disorder? a phenomenological comparison. *Compr Psychiatry.* 1995;36:77–81

8. Marks MN. Infanticide in Britain. In: *Infanticide: Psychosocial and Legal Perspectives on Mothers Who Kill.* Edited by Spinelli MG. Washington, DC: American Psychiatric Publishing; 2002:185–200.

9. M'Naghten's Case, 10 Clark and Finnelly 200 (1843).

10. Wisner KL, Peindl KS, Hanusa BH. Symptomatology of affective and psychotic illnesses related to childbearing. *J Affect Disord.*1994;30:77–87.

11. Wisner KL, Gracious BL, Piontek CM, PeindlK, Perel JM. Postpartum disorders: phenomenology, treatment approaches, and relationship to infanticide. In: *Infanticide: Psychosocial and Legal Perspectives on Mothers Who Kill.* Edited by Spinelli MG. Washington DC: American Psychiatric Publishing; 2002,36–60.

12. Casey R. Devils: on the head of a pin. *Houston Chronicle.* April 7, 2004.

☱ ☲ ☲ ☱

DENA S. DAVIS, JD, PHD

Informed Consent for Stem Cell Research Using Frozen Embryos

Almost every day brings fresh news about stem cells, the undifferentiated cells that appear to have the ability to evolve into many types of cells. On the scientific front, stem cells of all types—those obtained from early embryos, aborted fetuses and umbilical cord blood and other body tissues—have shown exciting potential to take on differentiated tasks. The possibilities seem infinite and could include the repair of heart and brain tissue, a cure for juvenile diabetes, the amelioration of multiple sclerosis, and more.[1]

On the legal and political front, we see a complex situation. The conflict is over the use of public monies for research with stem cells derived from very early embryos. Many scientists believe that these stem cells, being the least developed and the least "committed," have the greatest potency. The embryos under discussion are those frozen by couples in the course of infertility treatment and which they no longer wish to use. Because it is necessary to destroy the embryos to obtain the cells, many antiabortion lawmakers are opposed to using public funds for this research. U.S. Department of Health and Human Services Secretary Tommy Thompson has not yet said whether he will back public financing of stem cell research. Letters urging the president to back stem cell research have come from members of Congress, Nobel laureates, and university presidents. But 20 Republican senators sent a letter opposing the use of federal funds for studies using stem cells derived from human embryos.[2,3]

Whatever happens on the federal level, private research with embryonic stem cells will continue. Because the donors (the embryos' progenitors) are human, it is considered research with human subjects. Does this research raise issues of informed consent that are more problematic than other forms of research? In deliberations published by the American Association for the Advancement of Science,[4] the National Bioethics Advisory Commission[5] and the National Institutes of Health (NIH)[6] itself, one hears strong echoes of two other situations in which consent has been considered problematic enough to require special safeguards: consent for donation of fetal tissue following planned abortion, and consent for donation of cadaver organs for transplant.

In both cases, extra safeguards have been put into place. Women contemplating abortion can be asked to donate fetal tissue only after they have made the decision to abort so that their decision is not influenced by the possibility of donation. In the organ transplant scenario, a "wall" is put up between the people caring for the dying person and the people who ask families to consent to donation. This is to protect healthcare providers from conflict of interest, and to reassure families that their loved one's care was not negatively influenced by the possibility that he might become an organ donor.

Does consent to donation of frozen embryos for research purposes also require special safeguards? One might think so. Couples struggling with infertility are famously vulnerable, experiencing stress in almost every sphere of their lives. Further, one might argue that the sensitive status of human embryos gives society a stake in ensuring that couples donate them only after the most rigorous process of voluntary and informed consent. The proposed NIH guidelines include the following safeguards:

- There should be no inducements for donation, "monetary or otherwise."
- There should be a "clear separation" between the initial decision to create the embryos and the subsequent decision to donate excess embryos. Individuals should be approached about the possibility of donation only after they have completed their fertility efforts and determined that they have no more use for the embryos.
- Individuals should understand that they have other choices for their embryos.

· The physician responsible for treating the individuals should not be the same one who seeks to acquire embryos for research.

On the other hand, potential embryo donors are, in fact, practically ideal subjects of the consent process. People who have gone through in vitro fertilization (IVF) as a treatment for infertility are at least in their 20s and often older. Because in many states insurance does not cover IVF, they are likely to be middle class and reasonably well educated. By the time they have reached closure on the IVF process, either by successfully procreating or by deciding to complete their family in another manner, they are likely to be extremely well informed. Second, the decision can be made in a leisurely fashion, as embryos can be stored for an indefinite period of time. Further, their options include donation for research, donation to another infertile couple, and disposal (which can be accomplished in a dignified way with whatever rituals the couple finds comforting).

Compare this with a typical woman having an abortion and being asked to donate fetal tissue. This woman might be young, poor, and uneducated, and is certainly under stress and racing the clock. Again, if we compare the situation of a family being asked to donate organs, we see people who are grieving and stressed and who must make a decision quickly. Thus, although donation of fetal tissue and of cadaver organs may superficially appear to have similarities with donation of embryos for research, in fact the differences outweigh the similarities.

Finally, people being asked to donate embryos have probably thought long and hard about the meaning of those embryos and their potential for human life. After all, the embryos were originally created for transfer to the uterus. In at least some of the families, a "brother" or "sister" of these embryos has now completed the process of transformation into personhood and is a member of the family. This should reassure those who worry about thoughtless disposition of embryos. RESOLVE, the support group for people facing infertility, has come out in support of federally funded stem cell research.

In sum, if it becomes possible to use public money for stem cell research, the NIH rules that would apply are, if anything, overprotective of potential donors. In the private sphere, the standard protections for informed consent that pertain to any research setting are sufficient to ensure that couples are making the decision whether or not to donate their spare embryos in ways that are consonant with their values.

NOTES

1. Kaji EH, Leiden JM. Gene and stem cell therapies. *JAMA* 2001;285:545–50.

2. Southwick R. 95 Lawmakers ask Bush to allow federal aid for stem-cell studies. *Chronicle of Higher Education* March 30, 2001.

3. Southwick R. College presidents back stem-cell research. *Chronicle of Higher Education* April 6, 2001.

4. American Association for the Advancement of Science, Institute for Civil Society. *Stem Cell Research and Applications: Monitoring the Frontiers of Biomedical Research.* Washington, DC:AAAS, 1999.

5. *Ethical Issues in Human Stem Cell Research,* Executive Summary. Rockville, MD: National Bioethics Advisory Commission, 1999. http://www.bioethics.gov

6. *Draft National Institutes of Health Guidelines for Research Involving Human Pluripotent Stem Cells.* Rockville, MD: National Institutes of Health, 1999. http://stemcells.nih.gov/ news/news Archives/draftguidelines.asp

☷ ☶ ☵ ☳

REBECCA DRESSER, JD

Financial Interests and Research Protections: Can They Coexist?

By now, nearly every clinician and researcher knows about the Jesse Gelsinger case. Gelsinger died in 1999 after volunteering to participate in a University of Pennsylvania study assessing the safety of a genetically altered adenovirus. In the aftermath of Gelsinger's death, government officials and a university review committee found several problems with the study. One major concern was the financial arrangements underlying the research.

James Wilson, MD, was the director of the university institute that conducted the Gelsinger study and was also the founder of Genovo, a biotechnology company that had attracted investments from two larger biotechnology companies. Some of the funds invested in Genovo were used to support research at Wilson's university institute. In turn, Genovo and the other biotechnology companies held commercial rights to discoveries related to research at the institute. If Genovo and the other companies did well, more money would be available to fund institute research. In addition, both Wilson and the University of Pennsylvania owned stock in Genovo. If the study results proved promising, the stocks value could go up, thus benefiting the institute director and the university.[1,2]

These financial arrangements were not unique. The private sector now supplies a significant portion of US funding for biomedical research. Laws granting intellectual property rights for biomedical inventions have encouraged more commercial activities among academic scientists and institutions. Many academic and community physicians recruit patients and conduct studies for commercial sponsors. The general view is that industry funding and intellectual property rights are good for society because they increase the chance that research findings will be translated into actual clinical improvements. At the same time, these financial arrangements create incentives that could lead some investigators to compromise their responsibilities to human research participants.

During the 1990s, the US Public Health Service and the Food and Drug Administration issued regulations requiring researchers, institutions, and companies sponsoring research to disclose and manage financial conflicts of interest. But the Gelsinger case, together with other indications that oversight was inadequate, prompted an examination of whether additional measures were needed.

As part of this examination, the US Department of Health and Human Services (HHS) sponsored a 2000 conference on financial conflicts of interest in research and their potential effect on protection of human study participants. After the conference, the HHS Office of Human Research Protections issued a "Draft Interim Guidance" entitled, "Financial Relationships in Clinical Research: Issues for Institutions, Clinical Investigators, and IRBs To Consider When Dealing With Issues of Financial Interests and Human Subject Protection."[3]

The guidance document urged clinical investigators, research institutions, and Institutional Review Boards (IRBs) to consider how financial incentives—such as payments to investigators who serve as consultants or speakers, bonuses for recruiting research participants, and fees to clinicians who refer their patients to study investigators—could "color the consent discussion in a manner that encourages participation by subtly minimizing the presentation of risks or overstating the benefits" or could "affect one's judgment, or willingness to report adverse reactions possibly related to the study article, or the analysis or interpretation of data." The document said that IRBs should ensure that prospective research participants are notified of a study's funding source and the payment arrangements for the investigator " whenever that information is considered to be material to the potential subject's decision making process."

The guidance document also remarked on the lack of a single prevailing approach to financial conflicts in human research. This observation was confirmed by speakers at the HHS conference and writers responding to the draft guidance. According to some commentators, clinical researchers should be prohibited from holding financial interests that could be affected by the results of a study they oversee or conduct. A related view is that universities and other nonprofit institutions should be prohibited from holding equity interests in companies that could profit from research conducted at the institution. Others say such prohibitions would be premature and potentially harmful. They argue that research institutions, sponsors, and professional organizations need more time to understand

and develop effective strategies to manage financial conflicts of interest. This group is worried that prohibitions on certain financial arrangements could impede development of new products that could benefit society.

Complex issues are raised by the heightened commercial presence in clinical research. I offer two general points that should be taken into account in efforts to create and implement policies in this area. First, investigators are human beings whose clinical research judgments may intentionally or inadvertently be shaped by the desire to benefit financially from their activities. Whether researchers hold stock in a company that will be affected by study results or are eligible for recruitment bonuses if they rapidly enroll participants, the potential for inadequate participant protection must be acknowledged. Moreover, even if no actual problems arise, such arrangements may create the appearance of a conflict of interest. If the general public perceives clinical investigators as primarily motivated by monetary gain, people could become less willing to enroll in research. Scientists and clinicians ask people to accept the risks and burdens associated with study participation so that patients in the future may benefit. But such appeals to altruism may seem hypocritical coming from a research community that appears more concerned with financial rewards than with helping future patients.

Policy makers considering conflicts of interest should also keep in mind a second general point. History demonstrates that financial interests are not the sole source of failures to protect research participants. In any research situation, investigators want to enroll participants, complete their trials, and collect interesting data. Desires for prestige, peer recognition, and scientific curiosity can also distract investigators from their responsibilities to research participants. Thus, the absence of a financial conflict does not eliminate the requirement to ensure that individuals receive accurate information and protection from undue harm in research.

Ideally, the inquiry into financial conflicts will highlight the need to protect participants in every research study. Without the volunteers, after all, neither scientists nor society could achieve any of the benefits available from biomedical research.

NOTES

1. Marshall E. Gene therapy's web of corporate connections. *Science* 2000;288:954–5.

2. Nelson D, Weiss R. Hasty decisions in the race to a cure? Gene therapy proceeded despite safety, ethics concerns. *Washington Post* November 21, 1999:A1.

3. http://www.fda.gov/opacom/factsheets/justthefacts/11subpr.html

ALEXANDER MORGAN CAPRON

Governmental Bioethics Commissions:
The Nature of the Beast

The topic of governmental bioethics commissions has little to do with the law (except for the statutes or executive orders under which they are typically established) and may seem too commonplace to deserve further thought. Yet many issues are imbedded in each of the topic's three parts: In what sense are such bodies governmental? How do they do bioethics? And what kinds of commissions are they? Let's start with this last question.

Public commissions come in a variety of forms, divided basically between permanent bodies to which Congress has delegated lawmaking functions and ad hoc panels that are convened to provide advice on a particular subject. At both the state and federal levels, panels of the former type have a history dating to the 19th century. Bodies such as the Interstate Commerce Commission and the Federal Trade Commission fill in the details of broad, general statutes that frame their respective fields by issuing rules and applying them in individual or categorical determinations. The members of such commissions are typically appointed by the chief executive and serve as full-time public officials, with expert advice from their staff. The members of ad hoc advisory panels—who may be appointed not only by the chief executive but by other executives or even legislative or judicial branch officials—typically do not enter full-time governmental employ, though they too may be supported by staff. In most cases, they do not issue regulations or adjudicate individual claims but may offer advice to officials who do.

The several dozen federal and state "bioethics commissions" that have functioned over the past three decades have all been of the latter type—ad hoc and advisory. Indeed, most have existed for relatively brief periods, though several were established in a fashion that would have allowed them to continue indefinitely, and at least one specialized board (the Recombinant DNA Advisory Committee, or RAC) has existed for more than a quarter century. Yet being merely advisory is not inherent in the task of doing "public bioethics." For example, the UK's Human Fertilisation and Embryology Authority (HFEA)—a mixed panel of experts and laypersons, like commissions in the US—not only licenses fertility clinics but decides on ethical grounds whether particular assisted reproductive technologies may be used. The HFEA recently permitted one couple to use preimplantation genetic diagnosis (PGD) to select embryos for implantation which were not only free of the genetic disease that affects the couple's first child but which would make well-matched donors of cord blood stem cells for the existing child. Conversely, PGD was denied to another couple because the condition affecting their existing child was extremely unlikely to recur and thus the only reason to select embryos would be to create a suitable donor.

The second aspect of these commissions is that they "do bioethics." Yet does it seem reasonable for a mixed group of laypersons and experts from a range of fields, meeting for a day or two each month or so, to produce "bioethics"? If it were an academic discipline (a subset of philosophy or theology) or even a professional field, the answer would probably be "no." Committees aren't known for great, original thinking, and the eclectic nature of bioethics commissioners makes that even less likely. But the roots of bioethics as an interdisciplinary field that arose in the late 1960s from collaborations among natural and social scientists, physicians, nurses, philosophers, theologians, lawyers, and others, make it an ideal field for a public commission.

Furthermore, while bioethics commissions do undertake or sponsor original studies (which not only influence their conclusions but are published as appendices to their reports), their most important contributions are typically synthetic: having clarified the issues and arguments, they draw together the best current thinking and move the field forward by formulating a new consensus. Two reports by the President's Commission for the Study of Ethical Problems in Medicine and Biomedical and Behavioral Research (1980 to 1983) illustrate this point.[1,2] Among the topics assigned by Congress, the commission decided to start with "the matter of defining death" precisely because it had been debated for more than a decade and a broad agreement existed on how it should be resolved both medically and legally.

The commission was able to bring the other groups whose competing statutory proposals had stymied action in most states to agree on a uniform proposal—which was then quickly adopted across the country—and to facilitate the leading medical authorities on the subject to promulgate what was recognized as the accepted medical criteria for declaring death.

As an offshoot to this assigned topic, the commission decided to undertake another large study on the situations in which patients, families, and physicians must decide whether to forgo life-sustaining treatment. Medical thinking, case law, and public awareness on this topic were all rather rudimentary at this time. "Living wills" had been around for about 15 years but few people had them and only 15 states had "Natural Death" statutes authorizing the use of "directives to physicians." Moreover, most people—including many healthcare providers—operated from the assumption that it was wrong (and even illegal) ever to discontinue life support, perhaps even when the patient's wishes to do so were known. Drawing on the best ethical and legal analysis, the commission articulated why this was not the case, provided a framework for hospital ethics committees (which were just being widely instituted), and urged states to formulate and adopt durable power of attorney for healthcare statutes (which nearly all of them did over the decade that followed).

These two reports also help flesh out the significance of the topic's third facet, namely, that the commissions are "governmental." Plainly, nongovernmental bodies also propose legislation as well as changes in professional practices. Governmental commissions—especially those appointed by US presidents—have two advantages, however, one is visibility (and, if they do their work well, a sense of legitimate authority), and the other is that their pronouncements are seen as "official" in a sense that is helpful in getting action from legislators and bureaucrats, even when the commission operates at a federal level and its recommendations are for state action (as was true of the two reports I just described). This is not to say that recommendations are never ignored—especially once a commission's charter has expired and it is not around to pester policy makers for a response—but the governmental commissions still have more leverage than private ones.

At the same time, these commissions are not governmental in the sense a federal agency or congressional committee is governmental. Indeed, several of the presidentially appointed commissions continued to function after a change of occupants at 1600 Pennsylvania Avenue, certainly straining the sense that they were part of the current administration. Even when they possess something close to decision-making power—as, for example, is true of the RAC for r-DNA research and gene transfer experiments that seek federal funding—bioethics commissions typically operate more like outsiders. Still, by virtue of their official status, they are more open and "transparent" in their processes than private bodies, which is a great virtue for those who favor democracy over rule by experts.

In the 30 years since the first steps were taken—in the wake of revelations of the Tuskegee experiment and other research scandals—to establish what became a succession of bioethics commissions, they have become familiar fixtures (not only in the US but around the world). Individually, they have had hits and misses in helping the public and policy makers understand modern biomedical science and practices and their ethical and social implications. Yet collectively these commissions—both at the national level and in a number of states—have succeeded in building a bridge connecting the legislative and executive branches, experts and academics in science, philosophy and law, and the general public, and in aiding the adoption of better governmental, organizational, and professional policies, and the making of more ethically enlightened individual decisions.

NOTES

1. President's Commission for the Study of Ethical Problems in Medicine and Biomedical and Behavioral Research. *Defining Death: A Report of the Medical, Legal and Ethical Issues in the Determinations of Death.* Washington DC: US Government Printing Office, July 1981.

2. President's Commission for the Study of Ethical Problems in Medicine and Biomedical and Behavioral Research. *Deciding to Forego Life-Sustaining Treatment: A Report on the Ethical, Medical, and Legal Issues in Treatment Decisions.* Washington DC: US Government Printing Office, March 1983.

☳ ☲ ☵ ☳

PART SIX

Ethics and the Humanities

Review by David Steinberg, MD

Wrongful Death: A Memoir, by Sandra M. Gilbert

W. W. Norton and Company, New York/London, 1995, 364 pages

Wrongful Death is the skillfully written, often poetic, story of the death of the author's husband due to medical malpractice. It is a tale of traumatic loss, unanticipated grief, loving recollections, and near vengeful anger. The two major protagonists—the culpable urologic surgeon who lied and trivialized, and the aggrieved widow who sued him for malpractice and then salted the wound by writing this book—leave little ground for reconciliation.

Elliot Gilbert was 60 years old, in robust health, and chairman of the English Department at the University of California at Davis when he was diagnosed with localized prostate cancer and admitted to his university's medical center for a radical prostatectomy. He jokingly reassured his family, "the chair of urology can't kill the chair of English." Unfortunately, he was wrong. A little more than 24 hours after he was admitted to the hospital, Elliot Gilbert was dead.

The urologic surgeon told the shocked, bereaved family that his patient had a heart attack. That was a lie, because Elliot Gilbert had bled to death. The surgeon's lie shapes Gilbert's story almost as much as the fact of her husband's death; anger is woven into her grief. She tells her dead husband, "they killed you sweetheart" and quotes Pliny the Elder, "Only a physician can commit homicide with complete impunity." Her anger is magnified because no one will accept the blame for her husband's death. She says, "Responsibility in the often miraculous but always highly technologized realm of modern medicine is so dispersed, so fragmented, that finally it accrues to no one."

In telephone calls to the depressed and traumatized woman, the urologic surgeon establishes himself as a monument to insensitivity. "For you this is unpleasant, awful, but believe me, for me it's shattering." And, "Just thought I'd call to tell you the surgery was a complete success . . . We got it all out." Gilbert comes closest to understanding the man who killed her husband when she allows that the surgeon's "anesthetized" response to her plight might be explained by an experience "perhaps too shattering to acknowledge."

Gilbert's personal mission, to find out what happened to her husband, is only partly successful. She blames "stonewalling," though by settling her lawsuit she gave up the chance for the trial that might have given her the missing answers. Nonetheless, she garnered enough information for a reasonably accurate formulation of the pivotal event.

After surgery, at about 2:15 p.m., Elliot Gilbert was transferred to the recovery room. At that time his hematocrit, a test that measures the volume of red blood cells, was a modestly low 32 percent. At 3:05 p.m. Elliot Gilbert's systolic blood pressure fell to a worrisome 72 mm Hg. Although another hematocrit was sent promptly to the laboratory and the result could have been available within minutes, no hematocrit was noted until 6:30 p.m.—an unexplained delay of more than three hours. That hematocrit was an alarming 17 percent, and shortly afterward a frightening 13 percent. The dramatic fall in hematocrit is best explained by massive bleeding. What isn't explained is the more than three-hour delay that probably cost Elliot Gilbert his life. Why didn't any of his doctors look for the result of the 3:05 p.m. hematocrit? It can't be because they didn't know better; all doctors know that a fall in blood pressure can mean bleeding. To explain the fatal delay we must, with the help of conjecture, probe the often banal nature of medical error.

The urologic surgeon could have been so overly confident of his skills that he was blinded to the possibility that he erred and left behind a bleeding, severed blood vessel. Or perhaps his mind was elsewhere. About two hours before Elliot Gilbert died the surgeon "walked away" to go to a meeting; it could have been an important meeting and thinking about it might have been distracting. Responsibility for Elliot Gilbert's care probably was delegated to residents or fellows in training. It's possible that one of them wrongly assumed one of the others had seen the hematocrit and said nothing because it was satisfactory. Or maybe when Elliot Gilbert's blood pressure temporarily rose after he got intravenous fluids they became complacent and simply forgot about the hematocrit. Elliot Gilbert probably died an "absurdly unnecessary death" because human weakness and fallibility allowed a small error, but one with awesome consequences—confirming for Gilbert "the randomness of life and death."

Gilbert's outraged feelings are understandable because she lost her husband and suffered grievously; but is hers the only legitimate perspective for judging the urologic surgeon? Elliot Gilbert's hypotension was but one problem for the surgeon who on any given day might also confront, in other patients, blood in the urine, flank pain, an obstructed ureter, a mass in the kidney, a tumor in the bladder, a lodged renal stone, a narrowed renal artery. To manage these problems he must make numerous decisions, many of them critical. Multiply his decisions of a day by his weeks, months, and years in practice and ask whether out of this enormous mass of doctoring we have the right to expect success in each and every instance. We should abhor medical error. We should establish systems to prevent it. We should set limits on what we will tolerate. But on judgment day, we need to acknowledge human fallibility, including the understandable but morally indefensible impulse to lie to cover up one's mistake.

Wrongful Death is an engrossing story and arguably the best starting point for an exploration of medical error. It reveals the burden on innately imperfect physicians not to err, the flesh and blood agonies of medical mistakes, and our often angry, litigious, and ultimately unsatisfying responses when things go wrong. It also reminds us of the power of the pen, which in aggrieved and skillful hands can immortalize our mistakes.

Review by Catherine Belling, MA

The Doctor Stories, by Richard Selzer
Picador, New York, 1998, 389 pages

A writer who is also a doctor is, according to Richard Selzer, "especially blessed in that he walks about all day in the middle of a short story." The stories in this new collection demonstrate Selzer's ability to produce a rich symbiosis between the storyteller's skill and the physician's material.

In "A Worm from my Notebook," Selzer says that "fine writing can spring from the most surprising sources," and demonstrates this by constructing a story about what must be one of the most disgusting parasites to afflict a human host, the Guinea worm (in whose deliciously ugly Latin name, *Dracunculus*, Selzer clearly delights). A man discovers the two-foot worm extending under his skin, "feeling the creature respond with slow pruritic vermiculation." That the source of such a detail is medical reality rather than fantasy makes the fate of the patient especially gripping.

In his introduction, Selzer admits to the pleasure of using "horror and the grotesque as instruments of illumination, as well as to produce a physiological effect." Here, I think, lies part of what it means to be both doctor and writer: a physician's access to the particulars of what can— and does—happen to the human body, when combined with a writer's ability to convey such things in visceral detail, makes for stories that have no trouble producing both fascination and a degree of revulsion. But more importantly, Selzer uses his exact evocations of somatic conditions to cast light on profound truths about our body-bound lives.

One of my favorite stories in this book, and one that seems not yet to have entered the canon of classic clinical tales such as "Imelda," "Mercy," and "Brute," is a concise picture of terminal illness that illuminates all the terrible complexity of taking care of the dying patient by focusing on the relatively minor procedure of its title, "Tube Feeding."

The story's only characters are a nameless couple. She is dying of cancer; he cares for her. The entire narrative encompasses the few minutes one morning when he feeds her, as he has done many times before, by pouring eggnog through a funnel into the gastrostomy tube that leads to her stomach. Selzer lulls us with evidence of the affection and efficiency with which this is done. The man is an ideal caregiver, she an uncomplaining patient. He kisses her and says she is lovely as he picks out a silk scarf for her chemotherapy-bald head. Then Selzer shows us, in terrible detail, "the great red beard" of her tumor, which has "burst

forth, exuberant . . . mounding upon her neck, twisting and pulling her features until she was nothing but a grimace trapped in a prow of flesh." We see the patient through her husband's eyes, in which she is still lovely, as long as he carefully sees "only her brow where the skin is still pale and smooth, nothing below her eyes."

This delicate balance of love and horror characterizes his care, too. He is "gallant," toasting her with the funnel as if he were feeding her champagne, but they both know his gallantry is a "device," a brave deception. So when things go wrong and the tube slips out of her stoma, the brutal recognition of despair is especially painful. He successfully inserts a new tube but then has to run to the bathroom to vomit. She hears him retching. Although neither acknowledges it aloud, "a limit has been reached." The reader shares both sources of nausea: gut-level loathing for what cancer can do (a nausea made vivid right from the first sentence's sickening juxtaposition of "eggnog" and "emesis basin"), and the subtler, guiltier horror of watching a husband having to keep his wife alive by funneling food through a rubber tube into a grotesque hole in her body.

In the last half-page of the story, the contentious ethical question of withholding nutrition is broached with the lightest touch. Struggling to insert the tube, the husband begins to panic about not getting it in: "She will starve." I came to a halt on that word; we've already been told of her pain, so bad that any moment without it is felt as nostalgia rather than reality, and the tumor is cutting her off at the throat. In her refusal of more eggnog and his packing away of the feeding equipment, we find Selzer-the-physician's quiet argument for a love that includes the acceptance—and even the welcoming—of death (and a strong counterpoint to "Mercy," in which a doctor learns he is not yet ready to hasten the death of his patient).

One piece of advice Selzer gives on writing fiction is to focus on the specific. His stories are anchored by the precise details of practiced clinical observation. A wasting patient "grows daily less differentiated until she is something rudimentary, a finger of flesh." A dislocated shoulder slips back into its socket with "a sudden muffled sound as though an apple had fallen from a tree into wet earth." A surgeon whose patient has died feels for the femoral artery but finds "only his own pulse hammering at the girl's flesh to be let in." *The Doctor Stories* demonstrates the attention with which Selzer has inhabited the fascinating world in which all physicians do their work, and the skill with which he can recreate it.

Review by Jack Coulehan, MD, MPH

End of the Line: Depression and Burnout in Ward No. 6

In *Chekhov's Doctors: A Collection of Chekhov's Medical Tales,* Jack Coulehan, MD, Editor; Kent State University Press, Kent, Ohio, 2003, 232 pages

When Anton Chekhov graduated from the University of Moscow Medical School in 1884, he had a decision to make. During the previous four years, the young man had supported himself and his family by writing humorous sketches and stories for Moscow weekly magazines. By that time Chekhov was so well regarded as a writer—at least 150 published pieces—his editors clamored for more. Why waste his time practicing medicine? Nevertheless, the newly minted Dr. Chekhov hung up his shingle and for the next five years or so practiced primary care medicine.

But he managed to avoid that either-or decision. At night and on weekends, he wrote as much as ever, publishing an additional 190 stories before 1890 and, along the way, winning the Pushkin Prize, the Russian equivalent of America's Pulitzer, by the age of 28. As Chekhov's fame grew, he closed his urban practice and moved to the country, where he continued to work as a district doctor and public health officer until incapacitated by tuberculosis in 1897. For example, in less than five months in 1891, Chekhov reported seeing 453 patients at a district clinic and making 576 house calls. He also busied himself with grassroots activism, building schools for peasants, raising money for famine victims, and, most famously, exposing inhuman living conditions in the czarist prison colonies on Sakhalin Island.

Chekhov always maintained that medicine was his lawful wife and literature, his mistress: "When one gets on my nerves, I spend the night with the other." But in reality, he never kept them separate; his professions interacted and enhanced each other, especially the influence of medicine on Chekhov's plays and stories. Obviously, one such influence was the author's deep insight into the medical life, which he conveyed in his numerous stories about physicians. Chekhov's doctors range from callow medical students to obnoxious, insensitive practitioners and from courageous public health workers to beloved village physicians. However, some of his most fascinating creations are the physician characters who suffer from disappointment, ennui, or burnout.

"Ward No. 6," a long story published in 1892, is a masterpiece of burnout. The protagonist is Dr. Ragin, the withdrawn and depressed director of a district hospital. He had arrived at the job 20 years earlier, as an energetic young doctor: "At first Dr. Ragin worked very hard. He received patients every day from morning to dinnertime, performed operations, and even did a certain amount of midwifery…" But over the years, his energy has dissipated. He now realizes how poorly equipped and out-of-date his hospital is. He professes the "palpable futility" of medical practice, because social and economic forces beyond medicine's control determine health and disease. Thus, Ragin has retreated into a shell, detached not only from his patients, but also from all human contact. While a junior doctor actually takes care of the hospital patients and runs the clinic, Ragin spends his days sitting in his study and drinking beer.

While heavy demands and poor working conditions contribute to Ragin's predicament, he faces a deeper problem as well. Is his sense of futility solely a consequence of medical practice? Or is something deeper missing? Ragin comes across to us as unreflective, apparently having suppressed his emotional life and replaced it with a set of abstract beliefs. Ragin's lack of self-knowledge has crystallized around a profound sense of emotional numbness. When he was younger, he evidently meant well and worked toward his professional ideals, but the commitment was superficial. In the long run, he never learned to look beyond the accumulation of day-to-day disappointments to find satisfaction in meaningful relationships with his patients and others.

Early in the story, Ragin visits the mental ward (Ward No. 6), where he meets Ivan Gromov, a brilliant paranoid who embraces life passionately. The passion attracts Ragin like a moth to a candle. Ragin yearns to feel something, anything, even to experience suffering, rather than to remain suspended in his emotionless cocoon. He develops an obsession that only by making himself suffer will he be able to experience an emotional life and, therefore, be truly human. Predictably, this new obsession makes him even more dysfunctional, a situation that allows the junior doctor to have him fired as hospital director and, ultimately, committed to Ward No. 6 as mentally ill. Once Ragin becomes a "nobody," his isolating cocoon disappears. The ward orderly hits him when he tries to escape, thereby giving Ragin an opportunity to suffer. Shortly thereafter, he has a stroke and dies.

A dismal story, perhaps, but full of psychological insight. Many healthcare professionals become vulnerable to depression and burnout, because we lack the inner resources to cope, day in and day out, year after year, with our difficult work. We learn during professional school and postgraduate training to distance ourselves emotionally from the situation at hand, to be "objective" and exhibit "detached concern" (an oxymoron, if you think about it). Too often, we learn the "detached" part very well, by suppressing our feelings and avoiding self-reflection. But we often tend to intellectualize the "concern" part, so that caring becomes a series of concepts and procedures, rather than a compassionate presence for the patient.

In medical education you frequently hear repeated Dr. Francis Peabody's famous one-liner: "… for the secret of the care of the patient is in caring for the patient." While this is true as far as it goes, a further step is necessary as well: the secret of caring for the patient is to develop self-awareness; that is, caring first for oneself. Dr. Ragin's plight is extreme, but the dynamics that led him eventually to withdraw from practice may threaten any healthcare professional who works so hard at detachment from patients that he or she also becomes detached from his or her own emotional life. "Ward No. 6" serves as fair warning of what can happen if we totally ignore the dictum, "Physician, heal thyself!"

Review by David Goldblatt, MD

Million dollar boo-boo

Million Dollar Baby, Warner Brothers Studio, 2004

Million Dollar Baby, a movie based on a short story by a former boxer and cut man, won four 2005 Academy Awards, including best picture, actress, supporting actor, and director (Clint Eastwood). I will discuss the ethical dilemma presented in the film. If you don't know the plot, you should decide whether you want to read on.

Maggie, a boxer, has been sucker-punched in a title fight. She has high cervical, ventilator-dependent quadriplegia. She transfers to a rehabilitation facility, all expenses paid by the Boxing Commission. Despite competent care, she loses a leg to infection. With her career at an end and no other interest in life (she has at last rid herself of her cartoonish trailer-trash family, and she has no desire to pursue an education), she asks her devoted manager and trainer, Frankie, played by Eastwood, to help her to die. She does *not* have that discussion with her doctor, whom we see only briefly.

When Frankie tells Maggie he can't do what she wants him to, she tries, twice, to kill herself by biting deeply into her own tongue. Her doctors respond by keeping her under sedation.

Frankie, a questioning Catholic, goes to his priest, who says that if Frankie does help Maggie to die, he will be irredeemably "lost." Nevertheless (in a strategy that works on the screen but would cause a patient suffering in real life), Frankie, in secret, first disconnects the ventilator, then administers a large dose of epinephrine through the IV.

This depiction of mercy killing has evoked much discussion, from persons partisan to the sanctity-of-life concept and from advocates for the disabled, some

of whom believe that the able-bodied are plotting to do away with the disabled by discounting their lives, failing to acknowledge that it's "all right" to be that way. Both factions appear to have accepted the film's tacit assumption: Maggie's doctor, who has kept her alive even at the cost of a leg, and has kept her from taking her own life even at the cost of her alertness, would, if he were to abandon the fight and let her have her wish, be no different from Frankie. He would be killing his patient. Because he can't do that, it's up to Maggie and Frankie.

Because I don't buy the story's premise, I don't—how else can I say it?—buy the punch line.

Euthanasia, suicide, and assisted suicide remain choices, legal or not, for persons who have the capacity to decide whether or not to live with either disability or illness. As a person who has undergone chemotherapy, I think about decisions I may or may not act on if my illness progresses despite treatment. These choices are important, but, in Maggie's situation, *they should be irrelevant.*

Persons who retain the ability to make decisions on their own behalf and who are receiving any form of treatment have the right to refuse it. That remains true even when forgoing treatment will surely result in death. When a person who is receiving life-sustaining treatment (usually, artificially administered hydration and nutrition, hemodialysis, or mechanical ventilation) had firmly made the decision not to "live this way," euthanasia or suicide, assisted or not, is neither appropriate nor required.

As a clinical ethicist, I have talked with competent, ventilator-dependent patients who had traumatic quadriplegia or amyotrophic lateral sclerosis, to help them decide about foregoing life-sustaining treatment. As an attending physician, I have withdrawn ventilatory support. Those experiences were difficult and deeply moving. My skills in both roles improved with experience. I do not regret my participation.

Maggie, as she was portrayed, had the capacity to make a valid refusal of treatment. Once she had made her decision, her doctor should have been the one to stop the ventilator, in accordance with a tested protocol. No physical suffering. No horrible self-mutilation. No clandestine, illegal mercy killing.

Whether or not good ethics and attention to established legal precedent could have made a good short story or a good movie is a question I shouldn't try to answer. Nevertheless, the movie had the opportunity to inform the public that, when a treatment is life-sustaining, another choice exists. Passing up that opportunity was a boo-boo.

As we were about to get into our cars outside the theater where we had just watched *Million Dollar Baby*, a man who recognized me and knew I am a doctor remarked on the ending. I gave him the 30-second version of this article. "That's good to know," he said.

Review by David Steinberg, MD

The Spirit Catches You and You Fall Down, by Anne Fadiman

Farrar Strauss and Giroux, New York, 1997, 339 pages

Foua and Nao Kao Lee and their daughter Lia's doctors could not have differed more strikingly in their understanding of Lia's epilepsy. For her comparatively unimaginative Western doctors, epilepsy was simply an overt manifestation of aberrant electrical activity that required treatment with medicine; for Lie's Homing parents, epilepsy, known to the Hmong as *quong dab peg,* was a distinguished illness understood in terms of spirits called dabs, fugitive souls, shamans, and the afterlife—not voltage. An arguably unnecessary "collision of two cultures" fragments Lia's medical care into suspicion, noncompliance, anger, distrust, court orders, and a tragic conclusion.

The Laotian Hmong were migrant, mountain people and tough fighters who, in the 1960s, were organized by the American Central Intelligence Agency into a clandestine anti-Communist army. When the war in Vietnam was lost, many of them ended up landless refugees in the US—a world so different from their ancestral home they might as well have been sent to another planet. The Hmong were called "the most primitive refugee group in America"; one study of Indochinese refugees found that the Hmong exhibited the highest degree of "alienation from their environment." Most Hmong had never seen a light switch, a telephone, or an air conditioner. These problems were addressed by a pamphlet, "Your New Life in the United States," that advised: never urinate in the street; do not stand on the toilet; the door of the refrigerator must be shut.

Dwarfing the formidable mundane challenges of everyday life, the widest chasm for the Hmong was conceptual and linguistic. Lia's doctors lived in the steely cold world of medical science; Lia's parents inhabited a phantasmagoric universe of spirits. The Hmong did not distinguish between mental and physical illness, between medicine and religion, or between language and music (their language is musical). There were no Hmong names for organs such as the pancreas. Anne Fadiman, in this fascinating and fair book, criticizes Lia's American doctors because they never tried to understand the nature and magnitude of the conceptual gulf that separated them from their patient's family.

Hmong theory on the nature of illness is an example of the width of that gulf. "Your soul is like your shadow. Sometimes it wanders off like a butterfly and that is when you are sad and that's when you get sick, and if it comes back to you, that is when you are happy and you are well again.... A twix neeh [a shaman] is needed to perform the ritual of animal sacrifice so the slaughtered animal's soul can be used as ransom for the fugitive soul of the sick person. Sickness is related to the soul and that's why spiritual healing is needed."

Finding American medicine incomplete, Lia's parents took her from Merced, California, to Minnesota to see a famous twix neeh who had himself suffered from epilepsy (epilepsy made Lia special because epileptics might themselves become a twix neeh). Lia did well after the twix neeh's ministrations; her doctors, unaware that they were not Lia's only caregiver, ascribed her improvement to the Depekene they had recently prescribed. Lia's family assumed she got better because of the trip to Minnesota.

Lia's parents did not give their daughter her medication; Lia's outraged doctors, confirming the Hmong's worst prejudices about the medical profession, had Lia put in foster care. She was taken from the "bad parents" we will come to know as extraor-

dinarily loving and caring. We taste the bitter fruit of cultural misunderstanding.

Fadiman resists the temptation to serve up a neatly wrapped package and helps us see the complexities of Lia's story. Foua and Nao Kao didn't withhold their daughter's medicines solely because of spirits and shamans; the drugs (which proved to be a poorly chosen regimen) made Lia sick and they didn't work. Any reasonable parent might have questioned their use. The story's disastrous denouement comes, not from parental neglect or "a very dense cultural barrier," but from a humbling diagnostic oversight.

In medicine, the extreme case often illuminates the commonplace. The typical clinical encounter may not be a massive cultural challenge; nonetheless, each patient has personal quirks, a unique cultural, religious, and family background and a different way of dealing with illness. Patients often see the world of illness differently than their caregivers and may be unhappy, noncompliant, or drawn to alternative therapies. Arthur Kleinman has made the distinction between disease and illness. Disease is narrow pathology; illness encompasses the meaning, the nature, and the implications of that pathology.[1]

The lesson of *The Spirit Catches You and You Fall Down* is that clinicians will do a better job if they try to understand what makes patients and their families tick.

NOTE

1. Kleinman A, Eisenberg L, Good B. Culture, illness and care: clinical lessons from anthropologic and cross cultural research. *Ann Intern Med* 1978; 88:251–58.

Review by Andrew G. Villanueva, MD

How We Die, By Sherwin B. Nuland

Vintage Books, A Division of Random House, Inc. NY, 1995, 278 pages

In *How We Die,* Dr. Nuland uses his skills and experiences as a surgeon, teacher, and author not only to pen a national best-selling book, but to offer a frank, yet compassionate, examination of a subject *all* people eventually face. He observes that "Poets, essayists, chroniclers, wags, and wise men write often about death but have rarely seen it. Physicians and nurses, who see it often, rarely write about it."

Dr. Nuland seems uniquely suited to bridge this gap. As a clinician he knows the scientific basis of the dying process and, over a long career, has personally observed the manifestations of this process in many patients. As a littérateur and medical historian, he knows how the great thinkers of the past viewed dying and can put the modern American method of dying into historical perspective.

As a man personally affected by death (his mother died of colon cancer when he was eleven years old and his brother recently died of the same disease at the age of 62), he understand the emotional impact on patients and their survivors. And, as an experienced teacher and skillful writer, he is able to blend these views into an informative and captivating book that is worth reading by laypersons and healthcare professionals alike.

Dr. Nuland strives to "de-mythologize the process of dying" by presenting it in stark biological and clinical detail. He quotes John Webster's observation that "death hath ten thousand doors for men to take their exits," but limits his descriptions to six disease categories that occur frequently and involve universal processes of dying. He describes coronary artery disease, stroke, dementia of the Alzheimer's type, violent deaths, AIDS, and cancer.

While he explains technical details of abnormalities found in these diseases—including atherosclerosis, derangements of neural connections in the brain, shock and organ dysfunction, destruction of white blood cells by the human immunodeficiency virus, and the growth and spread of cancer cells—his writing is neither pedantic nor stodgy. He introduces each chapter with memorable personal anecdotes and attaches human faces to disease and dying. We read about his bloody and unsuccessful attempt at resuscitating a heart attack victim when he was an unseasoned medical student. We observe his grandmother's aging and her inexorable physical decline before succumbing to the complications of a stroke. We share the pain of a close friend as she agonizes over the gradual loss of her spouse to Alzheimer's disease. We feel his helplessness as he describes his brother's travails with metastatic colon cancer and sense his guilt about having recommended toxic chemotherapy to treat what he knew was a terminal disease.

We also read of other people's experiences such as the mother who witnesses the brutal murder of her nine-year-old daughter and the friends and families who watch their loved ones suffer and die from the complications of AIDS.

The author serves as more than just a narrator or an expositor of the dying process. He recounts death's ancient place in human existence and cites pundits from the past who have written about death or have contributed to our knowledge about death: Virchow, Heberden, Osler, Montaigne, Tolstoy, and William Cullen Bryant. He decries the hubris of modern high-technology medicine and the emphasis on biomedical problem solving rather than humane patient care. He also discusses sensitive but important ethical issues such as the overtreatment of the seriously ill, medical futility, and assisted suicide.

Dr. Nuland demystifies dying without lessening its significance. He writes, "Only by a frank discussion of the very details of dying can we best deal with those aspects that frighten us the most."

He critiques the "method of modern dying," which avoids or hides death, often in a hospital, and which values the art of saving life over the art of dying. He teaches us that dying can be a time of hope—in many different forms—rather than hopelessness. In the end he wisely reminds us that, "The dignity that we seek in dying must be found in the dignity with which we have lived our lives. . . . The art of dying is the art of living."

Review by Delese Wear, PhD

The Sweet Hereafter, by Russell Banks

Harper Perennial, 1992, NY, 257 pages

I resisted the book for over a year in spite of my friends' insistence that I read it. No matter how much I loved Russell Banks' writing, I couldn't deal with a story that involved the death of children in a school bus accident. Finally, after listening to my reading companions insist over and over that there were no graphic accounts of how it happened, I picked up the book one evening and began to read. I finished this powerful, haunting novel hours later. Indeed, the book is not "about" the bus accident in Sam Dent, a small town in upstate New York. The circumstances leading up to the accident and the accident itself appear mostly in the first chapter, narrated by the bus driver, Dolores Driscoll. Dolores, matter-of-fact, talkative, "sanguine," according to Abott, her husband of 28 years, is an "optimist who acts like a pessimist" who treats her schoolchildren charges as if they were her own. A life resident of Sam Dent, she knows the family details of all the children who climb on board each morning, often chatting with their parents at the bus stops.

The remaining chapters have three different narrators: Billy Ansel, a widowed Vietnam veteran who lost a son and

daughter in the accident and now drinks himself into a less painful state; Mitchell Stephens, a negligence lawyer from New York City who appears quickly at the scene (with countless other litigators) fueled by his belief that there is no such thing as an accident; and Nichole Burnell, a teenage beauty queen cheerleader who survived the crash but not the psychological damage of incest. Nichole is now a paraplegic who holds the key to a huge settlement.

Thus, readers experience the story from inside the heads of the four narrators. The unique life events of the narrators influence how each experiences and makes meaning of the tragedy. Each tells the story of his or her life leading up to the accident, providing different angles and "facts" on the same event: the simple, forthright way Dolores describes the day of the accident—picking up children at bus stops, watching the sky lighten and noting the change in weather, drinking her second cup of coffee, swerving to avoid a dog; or Billy Ansel's terse, pain-ridden prose, "The only way I could go on living was to believe that I was not living." Nichole's account provides insight into profound changes in a young person who yesterday was a cheerleader, today a "wheelchair girl, a cripple." The contrast between her way of making sense of the accident and her parents' mercenary approach is profound, complicated by the secret Nichole has been hiding for years. For her, "before" and "after" not only was the division between an active, physically vibrant existence and life in a wheelchair, but also was the division between being victimized by her father's sexual advances and holding his secret over him. "The only truly valuable thing that I owned now happened to be Daddy's worst secret, and I meant to hold on to it. It was like I carried it in a locked box on my lap, with the key held tightly in my hand, and it made him afraid of me. Every time he saw me looking at him hard, he trembled." Indeed, her secret was the key to the unfolding of the story.

In choosing the voice of Nichole, Banks is also able to portray how family secrets like incest emerge in the midst of tragedy in the most unexpected ways. No one is immune from pain in this story—even the hugely successful, "permanently pissed off" lawyer Mitchell Stevens is dealing with his drug-addicted daughter Zoe who drops her HIV-positive status on him in one of her many phone calls during his months in Sam Dent.

As these stories intersect with each other and weave together how other families coped with this tragedy, Banks explores the complexities of grief, the various struggles to make meaning of something so "wickedly unnatural," and the human capacity for forgiveness and hope. Grief, we find, can never be predicted in its various enactments or neatly categorized by stages: "Death had permanently entered our lives with that accident . . . for us there was life, true life, real life, no matter how bad it seemed, before the accident and nothing that came after the accident resembled it in any important way." Some people respond with pure anger, like Wanda Otto's need to "blame" the accident on someone: "I want that person to go to prison for the rest of his life," she declared. "I want him to die there. I don't want his money." Some responded with a desire for money, like the Walkers: "They wanted money, not as compensation but because they had been broke for so long and had always wanted it." Others, like Billy Ansel, understood "the inescapable and endless reality of it" and had a desperate desire just to be left alone. As he said to his lawyer: "Leave me alone, Stephens. Leave the people of this town alone. You can't help any of us. No one can."

This is, in the end, a story that addresses through four narrators, each with something different at stake, one of life's most aching questions: When tragedy strikes, how is it to be explained? It is a question no one in medicine can avoid.

Review by James L. Bernat, MD

The Diagnosis, by Alan Lightman

Pantheon Books, New York, 2000, 373 pages

Literary depictions of illness have an illustrious heritage. Within the genre of novelists' descriptions of undiagnosed, fatal illness, Tolstoy's *The Death of Ivan Ilyitch* occupies the premier niche. Now, Alan

Lightman, Professor of Humanities and lecturer in physics at MIT, and author of *Einstein's Dreams,* has added *The Diagnosis.* This short novel depicts the personal agony of experiencing an undiagnosed illness within a 21st century context of high technology medicine and against a backdrop of the oppressive time pressure, materialism, anomie, and inhumanity of contemporary American urban life.

Bill Chalmers is a 40-year-old junior executive in a nondescript Boston financial district business with a suburban wife and teenage son. During a typical morning subway commute, he suddenly loses his orientation and memory and begins the descent into illness and the dissolution of his previously ordered life. The police believe him to be psychotic and take him to Boston City Hospital, from which he escapes. After losing his identity and dignity, his life further unravels with the loss of his job, his sense of self-worth, and his understanding of his place in the world.

Lightman's description of the time pressure of contemporary American urban professional life is anxiety provoking. Every task is timed and competitive. Those who are late become the losers. He punctuates each page by noting the time by the minute on clocks and watches. Wasted time is a source of frustration and disgust. Even exercise and relaxation must be timed. The reader becomes exhausted by the relentless march of seconds and minutes, Chalmers' futile rush to meet each accelerating deadline, and the continuous and unstoppable accumulation of e-mails, phone messages, memos, and in-box tasks. The time pressure portrayed in the first half of the book is reminiscent of the intense, unrelenting, and ultimately fatiguing rhythmic force of Ravel's *Bolero*.

Lightman portrays an inhuman, aggressive, uncaring society of people competing for money, prestige, and space, despite the meaninglessness of their work. Chalmers' company sells "efficiency management," and he describes his own role as "I process information." At best, his colleagues are indifferent to the needs of others; at worst, they are cruel and utterly lacking in warmth or caring. It is into this milieu that Chalmers seeks understanding and solace for his illness. Instead, those seeking his place in the hierarchy trample him. Eventually, he is fired for the most egregious failure possible: getting behind in his work. His illness is not a mitigating factor. Everyone in society is replaceable and those who fail to perform are expendable.

Chalmers responds with outbursts of anger directed against technology and the tragic futility of his wasted life. He sees the structure of society itself as a machine. In one remarkable chapter in which Chalmers and his wife are invited to a large party at the suburban mansion of Marbleworth—capitalist extraordinaire and owner of his downtown office building— Chalmers envisions Marbleworth as "the super machine who controls all the other machines." Chalmers fantasizes about destroying technology and even killing Marbleworth, evoking the spirit of the Luddites during the Industrial Revolution.

Lightman's depiction of physicians and academic medical practice is unflattering. Chalmers' physician, Armand Petrov, is a Massachusetts General Hospital internist who loves to order tests but hesitates to reach a diagnosis. As Chalmers inexorably deteriorates from limb numbness to outright paralysis, Petrov responds "we are making progress." This cryptic remark indicates only that he is excluding individual diagnoses by sequential testing but has not reached a specific diagnosis. The counterpoint of Petrov's diagnostic languor and the intense time pressure of the business world seems strangely ironic. Chalmers' evaluation by a MGH neurologist is particularly unhelpful. Eventually, he is referred to a psychiatrist who cryptically diagnoses unresolved anger.

Lightman treats the reader to several parallel subplots, including the conflicted relationship between Chalmers and his son and the virtual affair between Chalmers' wife and her unmet e-mail "lover." In an interesting and ultimately meaningful series of installments, Lightman retells from Plato's *Phaedra* the ancient story of the final few days of Socrates. He details the fascinating relationship between Socrates and his principal prosecutor, Anytus. The reader sees that, like

Socrates, Chalmers is condemned to die from "neglect of the gods," in this case, the gods of technology, money and power. By the end of the book, the two plots converge when Chalmers finally achieves the same degree of acceptance and equanimity toward his anticipated death from an undiagnosed illness as Socrates exhibited facing his own death from hemlock.

Review by David Steinberg, MD

An Unquiet Mind, by Kay Redfield Jamison

Vintage Books, New York, 1996, 240 pages

The brain is the repository of our consciousness and the locus of our personhood; this endows the already formidable torments of the mood and thought disorders with an intimate destructiveness. Kay Jamison, a psychologist and professor of psychiatry at Johns Hopkins Medical School, writes about one of these disorders—manic-depressive illness—from the dual perspective of a scientific scholar of the disease (when stabilized by lithium), and one of its victims. "Which of the me's is me?" she asks. "The wild, impulsive, chaotic, energetic, and crazy one? Or the shy, withdrawn, desperate, suicidal, doomed, and tired one?" *An Unquiet Mind* describes Jamison's roller coaster rides of exhilarating, glorious highs that degenerate into madness, and dark, brooding, black and gray depressive lows. Despite the chaos and agonies of her manic-depressive disorder Jamison is ambivalent about the lithium treatment that made a productive life possible. She loves the "glinting, glorious moments" of being mildly manic:

> The seductiveness of those unbridled and intense moods is powerful ... My awareness and experience of sounds in general and music in particular were intense. Individual

notes from a horn, an oboe or a cello became exquisitely poignant ... When you're high it's tremendous. The ideas and feelings are fast and frequent like shooting stars, and you follow them until you find better and brighter ones. Shyness goes, the right words and gestures are suddenly there, the power to captivate others a felt certainty. There are interests found in uninteresting people. Sensuality is pervasive and the desire to seduce and be seduced irresistible. Feelings of ease, intensity, power, well-being, financial omnipotence, and euphoria pervade one's marrow.

We are left to wonder, if so much of what we take as personality can be fashioned by illness with its near certain organicity, what that reveals about the nature of personality. Could our vaunted personal uniqueness simply be an epiphenomenon of our neural networks?

In the midst of her exuberant manic episodes something changes; the tempo accelerates dramatically. The mildly manic states Jamison found "powerfully inebriating and conducive to productivity" turn sinister. "The fast ideas are far too fast and there are too many; confusion replaces clarity." She doesn't sleep normally;

her memory fails. Relationships are damaged. Professional life becomes impossible. She engages in unrestrained buying sprees ("mania is not a luxury one can easily afford"). She becomes "wildly agitated, paranoid, and physically violent" and reaches a "definite point when I knew I was insane."

Jamison shares with other writers a difficulty in describing the depressive episodes that follow her mania. "Depression is awful beyond words or sounds or images." She tells us depression cannot be understood by extrapolation from the blue moods that follow the loss of a job or a divorce. True depression is different:

> It is a pitiless, unrelenting pain that affords no window of hope . . . there is nothing good to be said for it except it gives you the experience of how it must be to be old and sick and to be dying; to be slow of mind; to be ugly; to have no belief in the possibilities of life, the pleasures of sex, the exquisiteness of music, or the ability to make yourself or others laugh; it is flat, hollow, tiresome and unendurable; a gray bleak preoccupation with death, dying and decay.

One could imagine Jamison had made a deal with the devil: the intoxicating, productive, seductive bouts of controlled mania at the cost of madness and time spent in an unbearable depressive hell.

Most of us who are healthy do not appreciate the complexities of a life infiltrated by chronic illness. Each disease has its own personality and peculiar mischievousness. Jamison shares the global impact of manic-depressive illness on her life. Her need for secrecy. Her haunting worry—when will it happen again? Her struggles with lithium. Her disquietude over whether mental illness should disqualify her from treating patients. Her conflict over whether to have children and risk transmitting her genetically rooted disorder. Her need to pretend she was well when she wasn't.

Jamison says, "I have become fundamentally and deeply skeptical that anyone who does not have this illness can truly understand it." Most of us will thankfully accept that reading *An Unquiet Mind* is as good an understanding as we are likely to get or want.

Review by David Wykes, PhD

Darkness Visible: A Memoir of Madness, by William Styron

Random House, New York, 1990, 130 pages

Writers are prominent among the victims of depression, and the disease is particularly cruel because among the many things it tears away from its victims—self-esteem, sleep, the simple pleasures of existence, libido—is creativity. Most writers who survive a siege of depression know that the encirclement may resume, and understandably will show no desire to make the experience the subject of art. To write about it is surely to risk losing again the power to write.

William Styron's now famous essay is therefore, first of all, an act of bravery. He defied depression's long record of stealing writers' voices. (And it does so literally, as well as metaphorically; his own voice became "at times faint, wheezy and spasmodic—a friend observed later that it was the voice of a ninety-year-old.") For sound rhetorical purposes, Styron withholds until late, the fact that "By far the great majority of the people who who go through even the severest depression survive it," but, by its mere existence, his book asserts his own survival as a writer.

The generalization that "the horror of depression is so overwhelming as to be quite beyond expression" is triumphantly challenged on every page, and Styron places himself among the tiny group of artists who have contributed to the still elusive attainment of a clear representation of depression's meaning, "which sometimes, for those who have known it, is a simulacrum of all the evil of our world: of our everyday discord and chaos, our irrationality, warfare and crime, torture and violence, our impulse toward death and our flight from it held in the intolerable equipoise of history." Depression is not the sole property of our time, but it is our time's emblem.

Styron uses his blessedly restored voice to drive home the truths about depression that too few of the unimpacted public could then, in 1989, grasp and admit: that depression is truly madness; that it "can be as serious a medical affair as diabetes or cancer," that suicide for all victims is a contemplatable possibility, and for a few is truly the only end to simply unendurable torments; and that physicians and psychiatrists can (one hopes one should now write "could") be among the least comprehending of those to whom the depressive attempts to unburden him (or more often, her) self.

The poetry of Styron's descriptions is the index of his pain: "This leaden and poisonous mood the color of verdigris . . . melancholia's fecund self-humiliation . . . Now I was in the first stage—premonitory, like a flicker of sheet lightning barely perceived—of depression's black tempest." He protests tellingly against the disease's very name, "a true wimp of a word . . . for over seventy-five years [since being named by Adolf Meyer] the word has slithered innocuously through the language like a slug, leaving little trace of its intrinsic malevolence and preventing, by its very insipidity, a general awareness of the intensity of the disease when out of control." He even manages at times a twisted grin, as when warned of a drug's side effect of impotence: "Putting myself in Dr. Gold's shoes, I wondered if he seriously thought that this juiceless and ravaged semi-invalid with the shuffle and ancient wheeze woke up each morning from his Halcion sleep eager for carnal fun."

Styron takes his title from Milton's account of hell, but for me *Darkness Visible* is about another oxymoronic condition: death in life. When Styron reads again Coleridge's great poem, he will find that he too has been an Ancient Mariner, and that only Coleridge has written a better account of surviving depression, and of the cost of survival.

Review by David Steinberg, MD

Conquering Schizophrenia: A Father, His Son and a Medical Breakthrough,
by Peter Wyden

Alfred A. Knopf, New York, 1998, 335 pages

In 1972, Peter Wyden's 17-year-old son Jeff was diagnosed with schizophrenia. For more than a quarter of a century Wyden has persevered as his son's advocate and protector, and as a vigilant student of the mental disorder he was determined to see conquered. He tells his story with surprising clinical detachment, which can perhaps be explained by the alienating and emotionally draining nature of his son's illness. He writes, "facing Jeff for so long in his unreachable, demented incarnation was not easy to take. How do you keep loving a son who can be such an unpleasant stranger?" With few traces of self-pity, Wyden describes the harsh consequences of being the parent of a schizophrenic son.

Schizophrenia, he tells us, is an "impoverished man's disease that leaves all but the very rich penniless in the end, whatever the medical outcome." Despite his position as executive editor of the *Ladies Home Journal*, expenses, such as the $50,000 a year ("an enormous sum in those days") he paid the Menninger Clinic, left him bankrupt and his son a ward of the state.

Wyden also suffered a "guilt that never left." Jeff's earliest symptoms began when Wyden and Jeff's mother, Edith, were divorced. Wyden believed stress was a possible trigger for schizophrenia and blamed himself. This belief was reinforced by respected psychiatrists who maintained schizophrenia was a psychosocial disorder and the fault of dysfunctional families and "schizophrenogenic" parents.

Wyden was also plagued by physical exhaustion. He tells us that half of all schizophrenics attempt suicide and 13 percent succeed. Wyden points out that "many schizophrenics are secretive, live as social isolates and can kill themselves without warning." For a worried father, "the required level of alertness is quite tiring."

The book's only photograph, that of a smiling, 17-year-old boy radiating the vibrant promise of youth, reveals what can easily be imagined as Wyden's heaviest sorrow. What achievements awaited Jeff had mental illness not intruded? (Wyden's other son Ron is the United States senator from Oregon.) I was repeatedly drawn back to that haunting photograph knowing that its promise of unlimited possibility had been dashed by mental illness into

a vacant life spent "whiling away the years" in halfway houses and mental hospitals, often in restraints.

As a father trying to help a schizophrenic son, Wyden developed a keen appreciation of the hubris and failings of the medical profession. He illustrates this with a compilation of putative cures for schizophrenia that should send shudders down the sturdiest spine. Henry Cotton, a physician, believed the cause of schizophrenia was hidden bacterial infection and performed colectomies on hundreds of psychotic patients, and in 1921 alone, extracted 6,000 "infected" teeth. Another physician, John Rosen, tried beating schizophrenia out of his patients. Other proffered remedies on Wyden's list include emetics and purgatives, deliberate malaria, induced insulin shock, megadoses of LSD, and frontal lobotomies. The misguided doctors Wyden personally encountered were the "talking therapists" who believed that schizophrenia was a psychosocial condition that could not be treated with medicine. The influential psychoanalyst Silvano Arieti summed up that position, "One can no more treat so deeply an ingrained and emotionally internalized state of mind by drugs than one can take a pill to learn or unlearn French."

If Wyden's memoir has a hero, it is the German psychiatrist Emil Kraeplin who rejected the psychosocial and psychodynamic theories of his "arch competitor" Sigmund Freud. Kraeplin's detailed clinical observations led to the classification of schizophrenia as a brain disease. Wyden considers Kraeplin the father of biologic psychiatry and his achievements "the victory of scientific observation over philosophic and moral meditation." Sadly, Kraeplin proved to be a tainted hero with a dark side that championed racial purity and the German master race.

Students of drug development will find a lot of detailed material on the antipsychotics. Wyden carefully chronicles

the development of drugs to treat schizophrenia as he watches and waits for the
medicine that will make a difference for
Jeff. When it happened, the "breath-taking"
changes were "difficult to believe." On olan-
zapine, "His hands don't shake. The mental
hospital slouch is gone." For the first time
he is "tackling life issues maturely. . . . His

shell had dropped away. He was chatting,
trading gossip, obviously feeling comfortable on the outside." After more than 25
years, this is a significant, but incomplete
victory. Wyden tells us, "I kept thinking
that my long job of raising this son was
done. Instead, I am in my seventies, and
the task continues."

Review by Lois LaCivita Nixon, PhD, MPH

Wit: A Play, by Margaret Edson

Farrar, Straus and Giroux, 1999, New York, 96 pages

In 1999, when Margaret Edson's play, *Wit,*
opened off-Broadway, the buzz was immediate. Critics wrote of its power and intelligence; tickets sold out; the play soon moved
uptown to a larger house; the unknown
playwright (a kindergarten teacher!) was
courted and celebrated; and the play received not only the Drama Critics Award
for the Best Play and the Drama Desk
Award for Outstanding Play, but also the
Pulitzer Prize. The buzz continues.

Currently, the play is widely available
in regional theaters and a film version
with Emma Thompson has been produced by HBO. In addition, this play
about the final period in a woman's life
generates lively discussion in community
settings, hospital ethics committees, and
professional meetings. Entire classes of
medical students in Cleveland, Atlanta,
Washington, DC, Denver, and Tampa
have attended performances as well as
talkback sessions in which the dynamics
of the drama are reviewed and debated.

It is not surprising that critics, the
public, and healthcare professionals have
responded strongly to a play about a hospitalized woman struggling with end-
stage cancer. In an effort to understand
more about the nature of suffering, options, and choices, we continue to rely on
storytellers for meaning and comfort: the

novelists, the poets, filmmakers, and play-
wrights. Following in the tradition of *King
Lear, Lycidas, The Death of Ivan Ilyich, The
Wasteland,* and, most recently, the best-
seller, *Tuesdays with Morrie,* Margaret
Edson's tightly structured play provides
compelling insights into the conditions of
modern medicine, but, more importantly,
into the complexities and needs of human
beings journeying toward death.

Vivian Bearing, *Wit*'s 50-year-old protagonist, is a highly respected professor of
English literature whose work has cen-
tered on 17th century poet John Donne.
Accustomed to intellectual rigors associated with Donne's poetic intricacies, she
is uncompromising in research and teaching. Upon admission to the hospital's oncology unit with stage 4 metastatic ovarian cancer, Bearing encounters a research
unit and team that is similarly rigorous
and uncompromising. In unrelated
spheres of study, she and Harvey Kelekian,
the physician in charge of her experimental chemotherapy program, share a passion for aggressive probing and rationality. Both have been intensely focused on
their work and demonstrate a shared arrogance in their separate searches for
knowledge and excellence. Neither has
bothered with compassion or kindness in
their pursuits and relationships.

Bearing's status is unequaled; she is at the pinnacle of her profession. Now, dressed in the hospital-issue gown, the formerly proud woman must submit to the realm of medicine. In this setting, she feels more like a piece of meat or a bug than a human being.

Her first words are to the audience in which she mimics the routinized, vapid language patterns of healthcare workers while serving to draw viewers into the world she currently inhabits:

"Hi, how are you feeling today? Great. That's just great."

For Bearing, an erudite wordsmith, the line demonstrates medicine's reductive capabilities, its power to diminish. The question is an empty formality. Because the answer, "great," completes a meaningless hospital ritual, her presentation of both question and answer establishes the situation she is in and demonstrates the unexpected transformation of language—her tool—from power to meaninglessness. A few lines later, feelings of loss are underscored when this professor of linguistic riches presents an uncharacteristically spare summary to the audience:

"It is not my intention to give away the plot; but I think I die in the end. They've given me less than two hours. "

The next 75 minutes cannot be reduced to such simple terms for viewers brought into the gripping drama. When the curtain does fall, an engaged but hushed audience struggles to interpret the emotional impact of the succinctly wrought play. The audience becomes her confidante, perhaps the only confidante this self-armored woman has had during her life. It is through this tragic device that her losses are revealed and her commonly human feelings are articulated. Bearing understands her situation:

"I have cancer, insidious cancer, pernicious side effects—no, the treatment has pernicious side effects.... I know all about life and death. I am, after all, a scholar of Donne's Holy Sonnets, which explore mortality in greater depth than any other body of work in the English language."

Indeed, her professional competencies are as sharply honed as those of her oncologist. Both are familiar with death, both are tough and both are unyielding. Unfortunately, while exhibiting impressive professional skills, Bearing and Kelekian are clumsy and inept in their relationships with people, especially students and patients. Only when Vivian Bearing begins to see how little room was left in her life for meaningful relationships with students and others, does she begin to recognize her human needs and also those she failed to respond to in others.

Review by Jack Coulehan, MD, MPH

Travels with the Wolf: A Story of Chronic Illness, by Melissa Anne Goldstein

Ohio State University Press, Columbus, 2000, 264 pages

In *Travels with the Wolf,* a young woman develops a persistent and unexplained illness during her first year at college. Her doctors consider various diagnoses, including atypical appendicitis, for which surgery is performed, but the patient continues to suffer from aching, fatigue, and low-grade fever. Eventually she acquires the diagnosis of lupus, the wolf, but simply naming the beast fails to tame it. For the next ten years, Melissa Anne Goldstein experiences exacerbations and remissions, including lupus myelopathy, which leaves her too weak to walk. In the world of chronic illness, Melissa encounters numerous doctors who hold the reins of authority, yet live in a different world. Some fail to listen, others betray and abandon her. Only a few are willing to trust Melissa and walk with her.

Goldstein's well-written account of these events belongs to the relatively new literary genre called pathography, biography of illness. However, *Travels with the Wolf* is also an account of Melissa's quest for self-awareness. She converts her personal experience into the more general investigation of narrative in healing, both through creative writing—Melissa's illness experience is illustrated by her fine poems—and her professional work in the fields of literature and medicine.

Toward the end of the book, the author asks, "Why, I wondered, do physicians harbor such strong feelings about lupus?" I have to admit that long before page 247, I struggled with those strong feelings. At a few points, I wanted to take Melissa by the shoulders and yell, "Come on, stop whining! Surely, it couldn't have been that bad!" I'm ashamed to admit this, but such feelings show how I am vulnerable to the same disheartening conflict that Melissa describes. Physicians often have difficulty empathizing with patients who threaten the comfortable belief that "objective" categories and numbers accurately reflect patient experience. While this empathy gap is especially prominent in lupus and other autoimmune disorders, it may occur in all forms of chronic or recurrent illness. The culture of medicine tells us that we must trust the dictates of textbooks and machines. When patient experience comes into conflict with these dictates, we tend to cock our eyebrows in skepticism. Should we believe the patient whose reports, after all, are only "subjective," or put our faith in the more "objective" data, which, incidentally, is under our control?

We often solve this quandary by attributing the patient's discomfort to mysterious psychological factors, rather than clear-cut disease.

Melissa finds herself plagued by distrust, defensiveness, and betrayal. In 1988 when she questioned Dr. Smith's conclusion that her disability was caused by "excessive anxiety, not disease," the doctor "stood up, pulled the door open, then spat out, 'Our time is up.'" Two years later, Dr. Kostos, her second rheumatologist, responded to Melissa's persistent weakness after she completed a course of pulse steroids with a curt command, "Out of bed. On your feet." He attributed Melissa's symptoms to a stress reaction, but offered no help. Later still, Dr. Fields, a neurologist with whom she had had a good relationship for several years, diagnosed Melissa's fits as "pseudoseizures," yet never informed her of that diagnosis. Moreover, when questioned by other specialists, Dr. Fields insisted, "she's fooled us before" and refused to evaluate the seizures. When her rehab physicians sought a further workup, Dr. Fields responded by discharging Melissa from her service, again without explanation or acknowledgement.

Yet the news is not all bad. Other physicians emerge from these pages as sympathetic characters. How do these doctors differ from the betrayers? First, they are respectful of Melissa and willing to listen to her. Second, they enlist the patient as a partner in working toward a satisfactory result. Finally, they seem to be more concerned with doing whatever it takes to get Melissa back on her feet, than they are with defending medical theory or authority. In other words, these doctors are willing to enter the world of chronic illness as sympathetic helpers, rather than authoritarian policemen.

Travels with the Wolf also contains an interesting aside on the popular cultural belief in the mind's power to heal the body. This belief, which in its extreme form might be called "Bernie Siegelism," holds that "If you heal your life by improving your attitude, resolving conflicts, and letting go of anger and bitterness, then you can heal your body." The problem with the gospel of positive attitude lies in the implication that chronic illness is the sick person's fault. One could even attribute the etiology of a poorly understood disease like lupus to "bad thinking" that generates self-destruction. In any case, if you adopt the positive attitude described in Siegel's *Love, Medicine and Miracles*, you ought to get better. It is easy to see how a confirmed Siegelist might actually

blame Melissa for continuing to be sick. She just isn't positive, or holistic, or spiritual enough to get well! Unfortunately, at the core of much of our popular New Age healing lies this unspoken fillip of guilt.

Melissa Anne Goldstein is a fine writer. Readers who suffer from chronic illness themselves will likely cheer the very features of her story that made me, as a physician, uncomfortable. Yet it is precisely to experience this discomfort—and to reflect thoughtfully upon it—that I recommend *Travels with the Wolf* to physicians and other health professionals.

Review by Felice Aull, PHD, MA

Death of the Good Doctor: Lessons from the Heart of the AIDS Epidemic,
by Kate Scannell, MD

Cleis Press, Inc., San Francisco, 1999, 240 pages

Death of the good doctor? Is this a biography—in memoriam—extolling the life while mourning the demise of a beloved physician? Did the physician die of AIDS? Such might be your thoughts when first encountering this title. Yes, the book's author, physician Kate Scannell, did die—a figurative death. Under the medical imperative prevailing when she trained (she entered medical school in 1976), the "good" doctor provided cutting-edge interventions to save lives; a patient's death represented failure. Then came AIDS, a disease that transformed not only those infected but also many of those who treated these patients, who watched their extended sufferings and deaths.

Scannell was one of those transformed. She realized that her version of the "good doctor" as a "seasoned gunfighter, ready for medical challenges" who offered "aggressive, full-service, state-of-the-art care" was simply inappropriate in

the face of such prolonged suffering and inevitable death. In one particular case, she ordered all-out heroics, misinterpreting a dying AIDS patient's plea for help—in retrospect, "my unconscious denial of his dying." The next day she was told that the patient had died thanking the night shift doctor who discontinued his intravenous fluids and injected extra morphine. "I have never practiced medicine in the same way since his death," writes Scannell in the prologue to the book. *Death of the Good Doctor* chronicles how Kate Scannell learned a different way of practicing medicine from her patients. Each chapter tells the story of a particular patient with whom she interacted. At the same time, each chapter reveals a life—her life—fundamentally changed and changing.

Trained in rheumatology and immunology, Scannell in 1985 was attempting to move from an academic career to clinical practice in general internal medicine. Unexpectedly, she found herself in charge of the AIDS ward of a county hospital serving Oakland and Berkeley, California. She began her work there with great ambivalence, wary of drug-addicted patients and fearful of the dying. For five years Scannell took care of the sickest, most stigmatized members of society. Overwhelmed initially by the severity of illness in those for whom she was responsible, she gradually allowed herself to become emotionally connected to them in mutually therapeutic relationships. These remarkable relationships are detailed in the book.

Take for example, the belligerent drug addict, Jay, whose story Scannell relates in "Sleeping with the Fishes." Jay is thoroughly unlikable, abusive to the staff, deceitful, and mean. Most disturbing to Scannell was that "I hated the way that I experienced myself in his presence, as somewhat less than fully human, lacking any compassion for him." One fateful day Scannell loses her temper and asks Jay in frustration, "isn't there anyone or anything you have ever cared for besides yourself?" "Fishes," says Jay tearfully. Scannell buys him a bowl of fish. Jay watches the fish from his bed. Scannell doesn't understand what could possibly be of interest in watching fish, but at one point she joins Jay. She finds herself mesmerized, "floating with them, relinquishing to unpredictable currents . . . I felt peaceful." Jay notices Scannell's reaction, saying to her, "You get it now, don't you?"

This shared experience affects both physician and patient. Jay becomes more considerate and calm; Scannell takes greater notice of her surroundings, of other people—in her personal life as well as at the hospital. "I thought of how my own sense of belonging was expanding, too, through a succession of patients' lives

inviting me into the world . . . [a]nd how it was more than that—it was the very trees around my home, the sounds of the forest, the breakers in the bay."

But why would "belonging" be an issue for Kate Scannell? Because, the reader learns gradually, Scannell felt alienated socially and professionally—an alienation she hardly admitted to herself. When she entered medical school, she was one of few women in her class and had never encountered a woman physician. The male medical model, she felt, was one that had no room for empathic, intuitive interactions with patients. There seemed to be no tolerance for human frailty and uncertainty. "And this woman and physician was also a lesbian, someone whose identity was overtly pathologized by the medical profession and represented in psychiatric literature as 'deviant.'" Then, directing the AIDS ward, she slowly gave herself permission to follow her instincts, to become emotionally connected with patients, to tolerate and learn from their (to her) unfamiliar and sometimes quirky lifestyles and behaviors. There was a price to pay, however: most of her patients died. It took five more years before Scannell felt able to revisit that experience and to write about it.

This memoir, then, is a kind of illness narrative—by a physician who suffered from soul sickness, who had been unable to articulate her sense of personal and professional unease, whose life was altered by the dying patients in her care over whom she grieved. Like most narratives, especially illness narratives, the writing of this memoir was a way to make sense of and give meaning to experience. Kate Scannell's poetically rendered vignettes tell a tale of discovery and healing through powerful engagement with patients. At the same time, her book honors the memory of those patients.

Review by Richard M. Ratzan, MD

His Brother's Keeper: A Story from the Edge of Medicine,
by Jonathan Weiner

Ecco, an Imprint of HarperCollins, New York, 2004, 354 pages

Imagine you are the dean of a medical school, the chief operating officer of a corporation or a skilled programmer for IBM. Imagine yourself any of these and you learn, at the age of 31, that your 29-year-old kid brother has just been diagnosed with amyotrophic lateral sclerosis (ALS, also known as Lou Gehrig's disease). Certainly you would call, commiserate, try to help as much as you can. But would you quit your job, reinvent yourself as a manager of scientists—all strangers to you at the time—working in this and related fields of neurobiology, and embark on a financial and entrepreneurial crusade to try to save your brother?

Jamie Heywood was a 31-year-old mechanical engineer working for the Neurosciences Institute—the prestigious think tank of Gerald Edelman, the 1972 Nobel Laureate in Medicine, in La Jolla, California—when he and his tight Boston family of five, heard the news in the beginning of 1998. He handed in his resignation and began a marathon of activity all geared towards preventing his brother Stephen from becoming the wheelchair-bound shell of a man we see in Stephen Hawkings, the famous astrophysicist with ALS. Leaving California, Jamie sets up a 24–7 headquarters for ALS-related activities in, and later near, his family home in Newtonville, a suburb of Boston. *His Brother's Keeper* is the story of this crusade as told by the Pulitzer-winning science writer, Jonathan Weiner. (It first appeared in *The New Yorker* in 1999 in a shorter version.)

Stephen, the middle son of a South Dakota therapist and a British professor of

mechanical engineering at MIT, was the renegade of the three boys. Jamie and Ben went to MIT and graduated with degrees in engineering, which is the operative worldview of this book, since both the Heywoods' father, John, and the author's father, Jerome (at Brown University), are university engineers and the authors of highly technical books, respectively: *Internal Combustion Machine Fundamentals* and *Statistical Mechanics of Elasticity.*

Stephen, a carpenter, was restoring a house in Palo Alto, in December of 1997. He realized something was wrong when he had trouble turning a key. Almost exactly a year later Robert Brown, a neurologist at Massachusetts General Hospital, diagnosed Stephen with ALS. In May of 2000, a neurosurgeon injects Stephen's cervical spinal canal with stem cells (to no effect, but also with no harm). Exactly a year later, Stephen is in a motorized wheelchair with a voice so soft Jamie has to translate for the author.

Between the turn of the key in December 1997 and the wheelchair in May 2001, we watch as the author expertly narrates three stories: Stephen's illness and the Heywood family's reaction to it; his own mother's eerily similar neurodegenerative disease, progressive supranuclear palsy, or PSP (actor Dudley Moore died of PSP in March 2002); and the ongoing development—scientifically, politically and ethically—of gene therapy and what Weiner calls both "regenerative medicine" and "futuristic medicine."

This book creates a rich tapestry from the woof and warp of these narratives and the reader gets the macro and microscopic pictures of all three stories by the last page. Interwoven is the angst of Weiner's mother, Ponnie, as her mind slips and slides into cognitive decay; the history of Guam field research by John Steele on a fascinating variant of PSP (with generous and typically insightful comments by Oliver Sacks); the personal interviews with and revealing profiles of the major players in molecular genetics and "regenerative medicine." There are also literary references to Donne and Kafka, among others. Quite relevantly, when the author relates that a neurologist had told his family that his mother had a rare and incurable disease (Lewy body dementia), Weiner cites John Donne, from the XIIIth Meditation of his *Devotions Upon Emergent Occasions:* "It is a faint comfort to know the worst, when the worst is *remediless.*" Such references sometimes blind with their clarity, like the inclusion of Kafka's short parable, "An Imperial Message," a 250-word short story that begins, "The emperor, so a parable runs, has sent a message to you, the humble subject, the insignificant shadow cowering in the remotest distance before the imperial sun." Of course the message never makes it past all the obstacles to the humble subject. As a unifying parable of well-intentioned signals gone awry, the parable is brilliant in illuminating the neuropathology of ALS.

The dominant thread throughout, however, is the Heywood story and especially the driving force that is Jamie Heywood. Jamie quickly becomes the focus, the tapestry's overarching pattern as the dynamic ubermensch who oversees (having never been asked) his brother's scientific and clinical care, organizes a new co-operative initiative into the field of ALS research, and coordinates gene therapists, molecular biologists, clinicians, family members, and philanthropists at a cost. By story's end, Jamie is separated from his wife. Although we are given signals (paradoxically, the author seems to have gotten them but Jamie, like Kafka's humble subject, did not) by Melinda, Jamie's wife, of the toll such a frenetic life was exacting prior to the separation, we do not get the details of the breakup, just the aftermath of a deserted house. Is Jamie sad? Apparently. Remorseful? No. "When I asked Jamie if looking back he would do anything differently, he said, 'If you ask me would I prioritize Melinda above those life-and-death decisions—no.'"

Stephen, on the other hand, is happily married and playing with his child using hardware and software. How else would the ALS-stricken son and brother of engineers play with his child? And Stephen's response, typed on his keyboard amidst his family, "I FEEL LIKE A KING" says it all about the mind-body drama we have just read.

It is no minor accomplishment that Weiner, amongst the personal, political, and medical stories, clarifies almost effortlessly and transparently the mechanics—he is, after all, also the son of an engineer—of gene therapy and the pathophysiology of ALS. His explanation of science is painless and always carefully related to the patient and symptoms at hand.

Review by David Steinberg, MD

The Tyranny of the Normal: An Anthology,
Edited by Carol Donley and Sheryl Buckley

The Kent State University Press, Kent, Ohio and London, England, 1996, 406 pages

The normal, a useful concept in the daily practice of medicine, harbors a hidden seed of perversity which can germinate when our inner psychic insecurities are ignited or when the distinction between what is different and what is abnormal goes unappreciated. That is the message of this fascinating anthology of essays, fiction and poetry.

Leslie Fiedler's unsettling analysis of our ambivalent response to freaks, "those wretched caricatures of our idealized body image," deceptively casts doubt on the general relevance of this book. These human oddities, stars of the Barnum and Bailey sideshow—giants, dwarfs, Siamese twins, bearded ladies—stir the depths of our psyche where the "developmental insecurities of childhood and adolescence never die."

Each of us knows we are flawed and a freak to someone else. Freaks, distorted in the extreme, are reassuring testaments. They are abnormal: "Not us! Not us!" But they are simultaneously frightening and challenge the "conventional boundaries between male and female, between sexed and sexless and between large and small." This ambivalence has historically translated into both the destruction (the dwarfs were one of Hitler's earliest victims) and the deification of freaks.

Jonathan Sinclair Carey's scholarly essay, "The Quasimodo Complex," can be summarized succinctly: every society has its ideal body image, pressure to conform to that image has always been pervasive and powerful, and those who deviate too far from the standard suffer. Body image has been elevated to a high pedestal by its equation with inner moral virtue. "The

morally best, the most beautiful. The morally worst, the most deformed." Prejudice against the deformed is documented in the "ugly laws." Until 1974, Chicago, like other American cities, could fine anyone appearing in public who was "diseased, maimed, mutilated, or in any way deformed so as to be an unsightly or disquieting object."

The Quasimodo Complex, named after Victor Hugo's horribly deformed hunchback, is defined as "the self perception and identity formation of concealed and unconcealed deformities engendered from the implicit and explicit reaction of others." We are told that "whether in employment or daily social exchanges, discrimination or prejudice based on the stigma of deformity may be a far more intolerable hell and reality than any other imaginable."

The widespread relevance of this work becomes evident as the list of "freaks" blossoms to include people with cerebral palsy, spina bifida, cleft palate, port wine stain, a missing limb, a missing breast, and epilepsy (an unseen deformity). It also includes the overweight (anorexics and bulimics strive to conform to the image of beauty as thinness) and the aging, whose wrinkles have become the object of cosmetic surgery in a society that idolizes youthful appearance.

The superb literary selections supplement and enliven the essays with stories and poems.

John Updike's leper, a potter whose ceramics are perfectly smooth, describes his affliction: "Spots, plaques, and avalanches of excess skin . . . expand and slowly migrate across the body, like lichen on a tombstone. I am silvery, scaly. Puddles of flakes form wherever I rest my flesh. My torture is skin deep: there is no pain, not even itching. We lepers are ironically healthy in other respects. Lusty, though we are loathsome to love. Keen sighted, though we hate to look upon ourselves. The name of the disease, spiritually speaking, is Humiliation."

Every night, Ray Bradbury's dwarf goes to the carnival's mirror maze. "Now, now he opened his eyelids and looked at a large mirror before him. And what he saw in the mirror made him smile. He winked, he pirouetted, he stood sidewise, he waved, he bowed, he did a little clumsy dance.

"And the mirror repeated each motion with long thin arms, with a tall, tall body, with a huge wink and an enormous repetition of the dance, ending in a gigantic bow!"

This book about freaks, the deformed, the maimed, and the misfits, in the end, says the most about the rest of us.

Review by Lois LaCivita Nixon, PHD, MLITT, MPH

Dirty Pretty Things: A Narrative Frame for Black Market Organ Sale
Written by Steven Knight, directed by Stephen Frears, Miramax Films, 2002: available on DVD

> Self-styled "brokers" arrange the sale of organs to patients who can pay. Kidneys are the most commonly traded organs, and in most cases, poor persons in developing nations sell their kidney to a wealthy patient. The cost . . . can run over $100,000 but the person actually selling an organ often sees very little of what amounts to a tremendous fortune.
>
> —"The Black Market in Organs"
> *Express News,* University of Alberta

In dark theaters many films force audiences to pay attention to ideas on the periphery, to examine ourselves and our society, and to be moved by potent moral issues. Swirling currents of change give rise to debates about new conditions, social movements, postcolonial studies, and speeded-up access of information and transportation. Not all images or outcomes are positive or hopeful but a good film story, such as the one described below, can function as a powerful tool for exposing problems affecting marginalized persons that ultimately affect all levels of society.

Dirty Pretty Things, a film directed by Stephen Frears, exemplifies some disturbing intersections of globalism, biotechnology, and amoral behaviors brought about by abuse and greed. This story, like others including *Death and the Maiden, Lone Star, Philadelphia, Whose Life Is It Anyway, Requiem for a Dream,* and *Traffic,* utilizes the postmodern genre of film to concretize social and ethical dilemmas also considered in tabloid headlines, textbooks, and at professional conferences. The film's astonishing revelations about black market organ trafficking and views of gritty reality for society's poorest, most vulnerable, and barely visible populations, invite audiences to see, sort through details, formulate explanations, question motivations, and understand more fully political, social, and ethical choices and consequences.

A very dark side of London is depicted in the film, a place where everything is for sale, at a price: prostitution, drugs, and most central to the story, black market sale of human organs. The compelling and suspenseful narrative focuses on five characters connected in one way or another to Hotel Baltic, a seemingly proper hotel by day, a site of depravity at night. Okwe, an illegal immigrant physician from Nigeria with no work papers, who has left home under harrowing circumstances, struggles with two menial jobs—driving a taxi during the day and working at night as the hotel's front desk clerk. At the hotel he befriends and assists one of the chambermaids, Senday, another immigrant from Turkey, also without papers and at risk of deportation, but also subject to sexual compromise and abuse.

Other figures include the hotel manager, the Russian doorman, and the Croatian prostitute. That they all have roots in places other than London underscores the overriding theme of alienation and loss of identity. In one way or another all are immigrants, alien figures in the substrata of London's vast underbelly, the people nobody sees. "Our guests," observes the sleazy manager, "are strangers—they leave dirty things, we make them pretty." Without the work performed by the constant churning groups of lower-class workers cleaning toilets, washing dishes, and sewing in sweatshops—in the hopes of gaining first-class citizenship—our own lives in London, New York, Paris, or Miami would be quite different and less "pretty" than what we now experience.

For some time into the film the director uses his lens to focus audience attention on the nightmarish settings of lower-class workers living at the edge, people living in a dirty, dark, and frightening world just below the surface we occupy. After spending time exploring the subterranean abyss with characters whose lives seem hopelessly lost, the film story moves in another direction to show just how vulnerable—and valuable—these people are to those who seize on opportunities to profit.

During the night, while checking on an obstructed and overflowing toilet in one of the hotel rooms, Okwe's unclogging efforts produce a removed human organ. Shocked by this discovery but in no position to alert authorities, he and other staff engage in whispered conversations. Soon they learn about secret operations arranged by the hotel's manager, the procuring middleman in the deal, who has taken advantage of hotel rooms and his employee pool of illegal immigrants to establish a lucrative organ-for-passport trade. Unqualified figures function as incompetent surgeons succeeding—or sometimes failing—in their closeted labors. All donors, of course, are undocumented, invisible, expendable, and beyond the knowledge and jurisdiction of the law. They, but particularly their desired "spare" part, are reduced to commodity status for those willing to pay large sums of money.

Frears' story, however horrible, is not science fiction. When we fail to ignore the poor, provide education and health care, and support human worth and dignity, we can expect the quality of our own lives to diminish. When we read about organ cannibalism or the sale of "body parts" in Iran, Tokyo, and California, we should be grateful to Stephen Frears for providing ethicists with a grim but useful framework for discussions that must occur.

George J. Annas, MPH, JD, is the Utley Professor of Health Law, and Chairman of Health Law Department at the Boston University School of Public Health.

Paul S. Appelbaum, MD, is Professor of Psychiatry and Director, Division of Psychiatry, Law and Ethics, Department of Psychiatry College of Physicians and Surgeons of Columbia University.

Robert M. Arnold, MD, is the Criep Chair in Patient Care, Professor of Medicine in the Division of General Internal Medicine and Chief, Section of Palliative Care and Medical Ethics at the University of Pittsburgh Medical Center.

Felice Aull, PhD, MA, is Associate Professor of Physiology and Neuroscience at New York University School of Medicine.

John A. Balint, MD, is Professor of Medicine and Director Emeritus of the Center for Medical Ethics at Albany Medical College.

Diane Beeson, PhD, is Professor of Sociology in the Department of Sociology and Social Services at California State University, East Bay.

Catherine Belling, PhD, is Assistant Professor, Preventive Medicine and Associate Director, Institute for Medicine in Contemporary Society Stony Brook University School of Medicine, Stony Brook, NY.

James L. Bernat, MD, is Professor of Medicine (Neurology) at Dartmouth Medical School and Associate Editor of the *Lahey Clinic Journal of Medical Ethics.*

Susan D. Block, MD, is Chief of the Adult Psychosocial Oncology Program at Dana Farber Cancer Institute Cancer Institute and Associate Professor of Psychiatry and Medicine at Harvard Medical School.

Sarah-Vaughan Brakman, PhD, is Director of the Ethics Program and Professor of Philosophy at Villanova University.

Allan M. Brandt, PhD, is the Kass Professor of The History of Medicine in the Department of Social Medicine at Harvard Medical School and Professor and Chair in the Department of the History of Science in the Faculty of Arts and Science at Harvard University.

Dan W. Brock, PhD, is the Lee Professor of Medical Ethics and Director of the Division of Medical Ethics at Harvard Medical School. He is Director of the Harvard University Program in Ethics and Health.

Howard Brody, MD, PhD, is Director of the Institute for the Medical Humanities and Professor, Family Medicine at the University of Texas Medical Branch.

Jeffrey Burns, MD, is Chief, Division of Critical Care Medicine and Director of the Medical-Surgical Intensive Care Unit at Children's Hospital Boston and Shapiro Chair of Critical Care Medicine and Associate Professor of Anesthesia, Harvard Medical School.

Daniel Callahan, PhD, is cofounder of The Hastings Center and Director, The International Program at The Hastings Center, Garrison, New York.

Sidney Callahan, PhD, is an author, lecturer, and psychologist and has held the McKeever Chair of Moral Theology, St. John's University, New York.

Alexander Morgan Capron, LLB, is Director, Ethics, Trade, Human Rights and Health Law at the World Health Organization, Geneva, Switzerland, and Professor of Law at the University of Southern California Law School.

Frank A. Chervenak, MD, is Professor, Chairman and Director of Maternal Fetal Medicine, Department of Obstetrics and Gynecology, New York Presbyterian Hospital, Weill Medical College of Cornell University.

Cynthia B. Cohen, PhD, JD, is a member of the Affiliated Faculty of the Kennedy Institute of Ethics at Georgetown University and a Fellow at The Hastings Center.

Yali Cong, PhD, is Associate Professor of Medical Ethics, Department of Medical Ethics at Peking University Health Science Center, Beijing, China.

Jack Coulehan, MD, MPH, is Professor, Preventive Medicine and Director, Institute for Medicine in Contemporary Society, Stony Brook University School of Medicine, Stony Brook, NY.

Dena S. Davis, JD, PhD, is a Professor of Law at Cleveland-Marshall College of Law, Cleveland State University.

Daniel C. Dennett, PhD, is University Professor and Fletcher Professor of Philosophy, and Director of the Center for Cognitive Studies at Tufts University.

Michael DeVita, MD, is Assistant Professor of Anesthesiology/Critical Care Medicine and Internal Medicine, University of Pittsburgh School of Medicine.

Rebecca Dresser, JD, is the Kirby Professor of Law and Professor of Ethics in Medicine, Washington University, Saint Louis.

Joseph J. Fins, MD, is Professor of Medicine and Public Health and Chief, Division of Medical Ethics at New York Weill Medical Center of Cornell University.

Gary S. Fischer, MD, is Assistant Professor of Medicine and Faculty, University of Pittsburgh Center for Bioethics and Health Law.

Anne L. Flamm, JD, is Clinical Assistant Professor in the Department of Critical Care at the University of Texas M.D. Anderson Cancer Center in Houston, TX.

Mandy Garber, MD, MPH, is a fellow in medical ethics within the Section of Palliative Care and Medical Ethics in the Division of General Internal Medicine, at the University of Pittsburgh Medical Center.

Bernard Gert, PhD, is the Stone Professor of Intellectual and Moral Philosophy at Dartmouth College.

Heather J. Gert, PhD, is Associate Professor of Philosophy at University of North Carolina, Greensboro.

Leonard H. Glantz, JD, is Professor of Health Law and Associate Dean for Academic Affairs at Boston University School of Public Health.

David Goldblatt, MD, is Professor Emeritus of Neurology and of Medical Humanities, University of Rochester School of Medicine and Dentistry, NY.

Jane Greenlaw, JD, is Associate Professor and Co-Director of the Center for Ethics, Humanities and Palliative Care at the University of Rochester Medical Center.

Thomas Gutheil, MD, is Professor of Psychiatry, Harvard Medical School and Co-Director, Program in Psychiatry and the Law, Massachusetts Mental Health Center.

David Haig, PhD, is Professor of Biology in the Department of Organismic and Evolutionary Biology at Harvard University.

Herbert Hendin, MD, is Executive Director of the American Suicide Foundation and Professor of Psychiatry at New York Medical College.

James J. Hughes, PhD, is Associate Director of Institutional Research and Planning at Trinity College, Hartford, Connecticut, and Executive Director of the Institute for Ethics and Emerging Technologies.

Susan C. Hunt, MD, is Professor of Medicine at the University of Pittsburgh School of Medicine.

Albert R. Jonsen, PhD, is Emeritus Professor of Ethics in Medicine at the School of Medicine, University of Washington.

Eric T. Juengst, PhD, is Professor of Bioethics, and Associate Professor of Oncology at the Case Western Reserve University School of Medicine in Cleveland, Ohio.

Jerome Kagan, PhD, is the Starch Professor of Psychology Emeritus at Harvard University.

Robert A. Katz, JD, is Associate Professor of Law and Dean's Fellow at the Indiana University School of Law, Indianapolis.

Nuala Kenny, OC, MD, is Professor, Departments of Bioethics and Pediatrics at Dalhousie University, Halifax, Nova Scotia.

Gerrit K. Kimsma, MD, PhD, is on the medical faculty and a member of the Center for Ethics and the Philosophy of Life at the Vrije Universiteit Medical Center, Amsterdam, Netherlands.

Paul Lauritzen, PhD, is Professor of Religious Studies and Director of the Program in Applied Ethics at John Carroll University in University Heights, Ohio.

Benfu Li, MD, is Professor, Department of Medical Ethics and Director of Division of Medical Ethics at the Peking University Health Science Center, Beijing, China, and Chair, Chinese Medical Ethics Association.

Ruth Macklin, PhD, is Professor, Department of Epidemiology & Population Health, Division Head, Division of Philosophy and History of Medicine and the Trachtenberg Faculty Scholar in Biomedical Ethics and Professor of Bioethics in the Department of Epidemiology and Population Health at the Albert Einstein College of Medicine.

David Magnus, PhD, is Associate Professor of Pediatrics, Medicine, and Philosophy at Stanford University, and Director of the Stanford Center for Biomedical Ethics.

Gerald Q. Maguire, Jr, PhD, is Professor of Computer Communication at the Royal Institute of Technology in Stockholm, Sweden.

Mary Anderlik Majumder, JD, PhD, is Assistant Professor of Medicine with the Center for Medical Ethics and Health Policy at the Baylor College of Medicine.

Wendy K. Mariner, JD, is Professor of Law, Boston University School of Law, Professor of Health Law and Director, Patient Rights Program, Boston University School of Public Health, and Professor of Socio-Medical Sciences and Community Medicine, Boston University School of Medicine.

Laurence B. McCullough, PhD, is Professor of Medicine and Medical Ethics in the Center for Ethics and Health Policy at the Baylor College of Medicine in Houston, Texas.

Ellen M. McGee, PhD, is Director Emerita of The Long Island Center for Ethics.

Glenn McGee, PhD, is Professor of Medicine and Director of the Alden March Bioethics Institute at Albany Medical College.

Maxwell J. Mehlman, JD, is the Petersilge Professor of Law and Director of the Law-Medicine Center at Case Western Reserve University School of Law and Professor of Bioethics at the Case Western School of Medicine.

Gilbert Meilaender, PhD, is Professor of Theology and Duesenberg Chair in Christian Ethics at Valparaiso University in Valparaiso, Indiana.

Jon F. Merz, MBA, JD, PhD, is Associate Professor in the Department of Medical Ethics in the School of Medicine and Senior Fellow in the Center for Bioethics at the University of Pennsylvania.

Frances H. Miller, JD, is Professor of Law, Boston University School of Law and Professor of Public Health, Boston University School of Public Health, and Professor of Health Care Management, Boston University School of Management.

Thomas H. Murray, PhD, is President of The Hastings Center in Garrison, New York.

Lawrence J. Nelson, PhD, JD, is Senior Lecturer, Philosophy Department at Santa Clara University.

Stuart A. Newman, PhD, is Professor, Cell Biology and Anatomy at New York Medical College.

Lois LaCivita Nixon, PhD, MPH, is Professor in Medical Ethics and Humanities, College of Medicine and College of Public Health, University of South Florida, Tampa.

Robert D. Orr, MD, CM, is Clinical Professor in the Department of Family Medicine and Director of Ethics at Fletcher Allen Health Care at the University of Vermont College of Medicine in Burlington, Vermont.

David Ozar, PhD, is Professor, Department of Philosophy, Loyola University, Chicago.

Erik Parens, PhD, is a Senior Research Scholar at The Hastings Center and Adjunct Associate Professor in the Program in Science, Technology, and Society of Vassar College.

Robert A. Pearlman, MD, MPH, is a Professor of Medicine, Health Services, and Medical History and Ethics at the University of Washington and Chief, Ethics Evaluation Service, National Center for Ethics in Health Care.

Timothy E. Quill, MD, is Professor of Medicine, Psychiatry, and Medical Humanities and Director, Center for Palliative Care and Clinical Ethics at the University of Rochester, School of Medicine and Dentistry.

Richard M. Ratzan, MD, is Associate Professor, Department of Traumatology and Emergency Medicine, University of Connecticut School of Medicine.

Paul J. Reitemeier, PhD, is Associate Professor, Research and Development Division of the Graduate College and Chair of the Research Review Committee at Grand Valley State University in Allendale, Michigan.

John A. Robertson, JD, holds the Vinson and Elkins Chair at The University of Texas School of Law at Austin.

Walter M. Robinson, MD, MPH, is Senior Associate in Medicine, Center for Applied Ethics and Professional Practice, Education Development Center, Newton, MA; and Associate Professor of Pediatrics, Medicine and Bioethics, Dalhousie University, Halifax, Nova Scotia.

Lainie Friedman Ross, MD, PhD, is Associate Director, MacLean Center for Clinical Medical Ethics and Professor of Medicine at the University of Chicago.

James E. Sabin, MD, is Clinical Professor in the Department of Psychiatry and the Department of Ambulatory Care and Prevention at Harvard Medical School and Director of the Harvard Pilgrim Health Care Ethics Program.

Lawrence J. Schneiderman, MD, is Professor, Medicine and Family and Preventive Medicine at the School of Medicine, University of California, San Diego.

Richard A. Shweder is the Reavis Distinguished Service Professor of Human Development at the University of Chicago.

Peter Singer, MA, BPHIL, is the DeCamp Professor of Bioethics, University Center for Human Values, Princeton University.

Norman P. Spack, MD, is Clinical Director, Department of Endocrinology at Children's Hospital Boston and Assistant Professor in Pediatrics, Harvard Medical School.

Margaret Gail Spinelli, MD, is Associate Professor of Clinical Psychiatry, Columbia University College of Physicians and Surgeons and Director of the Maternal Mental Health Program, New York State Psychiatric Institute.

David Steinberg, MD, is Chief, Section of Medical Ethics at the Lahey Clinic Medical Center in Burlington, Massachusetts, and Assistant Clinical Professor of Medicine at Harvard Medical School.

Sharon Steinberg, RN, MS, CS, is mental health consultant in the Center for Fertility and Reproductive Health, Harvard Vanguard Medical Associates and Lecturer in the Department of Ambulatory Care and Prevention, Harvard Medical School.

Robert M. Taylor, MD, is Associate Professor of Neurology, Ohio State University College of Medicine.

Nicholas P. Terry, LLM, is Myers Professor of Law and Co-Director, Center for Health Law Studies, Saint Louis University School of Law.

Rosemarie Tong, PhD, is Distinguished Professor of Health Care Ethics at the University of North Carolina.

Leigh Turner, PhD, is an Associate Professor, Biomedical Ethics Unit and Chair of the Master's Specialization in Bioethics Program at McGill University in Montreal.

Robert M. Veatch, PhD, is Professor of Medical Ethics and the former Director of the Kennedy Institute of Ethics at Georgetown University.

Andrew G. Villanueva, MD, is Clinical Instructor of Medicine, Harvard Medical School, Clinical Assistant Professor of Medicine, Tufts University School of Medicine, and a member of the Pulmonary and Critical Care Department, Lahey Clinic Medical Center, Burlington, MA.

Delese Wear, PhD, is Professor of Behavioral Sciences, Northeastern Ohio Universities College of Medicine.

Garrath Williams, PhD, is Lecturer in Philosophy at the Institute for Philosophy and Public Policy at Lancaster University, Lancaster, UK.

David Sloan Wilson, PhD, is Professor, Departments of Biology and Anthropology at Binghamton University in Binghamton, NY.

William J. Winslade, PhD, JD, is the Rockwell Professor of Philosophy of Medicine, The Institute for the Medical Humanities at The University of Texas Medical Branch, Galveston.

Arthur P. Wolf, PhD, is the Packard Foundation Professor in Human Biology in the Anthropological Sciences Department at Stanford University.

Paul Root Wolpe, PhD, is Professor in the Department of Psychiatry and Senior Fellow at the Center for Bioethics at the University of Pennsylvania.

David Wykes, PhD, is Professor of English at Dartmouth College.

Xiuyun Yin, PhD, is Assistant Professor, Peking University Health Science Center, Beijing, China.

Stuart J. Youngner, MD, is the Watson Professor of Bioethics, Professor of Psychiatry and Chair, Department of Bioethics at Case Western Reserve University.

Laurie Zoloth, PhD, is Professor of Medical Humanities & Bioethics and Religion and Director of the Center for Bioethics, Science and Society at Northwestern University.

autonomy *(continued)*
183–84, 201, 203, 208, 279; science and technology as opposed to, 29; unfettered, 143
auto-resuscitation, 84, 86
availability of interventions, and information disclosure to patients, 201, 203, 204
avoiding unsurprising surprises, principle of, 202–3, 204, 205, 206

B

bacteria, genetically engineered, 152
Bailey, Michael, 99–100
Balint, John A., 207
Banks, Russell, 342–43
Baylor University Medical Center, 298
Beauchamp, Tom L., 5, 43–44, 47, 220
Beecher, Henry, 7
Beeson, Diane, 128, 132–33, 134
behavioral genetics, crime prevention as aim of, 312–15
Being Human (President's Council on Bioethics), 107
Bellah, Robert, 20
Belling, Catherine, 334
beneficence: can HIV-positive woman be forced to take medication to protect her fetus?, 221; confidentiality conflicting with, 184; cross-cultural differences regarding, 257; in principlism, 5; toward fetus and pregnant woman, 262
Benjamin, Harry, International Gender Dysphoria Association, 96, 98, 101
bereavement, as grounds for euthanasia, 251, 254
Bernardin, Joseph Cardinal, 310
Bernat, James L.: Annas's response to, 237; on brain death, 56–57, 78–81; DeVita and Arnold's response to, 82–83, 84; on physicians overtreating seriously ill, 234–36; response to Annas, 238; response to DeVita and Arnold, 85; review of Lightman's *The Diagnosis*, 343
Better Than Well (Elliot), 100
Beyond Therapy: Biotechnology and the Pursuit of Happiness (President's Council on Bioethics), 100, 107
biodiversity, genetically modified organisms as threat to, 151
Bioethics: A Return to Fundamentals (Gert, Culver, Clouser), 47
biomedical ethics: in clinical arena, 181–276; conservative, 108–9; in culturally diverse societies, 42–52; decisions as unavoidable, 4;

discourse versus discipline of, 4, 13; emergence of, 7–13; feminist approaches to, 6, 35–42; governmental commissions on, 326–29; and the humanities, 331–58; institutional problems of, 9, 12–13; and language, 53–103; and the law, 279–81; limits of, 46, 47; nature of, 3–6; and novel technologies, 105–80; philosophers and theologians in, 4, 12, 35; President's Commission for the Study of Ethical Problems in Medicine and Biomedical and Behavioral Research, 327–28; President's Council on Bioethics, 45, 100, 107; religion and, 29–35; social and political influences on, 4, 8. *See also* ethics consultation
Birth-mark, The (Hawthorne), 107
black market organ trafficking, 357–58
Block, Susan D., 243, 247
blood transfusion, informing patient of possible transmission of Creutzfeldt-Jakob disease from, 199–201, 203–5
body image, 356–57
body modification technologies, 102
Bornstein, Kate, 101
Bradbury, Ray, 357
brain chips, implantable, 164–72
brain damage: death row inmates with, 280, 316; traumatic brain damage and criminal responsibility, 315–18
brain death, 78–86; defined, 78; grounds for abandoning concept of, 79; higher-brain criteria, 56–57, 80; as misleading term, 79, 82; must multiorgan donors be brain dead?, 271–74; and removal of artificial heart, 59–60, 63, 66; whole-brain death, 56–57, 80, 85–86
Brakman, Sarah-Vaughan, 55–56, 70, 74, 75, 77
Brandt, Allan M., 4, 7, 10
Brave New World (Huxley), 139–40
BRCA1 gene, 282
Brock, Dan W.: Callahan's response to, 117, 118; on human cloning, 57, 110–13; on incompetent patients, 208–10; on liver allocation, 176–79; Macklin's response to, 113–14; response to Callahan, 118; response to Macklin, 115–16; Veatch's response to, 179, 180
Brody, B. A., 88
Brody, Howard, 231
Bt corn, 151–52
Buchanan, Allen, 313–14
Buckley, Sheryl, 356–57
Buck v. Bell (1927), 281, 314

communication problems with care givers, rational suicide and, 244

community: ethics of, 19, 20; femininity associated with, 36

confidentiality: with alcohol use by school bus driver, 230–31; beneficence conflicting with, 184; disclosing results of genetic testing to others, 284; the law in protection of, 279; Minnesota "Crack Baby" law and, 280; should clinical trial coordinator blow the whistle if study integrity is compromised?, 231–34. See also privacy

conflict of ethical principles, 184

Cong, Yali, 259

Conquering Schizophrenia: A Father, His Son and a Medical Breakthrough (Wyden), 347–49

consent. See informed consent

consequentialism. See utilitarianism (consequentialism)

constitutional rights, behavioral genetics and, 314

consultation. See ethics consultation

contracting for quality healthcare, 303–6

controlled non-heart-beating organ donation, 83

Cook, Stephen, 310

Cotton, Henry, 348

Coulehan, Jack, 336, 350

covenant, 12

"Crack Baby" law (Minnesota), 280

credentialing, cybermedicine and, 302

Creutzfeldt-Jakob disease (CJD), informing patient of possible exposure to, 199–201, 203–5

crime: behavioral genetics for prevention of, 312–15; DNA analysis showing innocence of convicted criminals, 280–81; forensic gene databanks, 157–58, 160; traumatic brain damage and criminal responsibility, 315–18

cross-cultural issues: in doctor-patient relationship, 256–59; in Fadiman's The Spirit Catches You and You Fall Down, 339–40

cross-hormones, 97, 98

Cruzan v. Director, Missouri Department of Health, 279

cultural evolution, as multilevel process, 24

culturally diverse societies, biomedical ethics in, 42–52

Culver, Charles M., 80

cybermedicine, legal pitfalls of, 299–302

"cyberthink," 165

"cyborgs," 108, 164

cystic fibrosis, 136

D

Darkness Visible: A Memoir of Madness (Styron), 346–47

Data Protection authorities, 163

Davis, Dena S., 320

dead donor rule, 56, 81, 82, 86, 272–73

death: cardiac-based definition of, 56, 59–60, 63, 83, 84, 273; defining for organ donation, 56–57; direct versus indirect causes of, 58–60, 62–67; in Edson's Wit, 349–50; "most reasonable" definition of, 80, 82–83; in Nuland's How We Die, 341–42; optimal analysis of concept of, 80; statutory tests for, 78–79; values in criteria for, 82, 85. See also brain death; end-of-life care; killing

death-by-cardiac-determination (DCD) organ donation, 56

Death of the Good Doctor: Lessons from the Heart of the AIDS Epidemic (Scannell), 352–53

"death with dignity" movement, 234

decision making: components of ethical, 187; decision maker's perspective in information disclosure to patients, 201, 203, 204–5; non-medical values in clinical decisions, 183–86; parents' discretion in making decisions for their children, 218, 219, 221; as unavoidable in bioethics, 4. See also surrogate decision makers

deCode Genetics, 159, 160, 162–63

Definition of Death, The (Youngner, Arnold, Schapiro), 56

deformity, 356–57

deLeon, Dennis, 192

Dennett, Daniel C., 168, 171

deontological ethics, 5, 34, 175–76

Depo-Provera, 313

depression: in Jamison's An Unquiet Mind, 345–46; refusing treatment in case of suicide attempt by depressed patient, 215–17; in Styron's Darkness Visible: A Memoir of Madness, 346–47

determinism, 142

DeVita, Michael A., 57, 82, 85, 86

Dewey, John, 17

Diagnosis, The (Lightman), 343–45

"dialysis suicide," 11

Diamond v. Chakrabarty (1980), 291, 292

Dickey Amendment, 74

dignity. See human dignity

dilemmas, moral, 34

direct-to-consumer marketing of prescription drugs, 301–2

Dirty Pretty Things: A Narrative Frame for Black Market Organ Sale (film), 357–58

disabilities: allowing quadriplegics time for reflection before discontinuing life support, 213–15; in Banks's *The Sweet Hereafter*, 342–43; disability rights activists and family decision-making authority, 295; in Million Dollar Baby, 338–39; prenatal testing and abortion in cases of, 128–35; traumatic brain damage as cause of, 315

disease. *See* illness

divinity, ethics of, 19

DNA analysis: innocence of convicted criminals shown by, 280–81; for parentage determination, 285

DNA Sciences, 161

DNR (do-not-resuscitate) orders, 235, 236, 264

Dobelle Eye, 164–65

doctors. *See* physicians

Doctor Stories, The (Selzer), 334–36

Dolly (sheep), 110, 114, 152, 292

donation. *See* gamete donation; organ donation; tissue donation

Donley, Carol, 356–57

Donne, John, 349, 355

donor of last resort, 276

donor rights laws, 280

do-not-resuscitate (DNR) orders, 235, 236, 264

Dostoevsky, Feodor, 17

double effect, principle of, 34, 59, 64, 240

Down syndrome, 128, 130, 133, 191

Dresser, Rebecca, 323

DrKoop (Web site), 300

drugs, illegal. *See* illegal drugs

duodenal atresia, 191

Durable Power of Attorney for Health Care (DPAHC), 196–98, 294, 295, 328

Dutch Voluntary Euthanasia Society, 250

dwarfs, 357

E

eating disorders, 37, 39

Edson, Margaret, 349–50

egg (oocyte) donation, 120–28; for assessing new reproductive technologies, 119; legal protection lacking for donors, 280; for lesbian couple, 125–28; as reproductive freedom, 111; resource allocation in, 123; rights and responsibilities of gamete donors, 286–87; risks to donors of, 121–22, 124; uncertainties in unregulated, 123–25

Elliot, Carl, 100

emancipated minors, 218

embryos: adoption of excess, 55–56, 70–78; considered as children, 55–56, 71, 74–75, 77, 108, 136; human chimera patent initiative, 290–93; informed consent for stem cell research using frozen, 320–23; preimplantation genetic testing, 128, 135–44

emotions: versus reason in moral debate, 154–57. *See also* repugnance

emotivism, 4–5, 18–21, 44–45

empathy: emergence of sense of, 15; empathy gap between physicians and patients, 351

employers, contracting for quality healthcare with insurers, 303–6

end-of-life care: artificial heart raising new problem for, 58–60; do physicians overtreat the seriously ill?, 234–38; North American debates over, 45; rational suicide and terminal illness, 243–48; in Selzer's *The Doctor Stories*, 335; surrogates making seemingly irrational requests for, 241–42; uncertainties regarding end-of-life scenarios, 185–86. *See also* palliative (comfort) care

"ends justify the means," 25

enhancement: as abuse of medicine, 146; as cheating, 145–46, 148, 149; in gene therapy, 144–50; implantable brain chips for, 165, 166, 170; preimplantation genetic diagnosis and, 138, 140, 141; treatment-enhancement distinctions, 144–45, 147

epilepsy, 339–40

equity (fairness): in access to medical care, 8; for egg donors, 124; emotions associated with, 21; genetic enhancement and, 138, 146; law promoting, 280; for minorities, 16; in organ allocation, 173–80; in principlism, 5; strong reciprocity for enforcing, 26; technology and, 170

error, medical. *See* medical error

ethics: components of ethical decision making, 187; deontological, 5, 34, 175–76; dictionary definition of, 3; language as indispensable medium in, 55–58; philosophical disagreements over, 3; principlism, 5, 43–44, 47–48, 50. *See also* biomedical ethics; morality; utilitarianism (consequentialism)

ethics consultation: disvalue of, 193; measuring value of, 192–93; as not ethics police force, 189, 191; as not relieving clinicians of their professional responsibility, 186, 193; roles of, 192; value of, 186–90; who it serves, 190–94; why someone would ask for, 190

genetically modified organisms, 150–57
genetic counseling, 130
genetic enhancement. *See* enhancement
genetic fingerprint, 158
genetics, behavioral, crime prevention as aim of, 312–15
genetic testing: disclosing results to others, 281–84; preimplantation, 128, 135–44, 326–27
gene transfer techniques, 144–50
genitoplasty, 96, 97
genocide, 27
Genomics Collaborative, 161
Genovo, 323
germ-line therapy, 156, 312
Geron Corporation, 292
Gert, Bernard, 3, 5, 47, 50, 51, 80
Gert, Heather J., 186, 202, 206
Gilbert, Sandra M., 333–34
Gilligan, Carol, 35–36
Glantz, Leonard H., 281
globalization, 42, 357
global positioning systems (GPS), 168–69
GnRH analogues, 97, 98
Goldblatt, David, 196; review of *Million Dollar Baby,* 338–39
Goldstein, Melissa Anne, 350–52
"good dying," rational suicide and lack of vision of, 243, 245–46
governmental bioethics commissions, 326–29
graphical user interface, 170
Greenlaw, Jane, 287
Groopman, Jerome, 140–41
groupishness, 27
growth hormone for short children, 146
guilt, 15, 16, 17, 21
Gutheil, Thomas, 309

H

HAART (highly active antiretroviral therapy), 220–22
Haig, David, 5–6, 25, 28
Hallie, Philip, 155
harms of information disclosure, 201, 203, 204
Harry Benjamin International Gender Dysphoria Association, 96, 98, 101
Hastings Center, The, 155
Hawthorne, Nathaniel, 107
Health and Human Services, Department of, 324
health business models, cybermedicine affecting, 301
healthcare quality, contracting for, 303–6
Healtheon, 300

Health Plan Employer Data and Information Set (HEDIS), 304
heart, artificial. *See* artificial heart
heart transplants, cost of, 61
height (stature), 138, 146
Helft, P. R., 267
Hemlock Society, 243
hemodialysis. *See* renal dialysis
Hendin, Herbert, 247
hermaphrodites, 101
Heywood, Jamie, 354–55
Hippocratic tradition, 175
Hirihito (emperor of Japan), 183
His Brother's Keeper: A Story from the Edge of Medicine (Weiner), 354–55
HIV: can HIV-positive woman be forced to take medication to protect her fetus?, 220–22; patient confidentiality and informing spouse of, 184; rational suicide and AIDS, 247; in Scannell's *Death of the Good Doctor: Lessons from the Heart of the AIDS Epidemic,* 352–53
Hmong, 339–40
Hodgkin's disease, teenagers' refusal of assent to treatment for, 217–19
Hoffman La Roche, 159
Holmes, Oliver Wendell, Jr., 281, 314
Holocaust, 27, 29, 155
homosexuality: transsexualism and, 100. *See also* lesbians
Hooking Up (Wolfe), 142
hormonal replacement therapy, 96, 98
House of Commons Scientific and Technology Committee, 114
How We Die (Nuland), 341–42
Hughes, James J., 57, 99
human chimera patent initiative, 290–93
human cloning. *See* cloning of human beings
Human Cloning Prohibition Act, 290, 292
human dignity: cloning of human beings and, 57, 115; in conservative rhetoric, 108; "death with dignity" movement, 234; live organ donation from patient in persistent vegetative state seen as violation of, 276
Human Fertilisation and Embryology Authority (United Kingdom), 326–27
human gene banks, 157–64
humanities, biomedical ethics and the, 331–58
Human Performance in Extreme Environment (journal), 226
Hume, David, 18
Hunt, Susan C., 220
Huntington's disease, 158, 313
Huxley, Aldous, 139–40

hypnosis, recovered memories controversy and, 310
hypospadias, 101

I

iatrogenic injury, 303
Icelandic Health Sector Database, 158–59, 160, 161, 162–63
idolatry, 30
ileus-like syndrome, 223
illegal drugs: Minnesota "Crack Baby" law, 280; pregnant women using, 288
illness: do physicians overtreat the seriously ill?, 234–38; language in perception of, 57. *See also* mental illness; terminal illness; *and particular illnesses by name*
Illness as Metaphor (Sontag), 57
implantable brain chips, 164–72
implantable cardioverter-defribrillator (ICD), patient insists on removal of, 207–8
implementation of ethical decisions, 188–89
impulsive behavior, traumatic brain damage as cause of, 315–16
incest: in Banks's *The Sweet Hereafter,* 342, 343; defined, 68; emotional charge of term, 55; father's sperm for in vitro fertilization seen as, 67–70; taboo against, 68–69
incompetent patients, forgoing potentially lifesaving treatment for, 208–10
individuality, cloning of human beings seen as threat to, 112, 117–18, 119
infant adoption, 71, 72
infanticide, maternal, insanity defense and, 318–20
information disclosure to patients, 198–206
informed consent: allowing quadriplegics time for reflection before discontinuing life support, 213–15; for astronauts in clinical research, 224–28; in clinical medicine and research, 7–8; cross-cultural differences regarding, 257, 258; and disclosing results of genetic testing to others, 284; for experimental fetal surgery, 89, 90–94; for human gene banking, 159, 160, 163; for implantable brain chips, 166; in intensive care unit treatment, 237–38; the law in protection of, 279; in live organ donation from patient in persistent vegetative state, 275; mental age of consent for live organ donation, 210–12; physician's authority taken for granted in, 8; refusing treatment in case of suicide attempt by depressed patient, 215–17; socioeconomic gradient regarding, 8; for

sperm donation, 270; for stem cell research using frozen embryos, 320–23; teenagers' refusal of assent to treatment, 217–19
In re A.C. (1987), 221
In re Quinlan, 279
insanity defense: maternal infanticide and, 318–20; traumatic brain damage and criminal responsibility, 316, 317
Institute of Medicine, 84, 222, 226, 303
Institutional Review Boards (IRBs), 7, 324
insurers: employers contracting for quality healthcare with, 303–6; ethics of physicians lying to, 194–96
Intel-AMA initiative, 302
intellectual property rights: research and, 324. *See also* patents
intensive care units (ICUs): do physicians overtreat the seriously ill in?, 234–38; invoking medical futility policies, 266–68
intention, exculpating bad effects by appeal to, 63–64
Internet, legal pitfalls of cybermedicine, 299–302
intersexed births, 101
Intersex Society of North America, 101
in vitro fertilization: conservative opposition to, 109; embryo adoption, 55–56, 70–78; father as sperm donor seen as incest, 67–70; preimplantation genetic testing, 128, 135–44; as reproductive freedom, 111. *See also* gamete donation
ischemia, 83, 173, 177
Islam, on egg donation, 121

J

Jamison, Kay Redfield, 345–46
Japan, patient autonomy in, 183
Jensen, Lene, 20
job performance, quality of life and, 168–69
Joint Commission on Accreditation of Healthcare Organizations, 7
Jonas, Hans, 12
Jonsen, Albert R., 4, 10, 207, 279
judgment, ethical, 187–88
Juengst, Eric T., 144, 147, 148, 149
justice: care versus, 36, 40–41; masculinity associated with, 36; in organ allocation, 174, 179–80; in principlism, 5; religion on centrality of, 31–32. *See also* equity (fairness)

K

Kafka, Franz, 355
Kagan, Jerome, 4–5, 14, 18, 19, 20

Kahn, Jeffrey, 142

Kamm, Frances, 178

Kant, Immanuel, 5, 17, 137, 268

Kass, Leon R., 4, 45, 107, 114, 116, 119, 153, 154

Katz, Robert A., 306

Kenny, Nuala P., 217

kidney transplantation, mental age of consent for live organ donation, 210–12

killer bees, 152

killing: absolute rejection as not widespread, 63; direct versus indirect, 58–60, 62–67; murder distinguished from, 63; spectrum of, 63. *See also* euthanasia; suicide

Kimsma, G. K., 249, 252, 255

Knight, Steven, 357–58

Korein, Julius, 85

Koski, Sandra, 309

Kraeplin, Emil, 348

L

Lancet, The, 136

Laney, Deanna, 319

language: emotionally-charged, 55, 62; power of, 55–58

Lauritzen, Paul, 107, 139, 143

Law Review Procedures for Termination of Life on Request (Netherlands), 250

learned intermediary doctrine, 301–2

legal guardian, appointment of, 209–10

"legitimacy" of children, 285

leprosy, 356–57

lesbians: egg donation for lesbian couple, 125–28; in Scannell's *Death of the Good Doctor: Lessons from the Heart of the AIDS Epidemic,* 353

Lewis, Dorothy Otnow, 316

Li, Benfu, 259

liberal democracies, cultural diversity in, 42–43

licensure, cybermedicine and, 300, 302

life: lack of agreement over beginning of, 82; medically contingent, 64–65; "sanctity of life," 31, 263; wrongful life suits, 144. *See also* death; end-of-life care; life support; quality of life

life support: allowing quadriplegics time for reflection before discontinuing, 213–15; artificial heart and forgoing of, 58–60, 62–67; brain death and, 79, 83; cross-cultural differences regarding, 259–61; family demands for futile treatment, 264–66; President's Commission for the Study of Ethical Problems in Medicine and Biomedical and

Behavioral Research and discontinuing, 327; refusing treatment in case of suicide attempt by depressed patient, 215–17; Wendland case, 293–95. *See also* renal dialysis (hemodialysis); ventilator

Lightman, Alan, 343–45

Lilford, R. J., 88

Lippman, A., 130

live organ donation: mental age of consent for, 210–12; from persistent vegetative state patient, 274–76

livers, allocation of, 172–80

living wills, 184–85, 196, 327

Lo, Bernard, 235

Louisiana, 75, 173

Love, Medicine and Miracles (Siegel), 352

Lovejoy, Arthur, 20

Lucid, Shannon, 228

lupus erythematosus, 350–52

lying to insurance companies, ethics of, 194–96

Lynn, Joanne, 37–38, 40–41

M

Macklin, Ruth, 57, 108, 113, 116, 117, 118

mad cow disease, 152, 199

Magnus, David, 5, 150, 154, 155, 157

Maguire, Gerald Q., Jr., 164, 166, 168, 171

Majumder, Mary Anderlik, 56, 74, 77, 78

malpractice, cybermedicine and, 301

mammoplasty, reduction, 97

managed care: cybermedicine and malpractice liability in, 301; ethics of physicians lying to insurance companies, 194–96; physicians' autonomy eroded by, 9; and respect for patient rights, 237

manic-depressive illness, 345–46

Mann, Charles, 312

Mantle, Mickey, 172

Man Who Would Be Queen: The Science of Gender Bending and Transsexualism (Bailey), 99–100

Marshfield Clinic, 161, 162, 164

Massachusetts Group Insurance Commission, 305

Massachusetts Health Care Purchasers Group, 304

maternal infanticide, insanity defense and, 318–20

maternal serum screening, 128

mature minors, 218

Mayo, T. M., 298

Mayo Clinic, 175, 300

McCullough, Laurence B., 56, 91, 93, 262
McGee, Ellen M., 164, 166, 168, 171
McGee, Glenn, 147, 149
McHugh, Paul, 100
mechanical ventilator. *See* ventilator
Medicaid, quality issues in, 304
Medical Biobank of Umeå, 162
medical error: Gilbert's *Wrongful Death: A Memoir*, 333–34; iatrogenic injury, 303
medical futility: as among few controversial issues, 48; categories of discussion of, 267; defining, 265, 267; family demands for futile treatment, 264–66; invoking policies on, 266–68; living wills and, 185; North American debates over, 45; and removal of artificial heart, 60; Texas Advance Directives Act, 296–99; uncertainties regarding, 185
medically contingent life, 64–65
medical managers, increasing authority of, 12
medical research. *See* research
medical tourism, 101
Medicare, quality issues in, 304
medicine in extreme environments, 226
Mehlman, Maxwell J., 312
Meilaender, Gilbert, 6, 39
meiotic drive, 23–24
memories, recovered, 309–12
mental age of consent for live organ donation, 210–12
mental illness: postpartum psychosis, 318–19; in Wyden's *Conquering Schizophrenia*, 347–49. *See also* depression; insanity defense; psychiatry
Merz, Jon F., 161
microorganisms, genetically engineered, 152
Miller, Francis H., 303
Million Dollar Baby (film), 338–39
Minnesota "Crack Baby" law, 280
minor treatment statutes, 218
miracles, 264–65
M'Naghten Test, 318–19
monitoring boards, for experimental fetal surgery clinical trials, 88, 92
morality: amoral roots of, 25–29; biological basis of, 22–25; cross-cultural variability in, 19; as motivator, 27; nature of, 14–21; religion and moral awareness, 30; religion in shaping, 44, 45, 49; universal standards of, 19–20, 43; unresolvable moral disagreements, 49–50. *See also* ethics
moral relativism: acceptance of moral conflict and, 52; righteous anger and, 27

moral sense, emergence of, 14–15
motivation, ethical, 188
multilevel selection, 23–29
murder: killing distinguished from, 63; removal of artificial heart and, 55, 58–67
Murray, Thomas H., 135, 140, 141, 142
myotonic dystrophy, 136

N

NASA (National Aeronautics and Space Administration), 222–29
Nash, Molly and Adam, 137, 141–42
National Academy of Sciences, 292
National Advisory Board on Ethics in Reproduction, 127
National Bioethics Advisory Commission (NBAC), 110, 112, 114, 321
National Committee for Quality Assurance, 303
National Embryo Donation Center, 72, 76
National Institutes of Health (NIH), 162, 314, 321–22
National Organ Transplantation Act (NOTA) (1984), 280, 306–7
National Public Defenders Association, 316
"natural death" statutes, 327
naturalistic fallacy, 28
natural reason, 49, 51, 52
natural selection: as amoral, 25, 27; multilevel selection, 23–29
Nelson, Lawrence J., 293
Netherlands, 66, 248, 249–52, 255
neural interfacing, 165
neural tube defects, 128
New Age healing, 352
Newman, Stuart A., 290
New York State Task Force on Life and the Law, 286–87
Nietzsche, Friedrich, 309
Nightlight Christian Adoptions, 75, 76
Nixon, Lois LaCivita, 349, 357
Noddings, Nel, 35, 36
non-health-related traits, 138, 140, 141, 144–45
non-heart-beating organ donation, 56, 57, 81, 82, 83–84, 86, 273–74
nonmalificence, principle of, 5, 265
normality, 356–57
Norplant, 302
Novagen, 161
Nuland, Sherwin B., 341–42

O

Oasis (Web site), 300
Office of Human Research Protections, 228

Oncomouse, 292

Oregon, 13, 66, 249, 254–55, 280

organ donation: brain death associated with, 79; from cloned twins, 111; dead donor rule, 56, 81, 82, 86, 272–73; defining death for, 56–57; mental age of consent for live donation, 210–12; must multiorgan donors be brain dead?, 271–74; non-heart-beating organ donation, 56, 57, 81, 82, 83–84, 86, 273–74; Pittsburgh Protocol, 81, 83–84

organisms, genetically modified, 150–57

Organ Procurement and Transplant Network (OPTN), 280

organ procurement organizations (OPOs), 172–73, 175, 306

organ transplantation: allocation of livers for, 172–80; black market organ trafficking, 357–58; economics of, 174; heart transplant costs, 61. *See also* organ donation

Orr, Robert D., 190, 271

Orwell, George, 139

"ought and *is,"* 28

Our Posthuman Future: Consequences of the Biotechnology Revolution (Fukuyama), 139–40

ovarian hyperstimulation, 122

Ozar, David, 186, 191, 192

P

Pacific Business Group for Health, 304, 305

pacifism, 67

pain: in alleged overtreatment of the seriously ill, 235, 237; rational suicide and, 243–44, 247; terminal sedation and euthanasia, 55, 238–40

palliative care: increasing recognition of, 234; moving out of hospital setting, 237; as never futile, 265; and patients with intermediate prognosis of survival, 236; and rational suicide, 243–44

Parens, Erik, 135, 140, 141, 142

parents: discretion in making decisions for their children, 218, 219, 221; genetic testing reveals that apparent father is not biological father, 281–82; rights and responsibilities of gamete donors, 284–87; Uniform Parentage Act, 76, 285–86

patents: human chimera patent initiative, 290–93; on human genes, 163–64

paternity, common-law presumption of, 285

patient confidentiality. *See* confidentiality

patient rights: do physicians overtreat the seriously ill?, 234–38; early focus on psychiatry, 8; the law in protection of, 279; medical managers usurping authority of, 12

patients: biomedical ethics leading to patient-centered ethic, 8; cross-cultural conflict in doctor-patient relationship, 256–59; ethics consultation's value for, 193; forgoing potentially lifesaving treatment for incompetent, 208–10; information disclosure to, 198–206; refusal of beneficial care by, 207–8; respect for autonomy of, 183–84, 201, 203, 208. *See also* patient rights

Peabody, Francis, 337

Pearlman, Robert A., 256

Peirce, Charles Sanders, 17

Pence, Gregory, 154

Pennsylvania, University of, 323

Perez v. Wyeth Laboratories, Inc., 302

persistent vegetative state: live organ donation from patient in, 274–76; multiorgan donation in cases of, 272–74; in Wendland case, 294

personality changes, traumatic brain damage as cause of, 315, 317

Personalized Medicine Research Project (Marshfield Clinic), 161, 162, 164

phalloplasty, 101, 102

phenylketonuria, 136

phrenology, 312

physical suffering: rational suicide and, 243–44. *See also* pain

physician-assisted suicide: as controversial, 185; for existential reasons, 249–56; in the Netherlands, 66, 248, 249–52, 255; North American debates over, 45–46; Oregon law on, 13, 66, 249, 254–55, 280; and rational control, 30; rational suicide and terminal illness, 243–48; slippery slope arguments used against, 280; terminal sedation contrasted with, 239

physicians: in Chekhov's "Ward No. 6," 336–37; constraints on autonomy of, 8–9; cross-cultural conflict in doctor-patient relationship, 256–59; do they overtreat the seriously ill?, 234–38; ethical consequentialism of, 175; ethics of lying to insurance companies, 194–96; flight surgeons, 223, 224; in Goldstein's *Travels with the Wolf: A Story of Chronic Illness,* 351; in Lightman's *The Diagnosis,* 344; medical managers usurping authority of, 12; paternalism and authoritarianism of, 7–8, 10–11, 184; in Scannell's *Death of the Good Doctor: Lessons from the Heart of the AIDS Epidemic,* 352–53; in Selzer's *The Doctor Stories,* 334–36

Pittsburgh, University of, 174
Pittsburgh Protocol, 81, 83–84
Plato, 18
"playing god," 31, 108, 153
police gene databanks, 157–58, 160
population genetic screening, 160
positive attitude, 352
posthumous sperm retrieval, 269–71
postmenopausal women, egg donation for, 122
postmodern theory, 50–51
postpartum psychosis, 318–19
power-focused feminist approaches, 36–37, 39–40, 41–42
Powers, Madison, 109
pragmatism, 52
prayer, 30
precocious puberty, 98
pregnancy: can HIV-positive woman be forced to take medication to protect her fetus?, 220–22; experimental fetal surgery, 56, 87–94; legal and ethical issues for pregnant women, 287–90; Minnesota "Crack Baby" law and, 280; prenatal diagnosis, 128–35; with twins where one has compromised growth, 262–63. *See also* abortion; fetuses; surrogacy, gestational
preimplantation genetic diagnosis, 128, 135–44, 326–27
prenatal diagnosis, 128–35
prescription drugs, cybermedicine and, 300, 301–2
President's Commission for the Study of Ethical Problems in Medicine and Biomedical and Behavioral Research, 327–28
President's Council on Bioethics, 45, 100, 107
Principles of Biomedical Ethics (Beauchamp and Childress), 47
principlism, 5, 43–44, 47–48, 50
privacy: astronauts' medical, 223–24, 226–28; cybermedicine as threat to, 302; disclosing results of genetic testing to others, 282, 284; human gene banks and, 163; implantable brain chips and, 167, 171; the law protecting right of, 279. *See also* confidentiality
probability, and information disclosure to patients, 200, 203
procreative freedom. *See* reproductive (procreative) freedom
professional standard of information disclosure, 198
progressive supranuclear palsy, 354–55
prophetic tradition, 31–32
proportionality, principle of, 265

proxy. *See* surrogate decision makers
psychiatry: biologic, 348; early patient rights focusing on, 8; gender dysphoria seen as psychiatric condition, 57, 95–103; recovered memories controversy, 309–12; *Tarasoff v. The Regents of the University of California* and, 283. *See also* insanity defense; mental illness
psychological distress: cloning of human beings seen as causing, 112; gender dysphoria, 57, 95–103; informing patient of possible Creutzfeldt-Jakob disease exposure causing, 199, 200, 201, 204; rational suicide and, 244
puberty, transgenderism and, 96, 97–98
punishment, 14, 15

Q

quadriplegics: allowing time for reflection before discontinuing life support, 213–15; in *Million Dollar Baby*, 338–39
quality healthcare, contracting for, 303–6
quality of life: cross-cultural differences regarding, 260; in end-of-life decision making, 234, 237, 241, 246; in "four boxes" method, 207, 208; job performance and, 168–69
"Quasimodo Complex, The" (Carey), 356
Quill, Timothy, 252
Quill v. Vacco, 279
Quinlan, Karen, 279

R

Ramsey, Paul, 12
rankings of goods and evils, 49
rational suicide, 243–48
rationing of healthcare resources: artificial heart raising question of, 61; Oregon law on, 13
Ratzan, Richard M., 354
Rawls, John, 154
reason: control as goal of, 30; deductive-nomological style of, 36; and feeling in moral psychology, 20, 21; as ground of morality, 17; interpretive style of, 36; natural reason, 49, 51, 52; rational legitimacy of religious belief, 32–33; rational suicide and terminal illness, 243–48; religion versus, 29; versus repugnance in moral debate, 154–57; theoretical versus practical modes of, 36
reasonable person standard of information disclosure, 199, 200
Recombinant DNA Advisory Committee, 326, 328

technology: financing as important as medical need for, 12; new disadvantaged groups created by new, 170; novel technologies, 107–10; patients feeling oppressed by, 11; physicians' professional dominance enhanced by, 11; political schism over, 108–10; quality of life diminished by, 169. *See also* assisted reproductive technologies (ARTs); cloning of human beings; gene therapy; life support
teenagers, refusal of assent by, 217–19
Ten Commandments, 4, 33
termanasia, 64
terminal care. *See* end-of-life care
terminal illness: critical illness distinguished from, 235–36; rational suicide and, 243–48; in Wendland case, 294. *See also* end-of-life care
terminal sedation, 55, 238–40
Terry, Nicholas, 299
Texas: Texas Advance Directives Act, 296–99; Andrea Yates case, 318–19
thalassemias, 136
therapeutic trial of defined duration, 208
Thompson, Tommy, 321
tissue banks, 306, 307–8
tissue donation: profits made from, 280, 306; who should capture the value of donated tissue?, 306–9
tissue engineering, for transgenderism, 102
tissue processors, 306, 307, 308
Titmuss, R. M., 159
To Err is Human (Institute of Medicine), 303
Tomlinson, T., 84
Tong, Rosemarie, 6, 35, 39, 40, 41
total artificial heart. *See* artificial heart
totalitarianism, implantable brain chips facilitating, 167
transfusion, informing patient of possible transmission of Creutzfeldt-Jakob disease from, 199–201, 203–5
transgenderism, 57, 95–103
transplantation. *See* organ transplantation
traumatic brain injury: and criminal responsibility, 315–18; death row inmates with, 280, 316
"Travels in the Valley of the Shadow" (Lynn), 37–38
Travels with the Wolf: A Story of Chronic Illness (Goldstein), 350–52
triage, for space medicine, 225
Turner, Leigh, 5, 42, 47, 48, 49, 50

Tuskegee Syphilis Study, 7, 11, 328
Tyranny of the Normal, The: An Anthology (Donley and Buckley), 356–57

U
UK Biobank, 158, 159, 160, 161
UK National Police Database, 158
Uman Genetics, 162, 164
Umeå University, 162
unbearable suffering, euthanasia for, 251–55
uncertainty: of end-of-life scenarios, 185–86; and family demands for futile treatment, 264–65
Uniform Anatomical Gift Act, 273
Uniform Parentage Act, 76, 285–86
unifying systems, 24
United Network for Organ Sharing (UNOS), 172, 173–74, 175, 176
Unquiet Mind, An (Jamison), 345–46
unsurprising surprises, principle of avoiding, 202–3, 204, 205, 206
Updike, John, 356–57
urgency as criterion for organ allocation, 172, 177–78, 179
US Public Health Service, 324
utilitarianism (consequentialism): basic assumption of, 5; in medical futility disputes, 268; in organ allocation, 173–74, 175–76, 177, 178; religious approach to ethics contrasted with, 34

V
values: technical matters distinguished from, 3. *See also* morality
Västerbotten County Council, 162
Vatican Pontifical Academy for Life, 79
Veatch, Robert M.: Brock's response to, 176, 177, 178; on ethics as analysis of choices, 3; on liver allocation, 172–76; response to Brock, 179–80; response to Steinberg, 65–67; Steinberg's response to, 62–63, 64, 65; on total artificial heart and killing, 55, 58–62
vegetative state. *See* persistent vegetative state
ventilator: allowing quadriplegics time for reflection before removing, 213–15; cross-cultural differences regarding, 259–61; death determination changed by, 79; invoking medical futility policies, 266–68; for long-duration space flights, 225; in *Million Dollar Baby*, 338–39; stopping artificial heart compared with stopping, 60, 63; and uncertainty in end-of-life scenarios, 185

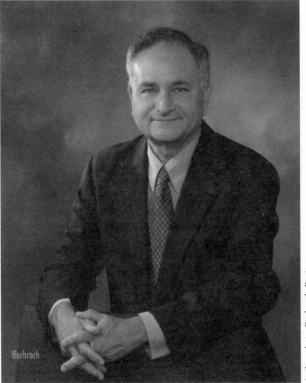

David Steinberg, M.D., is Director of the Section of Medical Ethics at Lahey Clinic Medical Center in Burlington, Massachusetts, where he practices hematology. He is editor of the journal *Lahey Clinic Medical Ethics* and is Clinical Assistant Professor of Medicine at Harvard Medical School.